Adenosine Receptors and Parkinson's Disease

Adenosine Receptors and Parkinson's Disease

Edited by

Hiroshi Kase
Kyowa Hakko Kogyo Co. Ltd.
Pharmaceutical Research and Development Division
Chiyoda-ku, Tokyo

Peter J. Richardson
Department of Pharmacology
University of Cambridge
Cambridge, England

Peter Jenner
Neurodegenerative Diseases Research Centre
Division of Pharmacology & Therapeutics
Guy's King's & St. Thomas' School of Biomedical Sciences
King's College London
London, UK

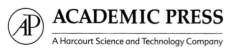

ACADEMIC PRESS
A Harcourt Science and Technology Company

San Diego   San Francisco   New York   Boston   London   Sydney   Tokyo

Academic Press
a division of Harcourt Brace & Company
525 B Street, Suite 1900, San Diego, California 92101-4495, USA
http://www.apnet.com

Academic Press
24-28 Oval Road, London NW1 7DX, UK
http://www.hbuk.co.uk/ap/

Library of Congress Catalog Card Number: 99-62783

International Standard Book Number: 0-12-400405-9

PRINTED IN THE UNITED STATES OF AMERICA
99 00 01 02 03 04 EB 9 8 7 6 5 4 3 2 1

CONTENTS

3 Medicinal Chemistry of Adenosine Receptors in Brain and Periphery

Junichi Shimada and Fumio Suzuki

4 Overview of the Physiology and Pharmacology of Adenosine in the Peripheral System

Akira Karasawa

5 Biochemical Characterization of Adenosine Agonists and Antagonists

Hiromi Nonaka and Michio Ichimura

8 Control of Gene Expression in Basal Ganglia by Adenosine Receptors

Alistair K. Dixon and Peter J. Richardson

9 Knockout Mice in the Study of Dopaminergic Diseases

Shiro Aoyama, Hiroshi Kase, Ja-Hyun Baik, and Emiliana Borrelli

10 Effects of Adenosine Receptors

Shizuo Shiozaki, Shunji Ichikawa, Joji Nakamura, and Yoshihisa Kuwana

11 Actions of Adenosine Antagonists in Primate Model of Parkinson's Disease

Tomoyuki Kanda and Peter Jenner

12 Selective Adenosine A_{2A} Receptor Antagonism as an Alternative Therapy for Parkinson's Disease

A. Hadj Tahar, R. Grondin, L. Grégoire, P. J. Bédard, A. Mori, and H. Kase

13 Neurobiology of Adenosine Receptors

Masahiro Nomoto

CONTRIBUTORS

Numbers in parentheses indicate the pages on which the authors' contributions begin.

SHIRO AOYAMA (171), Pharmaceutical Research Institute, Kyowa Hakko Kogyo Co., Ltd., Shizuoka, 411-8731 Japan

SARAH J. AUGOOD (17), Neurology Research, Massachusetts General Hospital and Harvard Medical School, Boston, Massachusetts 02114

JA-HYUN BAIK (171), Medical Research Center (Molecular Biology Section), College of Medicine, Yonsei University, Seoul, South Korea

P.J. BÉDARD (229), Neuroscience Research Unit, Laval University Research Center, Ste-Foy, Quebec, G1K 7P4 Canada

EMILIANA BORRELLI (171), Institut de Génetique et de Biologie Moléculaire et Cellulaire, C.U. de Strasbourg, France

ALISTAIR K. DIXON (149), Parke Davis Neuroscience Research Centre, Cambridge University Forvie Site, Cambridge, CB2 2QB United Kingdom

PIERS C. EMSON (17), Department of Neurobiology, The Babraham Institute, Cambridge, CB2 4AT United Kingdom

L. GRÉGOIRE (229), Neuroscience Research Unit, Laval University Research Center, Ste-Foy, Quebec, G1K 7P4 Canada

R. GRONDIN (229), Neuroscience Research Unit, Laval University Research Center, Ste-Foy, Quebec, G1K 7P4 Canada

SHUNJI ICHIKAWA (193), Pharmaceutical Research Institute, Kyowa Hakko Kogyo Co., Ltd., Nagaizumi-cho, Sunto-gun, Shizuoka, 411-8731 Japan

MICHIO ICHIMURA (77), Biochemistry, Pharmaceutical Research Institute, Kyowa Hakko Kogyo Co., Ltd., Sunto-gun, Shizuoka, 411-8731 Japan

PETER JENNER (211, 257), Neurodegenerative Diseases Research Centre, Division of Pharmacology & Therapeutics, Guy's King's & St Thomas' School of Biomedical Sciences, King's College London, London, SW3 6LX United Kingdom

TOMOYUKI KANDA (211), Department of Neurology, Pharmaceutical Research Institute, Kyowa Hakko Kogyo Co., Ltd., Sunto-Gun, Shizuoka, 411-8731 Japan

AKIRA KARASAWA (49), Pharmaceutical Research and Development Center, Kyowa Hakko Kogyo Co., Ltd., Tokyo, 100-8185 Japan

HIROSHI KASE (1, 171, 229), Pharmaceutical Research and Development Division, Kyowa Hakko Kogyo Co., Ltd., Chiyoda-ku, Tokyo, 100-8185 Japan

MASAKO KUROKAWA (129), Pharmaceutical Research Laboratories, Kyowa Hakko Kogyo Co., Ltd., Nagaizumi-cho, Sunto-gun, Shizuoka, 411-8731 Japan

YOSHIHISA KUWANA (211), Pharmaceutical Research Institute, Kyowa Hakko Kogyo Co., Ltd., Nagaizumi-cho, Sunto-gun, Shizuoka, 411-8731 Japan

AKIHISA MORI (107, 229), Pharmaceutical Research & Development Center, Kyowa Hakko Kogyo Co., Ltd., Chiyoda-ku, Tokyo, 100-8185 Japan

JOJI NAKAMURA (193), Pharmaceutical Research Institute, Kyowa Hakko Kogyo Co., Ltd., Nagaizumi-cho, Sunto-gun, Shizuoka, 411-8731 Japan

MASAHIRO NOMOTO (245), Department of Pharmacology and Clinical Pharmacology, Kagoshima University School of Medicine, Kagoshima, 890-8652 Japan

HIROMI NONAKA (77), Biochemistry, Pharmaceutical Research Institute, Kyowa Hakko Kogyo Co., Ltd., Sunto-gun, Shizuoka, 411-8731 Japan

PETER J. RICHARDSON (129, 149), Department of Pharmacology, University of Cambridge, Cambridge, CB2 1QJ United Kingdom

JUNICHI SHIMADA (31), Pharmaceutical Research Institute, Drug Discovery Research Laboratories, Kyowa Hakko Kogyo Co., Ltd., Nagaizumi-cho, Sunto-gun, Shizuoka, 411-8731 Japan

TOMOMI SHINDOU (107), Pharmaceutical Research Institute, Kyowa Hakko Kogyo Co., Ltd., Sunto-gun, Shizuoka, 411-8731 Japan

SHIZUO SHIOZAKI (193), Neurobiology, Pharmaceutical Research Institute, Kyowa Hakko Kogyo Co., Ltd., Nagaizumi-cho, Sunto-gun, Shizuoka, 411-8731 Japan

DAVID G. STANDAERT (17), Neurology Research, Massachusetts General Hospital and Harvard Medical School, Boston, Massachusetts 02114

FUMIO SUZUKI (31), Pharmaceutical Research Institute, Drug Discovery Research Laboratories, Kyowa Hakko Kogyo Co., Ltd., Nagaizumi-cho, Sunto-gun, Shizuoka, 411-8731 Japan

ABDAHLAH HADJ TAHAR (229), Neuroscience Research Unit, Laval University Research Center, Ste-Foy, Quebec, G1K 7P4 Canada

PREFACE

Diseases of the central nervous system represent the most challenging therapeutic area that remains in medicine and pharmacology. The degenerative disorders afflicting the brain, such as Parkinson's disease and Alzheimer's disease, are the most difficult to attack because only symptomatic therapy in the form of replacing neurotransmitters is available. Currently, nothing can be done to stop the onset or progression of the disease process. However, targeted pharmacological approaches are opening up new avenues of symptomatic treatment that are more effective than traditional therapies and that produce fewer side effects, thereby providing patients with improved quality of life.

Parkinson's disease was thought to have been solved once the depletion of striatal dopamine levels occurring as a consequence of nigral degeneration had been uncovered. The introduction of L-Dopa and, subsequently, dopamine agonist drugs revolutionized treatment and provided an effective reversal of symptoms, restoring mobility to previously severely disabled individuals. However, the honeymoon soon passed and it became obvious that L-Dopa's action waned with time and disease progression and that serious side effects such as dyskinesia and psychosis appeared. In addition, not all symptoms responded to treatment and the disease inevitably progressed. Clearly, other therapeutic approaches are required that relieve all symptoms throughout the illness and that do not cause the same inevitable side-effect profile.

The study of basal ganglia, in particular, the localization of cell surface receptor populations, has shown a way forward. The output neurons of basal ganglia possess a large number of transmitter receptors that are nondopaminergic and that lie beyond the damaged dopamine system. These targets also play a role in the control of motor function and so provide potential novel therapeutic approaches to treating Parkinson's disease. However, many of these neurotransmitter receptors are also found in other parts of the brain.

This means that they cannot be specifically targeted to control Parkinson's disease and inevitably their manipulation will cause a host of unwanted side effects.

Nevertheless, recent advances in the molecular biology of cell surface receptors has revealed previously unrecognized receptor subtypes and subunits, providing unique targets for pharmacological manipulation. The adenosine receptors are one such receptor system, with A_1, A_{2A} and A_{2B} and A_3 receptors being recognized. Whereas A_1 and A_3 receptors are widely distributed, the A_{2A} receptor population has a very discrete distribution in the brain, with a predominance of A_{2A} receptors found in basal ganglia associated with the indirect strio-pallidal output pathway. This raises the question of how these receptors can alter the function of basal ganglia with respect to motor activity and the future treatment of Parkinson's disease. In this volume we attempt to bring together current information indicating that the manipulation of A_{2A} receptors by selective antagonists such as KW-6002 may have an important role in treating Parkinson's disease.

Specifically, we have invited experts on a range of aspects of the chemistry, biochemistry, and pharmacology of adenosine receptors to present their views of the area and its relevance to the treatment of Parkinson's disease. The volume deals in depth with the structure–activity relationships that dictate selectivity for the A_{2A} receptor and the way in which the selective antagonism of this site alters motor behaviors through manipulation of the activity of acetylcholine and GABA containing neurons in the striatal output pathways. These actions are examined in relation to the distribution of A_{2A} receptors in brain and to the effect of A_{2A} antagonists in animal models of Parkinson's disease and in knockout mice. Specifically, the ability of KW-6002 to reverse parkinsonian motor deficits in MPTP-treated monkeys without provoking dyskinesia provides a major clue that A_{2A} antagonists may constitute a significant advance in the treatment of Parkinson's disease.

This volume will be of interest to anatomists, physiologists, biochemists, and pharmacologists studying basal ganglia function and to all clinicians and industrial scientists with an interest in Parkinson's disease and its treatment. It provides a unique in-depth assessment of the functions of A_{2A} receptors in brain and their relevance to a range of brain disorders, particularly Parkinson's disease. The content will stimulate further study of the adenosine receptor populations in brain and the exploitation of novel highly selective drug molecules for the treatment of basal ganglia diseases.

CHAPTER 1

Introductory Remarks

Adenosine A$_{2A}$ Receptor Antagonists: A Novel Approach to the Treatment of Parkinson's Disease

HIROSHI KASE

Pharmaceutical Research and Development Division, Kyowa Hakko Kogyo Co., Ltd., Chiyoda-ku, Tokyo 100-8185, Japan

Adenosine exerts a great variety of physiological effects on the nervous system and peripheral tissues. Drury and Szent-Györgyi first demonstrated the effects of adenosine on cardiovascular function in 1929 (Drury and Szent-Györgyi, 1929). Subsequently it became clear that adenosine, acting through specific receptors, is a potent biological mediator that modulates the activity of numerous cell types. These include various neuronal populations, platelets, neutrophils and mast cells, and smooth muscle cells in bronchi and vasculature. In the nervous system adenosine is released during cerebral ischemia, where it increases cerebral blood flow, inhibits synaptic activity, and decreases neuronal activity. Over the years, reports on possible functional roles for adenosine in the nervous system have increased steadily in number, with adenosine being implicated in epilepsy, cerebral ischemic preconditioning, sleep, and immune reactions within the brain (Brundege and Dunwiddie, 1997). A great deal of evidence shows that adenosine receptors are located throughout the nervous system and that extracellular adenosine can effectively modulate neuronal activity. There is however little evidence that adenosine is stored in synaptic vesicles or released from nerve terminals in response to an action potential in the manner of a classical neurotransmitter. Yet it is present in the extracellular space of the brain and can be released from neural cells by various stimuli, suggesting that adenosine is a neuromodulator that is released in unconventional ways (e.g., via nucleoside transporters) to interact with cell surface receptors. Despite many detailed investigations, the precise cellular mechanisms by which cells release adenosine, and so the neuromodulatory role of adenosine, remain to be elucidated (Brundege and Dunwiddie, 1997).

The most compelling evidence for a specific modulatory action of adenosine came after the molecular characterization of the known receptor subtypes, their intracellular signal transduction pathways, and their localization (Olah and Stiles, 1995). Of the four receptor subtypes (A_1, A_{2A}, A_{2B}, and A_3, Fredholm et al., 1994), the most extensively investigated have been the high-affinity A_1 and A_{2A} receptors. The use of selective agonists and antagonists for each receptor subtype has greatly contributed to the elucidation of adenosine function (Ongini and Fredholm, 1996). Recently, potent and selective A_{2A} receptor antagonists have been synthesized and investigation of their properties has led to advances in our understanding of basal ganglia function and in the development of a potential novel therapeutic approach to the treatment of Parkinson's disease (Richardson et al., 1997).

The main objective of this book is to present the current status of research on the adenosine A_{2A} receptor and its selective antagonists and to explain the use of A_{2A} receptor antagonists as a new symptomatic approach to the treatment of Parkinson's disease. For this purpose, Chapters 2–5 cover our current knowledge of the adenosine receptors in the brain and periphery and their selective agonists and antagonists.

In Chapter 2 Augood, Emson, and Standaert provide an overview of the microscopic and cellular localization of the four adenosine receptor subtypes in the brain and periphery and then attempt to highlight the potential functional roles of these receptors. Of particular importance is the selective localization of the adenosine A_{2A} receptor within the basal ganglia–thalamo–cortical circuits. The circuitry of the basal ganglia in primates serves as a basis for understanding the physiology underlying many basal ganglia-associated functions as well as the pathophysiology of disorders of movement associated with diseases of the basal ganglia (Albin et al, 1989; Alexander and Grutcher, 1990; DeLong, 1990; Obeso et al., 1997, Smith et al., 1998). An understanding of the model (shown in Fig. 1) provides insights into the functional role of this receptor in the striatum and the mechanism of action of its antagonists in models of Parkinson's disease which are discussed in the other chapters.

Shimada and Suzuki review the current status of medicinal chemistry of adenosine receptor antagonists, including the synthesis of the first A_{2A} receptor selective xanthine derivatives KF-17837 and KW-6002. They also

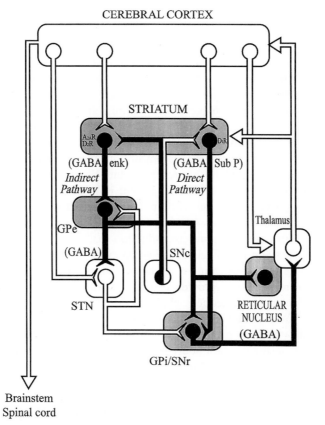

FIGURE 1. The circuitry of the basal ganglia in primates. Cortical information that reaches the striatum is conveyed to the basal ganglia output structures (Gpi/SNr) via two pathways, a direct inhibitory projection from the striatum to the Gpi/SNr and an indirect pathway, which involves an inhibitory projection from the striatum to the GPe, an inhibitory projection from the GPe to the STN and an excitatory projection from the STN to the Gpi/SNr. In addition, the Gpe projects directly to the Gpi/SNr and to the RTN. The information is then transmitted back to the cerebral cortex via the thalamus. The direct and indirect pathways largely arise from different populations of striatal medium spiny neurons. The striatonigral neurons of the direct pathway contain substance P and dynorphin and the striatopallidal neurons of the indirect pathway contain enkephalin. The striatonigral neurons express dopamine D_1 receptors while the striatopallidal neurons express dopamine D_2 and adenosine A_{2A} receptors. The striatal medium spiny neurons give rise to extensive local axon collaterals. The dopaminergic neurons of SNc exert an excitatory effect on the direct pathway via D_1 receptor activation and an inhibitory effect on the indirect pathway via D_2 receptor activation. Filled arrow shows inhibitory projection, open arrow excitatory. Abbreviations: GPe, the external segment of the globus pallicus; GPi, the internal segment of the globus pallidus; SNc, the substantia nigra pars compacta; SNr, the substantia nigra pars reticulata; STN, subthalamic nucleus; enk, enkephalin; subP, substance P. Modified from Fig. 12 in Smith *et al.*, 1998.

review the chemistry of adenosine A_1 receptor antagonists and discuss two promising therapeutic areas for such A_1 antagonists, cognitive deficit and acute renal failure. With respect to these topics, Karasawa reviews the pharmacology of the A_1 antagonists in renal failure (Chapter 4) while Shiozaki *et al.* deal with the potential of A_1 antagonists in increasing cognitive function (Chapter 10). Since adenosine acts on many cells and tissues, Karasawa has also covered current knowledge of the peripheral actions of adenosine in terms of the cardiovascular, renal, gastrointestinal, respiratory, pulmonary, inflammatory, and immune systems as well as the endocrine and exocrine systems (Chapter 4). This has relevance not only to the pharmacology of therapeutic agents acting on adenosine receptors but also to their safety. Nonaka and Ichimura, who discovered KF-17837 and KW-6002 as selective and potent A_{2A} antagonists, review the current status of the biochemical characterization of adenosine receptors and of A_1 and A_{2A} selective antagonists (Chapter 5). The intracellular signal transduction pathways of the adenosine receptor subtypes and the effects of the antagonists on these systems are also reviewed. These novel adenosine receptor compounds not only provide tools for basic research but also provide a means to develop related therapeutic agents, as covered in subsequent chapters. Mori and Shindou (Chapter 6) deal with the fundamental issue as to how striatal A_{2A} receptor stimulation by adenosine affects basal ganglia function, using electrophysiological techniques and adenosine receptor subtype selective agents. This chapter concentrates on new aspects of the A_{2A} receptor mediated inhibition of inhibitory GABAergic synaptic transmission. This discovery provided major clues as to the role of adenosine in the basal ganglia, leading to the development of a new hypothesis concerning the physiological and pathophysiological implications of adenosine action elicited via striatal A_{2A} receptors. In the subsequent chapter (Chapter 7), Richardson and Kurokawa describe the actions of adenosine A_1 and A_{2A} receptors on neurotransmitter release in the striatum using synaptosomes *in vitro* and intrastriatal microdialysis *in vivo*. In particular, the release of acetylcholine and GABA was found to be regulated by adenosine through A_{2A} receptors. These results are consistent with those obtained by electrophysiology described in Chapter 6. Dixon and Richardson (Chapter 8) subsequently deal with the ability of A_{2A} receptor antagonists to rectify abnormal gene expression in the two striatal output pathways caused by dopamine depletion or dopamine receptor blockade. The results are discussed in terms of the possible mechanisms by which blockade of the A_{2A} receptor normalizes neuronal activity in Parkinson's disease.

Analysis of the functional relationship between the A_{2A} and D_2 receptors is essential if we are to understand the roles of these two receptors and is central to the development of adenosine-based novel therapies for diseases affecting striatal dopaminergic function. In Chapter 9, Aoyama, Baik, Kase, and Borrelli, review the molecular biology and functions of dopamine receptor subtypes and then the use of knockout mice (in which members of the dopamine or adenosine receptor families have been deleted) to investigate the role of these receptors *in vivo*. An important finding by Borrelli and her colleagues is that D_2 receptor knockout results in a parkinsonian-like akinesia which is reversed by the selective A_{2A} receptor antagonist KW-6002.

Subsequent chapters (Chapters 10–12) highlight the effects of A_{2A} receptor antagonists on behavioral models, in particular those related to Parkinson's disease. Shiozaki, Ichikawa, Nakamura, and Kuwana describe the relationship of A_1 receptors to cognitive function and the A_{2A} receptors to sleep and motor function (Chapter 10). The adenosine A_{2A} receptor antagonists were also examined using MPTP-treated common marmoset as one of the most relevant pharmacological models of Parkinson's disease. A novel finding made by Kanda and Jenner was that KW-6002 improves motor disability without provoking dyskinesia (Chapter 11). Bédard and his collaborators further evaluated the antiparkinsonian and antidyskinetic effects of KW-6002 in MPTP-treated monkeys (Chapter 12). Oral administration of KW-6002 increased locomotion and improved parkinsonian symptoms in a manner comparable to that seen with levodopa. However, despite its ability to reverse motor disability, KW-6002 alone induced little or no dyskinesia. They concluded that selective A_{2A} antagonism improved parkinsonism in MPTP-treated monkeys and that A_{2A} receptor blockade is a potential nondopaminergic approach to treating parkinsonian patients, either alone or as an adjunct to levodopa or dopamine agonist therapy. Nomoto reviews the alterations in levels of extracellular adenosine and its metabolites in movement disorders (Chapter 13). Finally, drawing together all aspects of the basic and preclinical studies, Jenner and Marsden outline the prospects of adenosine A_{2A} receptor antagonists as potential therapeutic agents (Chapter 14).

I. A VIEW OF THE ACTION OF ADENOSINE IN THE STRIATUM

To provide a rational background to this book, it is necessary to show how adenosine produces its actions in the striatum, since this issue is important in the conceptual understanding of adenosine action and in drug development. First the hypothesis of adenosine A_{2A} receptor function in Parkinson's disease will be described. Then the concept of adenosine A_{2A}—dopamine D_2 receptor interactions proposed by Ferre *et al.*, will be discussed.

A. Adenosine A_{2A} Receptor Functions in Normal and Disease States

The basal concentration of adenosine in the extracellular space is between 20 and 300 nM. This is sufficient to tonically activate adenosine A_{2A} receptors to a modest extent (Nonaka *et al.*, 1994a, 1994b; also see Chapter 5) as evinced by the excitatory effects of adenosine receptor antagonists both *in vitro* and *in vivo* (Brundege and Dunwiddie, 1997). Similarly, the adenosine A_{2A} selective antagonist KF-17837 alone caused a significant increase of evoked and spontaneous GABAergic neurotransmission in striatal slices (Mori *et al.*, 1996). In addition to this tonic activity of adenosine, numerous conditions elevate the extracellular adenosine concentration, including hypoxia, ischemia, electrical stimulation, chemical depolarization, nonpathological nerve stimulation, and N-methyl-D-aspartate (NMDA) receptor activation (Brundege and Dunwiddie, 1997). Of particular relevance was the finding of Nomoto *et al.* (1998) who recently showed that the extracellular levels of adenosine (and its metabolite inosine) are higher in the striatum of MPTP-treated monkeys than in normal control monkeys. Recent evidence supports a role of adenosine in short-term synaptic modulation in hippocampal slices (Grover and Teyler, 1993; Michell *et al.*, 1993; Manzoni *et al.*, 1994; Brundege and Dunwiddie, 1996; Dunwiddie *et al.*, 1997) and in purinergic fibers of the medial habenula nucleus (Robertson and Edwards, 1998). These results suggest that adenosine may play a role as a feedback modulator of synaptic activity.

To explain the origins of extracellular adenosine, two major possible hypotheses have emerged: (1) Extracellular adenosine is formed from nucleotides, released into extracellular space, and catabolized to adenosine via a series of ectoenzymes (Zimmermann, 1992; Craig and White, 1993; Rosenberg *et al.*, 1994; Ziganshin *et al.*, 1994). Potential sources of extracellular adenine nucleotides include vesicular release of ATP that is colocalized with transmitters such as acetylcholine, norepinephrine, and 5HT (Silinsky, 1975; Burnstock, 1986; Richardson and Brown, 1987), nucleotide release after activation of NMDA receptors (Craig and White, 1992, 1993), and activation of adenylyl cyclase (Gereau and Conn, 1994; Rosenberg *et al.*, 1994; Rosenberg and Li, 1995). In purified cholinergic synapses from the striatum, ecto-ATPase (EC 3.6.1.15), ecto-ADPase (EC 3.6.1.6), and ecto-5′-nucleotidase (EC 3.1.3.5) have all been identified (James and Richardson, 1993). The conversion of AMP to adenosine by 5′-nucleotidase is the rate-limiting step in the extracellular conversion of nucleotides to adenosine in the brain (James and Richardson, 1993; Dunwiddie *et al.*, 1997). The release of ATP, ADP, and/or AMP into the extracellular space of the hippocampus results in rapid dephosphorylation to adenosine (within <1 s), and the adenosine formed then activates nearby A_1 receptors (Dunwiddie *et al.*, 1997). (2) Adenosine formed intracellularly is released into the extracellular space by a nonsynaptic mechanism (see Chapter 4). Intracellular formation of adenosine is directly related to cellular energetics and is oxygen dependent. Thus, hypoxia greatly increases adenosine production and its consequent release into the extracellular space via specific transporters, but only when energy metabolism is severely compromised (Brundege and Dunwiddie, 1997). However, it is still unclear how neuronal activation in nonhypoxic conditions induces the formation and increased release of adenosine. Also, despite detailed investigations into the effects exerted by adenosine and adenosine receptors, it is still not clear, in most cases, which cells are responsible for the release of adenosine.

B. New Aspects of Adenosine A_{2A} Receptor Function

The finding that activation of striatal adenosine A_{2A} receptors inhibits GABAergic neurotransmission (Mori *et al.*, 1996; see also Chapter 6) contrasts with the previous belief that adenosine suppresses synaptic transmission through the A_1 receptor. It also contradicts earlier literature in which activation of A_{2A} receptors enhanced transmitter release. This finding that presynaptic A_{2A} receptors, localized in striatal GABAergic medium spiny neurons, inhibit GABA release in the striatum suggested the following hypothesis: "Adenosine inhibits GABA release from the striatopallidal output neurons and thus reduces GABA-mediated intrastriatal recurrent feedback inhibition" (Mori *et al.*, 1996, Richardson, *et al.*, 1997; see Chapters 6 and 7).

In support of this hypothesis, experiments with striatal synaptosomes showed an adenosine A_{2A} receptor selective agonist to directly inhibit GABA release from striatal nerve terminals (Kurokawa *et al.*, 1994; see also Chapter 7). In addition, A_{2A} receptor mediated inhibition of neurotransmission has recently been reported in neurons cultured from the suprachiasmatic and arcuate nuclei (Chen and Van den Pol, 1997) and in purinergic fibers of the medial habenula (Robertson and Edwards, 1998). However, in contrast to the hypothesis, the A_{2A} receptor has been shown to enhance GABA release in both striatal and pallidal slices (Mayfield *et al.*, 1993, 1996; Fredholm and Svenningsson, 1998).

Consideration of the preparations and methodologies used suggests a means of reconciling the data from the electrophysiological (Mori *et al.*, 1996) and synaptosomal transmitter release experiments (Kurokawa *et al.*, 1994), with those of Mayfield and colleagues measuring release from brain slices (Mayfield et al., 1993, 1996). In the electrophysiological study using whole-cell patch-clamp recording (Mori et al., 1996), the membrane potential at a neuron was kept constant at the resting level ($-70\,\text{mV}$) by voltage clamp, and the effect of the A_{2A} receptor on GABAergic inputs into the voltage clamped neuron was assessed. Changes in the release of GABA within the slice would therefore have no apparent effect on the excitability of the neuron. In the synaptosomal release experiments (Kurokawa et al., 1994), the direct effects of the A_{2A} receptor on the GABA-containing nerve terminals of the striatum were assessed. However, transmitter release studies using slices estimate the release from all the components present, which still maintain their anatomical connections. Thus a reduction in GABA release from one component could, paradoxically, increase total release of GABA by relief of GABA-mediated inhibition. In this context it is interesting to note that striatal medium spiny neurons give rise to extensive local axon collaterals that arborize within, or close to, their dendritic field and form symmetric synapses with dendrites and spines (Smith et al., 1998). High levels of A_{2A} receptors are present on striatopallidal GABAergic neurons, located on dendritic shafts and spines, and on axon terminals (Rosin et al., 1997).

Given this anatomical organization in the striatum, an A_{2A} receptor mediated reduction in the release of GABA from collateral nerve terminals would reduce the GABA-mediated inhibitory effect on intrinsic GABA-containing neurons, so causing an increase in GABA release in intact preparations (Richardson et al., 1998). This recurrent feedback inhibition of the GABAergic output neurons could have a significant physiological effect in that an increase of GABA release from axon collateral terminals could set the GABAergic projection neurons into a less active state, resulting in reduced GABA release from the axon terminals. This decrease in collateral GABA release would, in turn, change the GABAergic output neurons into a more active state. Since A_{2A} receptors on the axon collateral terminals inhibit this recurrent feedback inhibition, activation of these receptors would cause overactivity of striatopallidal output neurons. Such an overactivity of these neurons is seen in models of Parkinson's disease. Hence, the increase in GABA release seen in slices (Mayfield et al., 1993, 1996) may be a consequence of reduced GABA output from A_{2A} receptor bearing nerve terminals. The microdialysis data in which adenosine receptor blockade in the striatum increased GABA release in the globus pallidus (Ferre et al., 1993) could be explained in the same way; i.e., the increase in GABA in the pallidum was a consequence of the reduced inhibitory striatopallidal output, itself a result of increased recurrent feedback inhibition within the striatum.

C. Intracellular Signal Transduction of Presynaptic A_{2A} Receptors in the Striatum

The inhibition of GABA release in the striatum was mimicked by application of the membrane-permeable cAMP analogues 8-bromo-cAMP and dibutyryl-cAMP (Mori *et al.*, 1996), suggesting the involvement of the cAMP pathway in the presynaptic modulation of GABA release by A_{2A} receptors (see Chapter 5). This is consistent with the well-characterized ability of A_{2A} receptors to stimulate G_s. Although an ability to stimulate protein kinase C has been reported (Gubitz *et al.*, 1996), there has so far been no direct evidence that A_{2A} receptors activate phospholipase C. It has also recently been reported that A_{2A} receptor activation results in inhibition of voltage-gated calcium channels (Chen and Van den Pol, 1997) via cAMP elevation (Park *et al.*, 1997, 1998). In synaptosomal preparations from the striatum, no evidence was found for cAMP mediating the inhibition of GABA release by activation of A_{2A} receptors, although the involvement of protein kinase C and N-type Ca^{2+} channels was suggested (Kirk and Richardson, 1995). The issue requires further investigation.

D. Adenosine A_{2A} Function in the Parkinsonian State

Increased activity of the direct pathway (Fig. 1) is associated with facilitation of movement and increased activity of the indirect pathway is associated with inhibition of movement, with Parkinson's disease arising as a result of an imbalance in the activity of these pathways in favor of the indirect pathway. Current models of the pathophysiology of parkinsonism emphasize increases in the overall activity in the striatopallidal indirect pathway (DeLong, 1990; Obeso *et al.*, 1997). Since A_{2A} antagonists block the striatal A_{2A} receptor induced disinhibition among striatopallidal cells, these compounds might suppress the excessive activity of the indirect pathway caused by denervation of the nigrostriatal dopaminergic system.

Striatal projection neurons receive inputs from a large number of cortical neurons, suggesting that a striatal neuron may increase its firing rate only if there is activation of convergent input from many different cortical neurons (Smith *et al.*, 1998). According to Kita (1996), the response mediated via GABAA receptors has a reversal potential near the spike threshold potential of the spiny projection neurons and acts mainly to shunt the glutamatergic inputs. Thus the above-described A_{2A} receptor mediated inhibition of recurrent feedback regulation of the GABAergic neurons might cause facilitation of the striatopallidal output (see Chapter 6).

Recent immunohistochemical data (Rosin *et al.*, 1997) show that A_{2A} receptors are located at axon collaterals of the medium spiny neurons, which is consistent with the electrophysiological and synaptosomal release data mentioned earlier, as well as with the possible disinhibitory modulation of striatopallidal neurons. This receptor could therefore selectively increase the neuronal activity of certain clusters of the striatopallidal neurons, although little evidence has been found for surround inhibition arising from the collaterals of these neurons (Jaeger *et al.*, 1994; Stern *et al.*, 1998). As already described, a low, tonic level of adenosine is usually present in the extracellular space, which may increase in Parkinson's disease (Nomoto *et al.*, 1998, Chapter 13) and attenuate recurrent inhibition between the projection cells via A_{2A} receptors. Another possibility is that these receptors regulate GABA release from interneurons, but as yet there has been no evidence for GABA interneurons expressing A_{2A} receptors.

Recently, Bergman *et al.* (1998) examined the basic mechanisms of information processing by the basal ganglia in health and disease. They developed the hypothesis that subcircuits of the basal ganglia are functionally segregated and that these subcircuits show independence of activity in normal neuronal processing. The firing of neurons in the globus pallidus of normal monkeys is almost always characterized by uncorrelated activity of their functional subcircuit. Despite a high degree of anatomical convergence or funneling from the striatum to the pallidum, pallidal neurons do not share many common inputs from the striatum and, in the normal state, pallidal neurons act independently. In this state, even the numerous lateral interconnections in the striatum are functionally weak. After dopamine depletion and the development of parkinsonism by treatment with MPTP, the networks of the basal ganglia lose their ability to keep the activity of pallidal neurons independent, and the previously inhibited cross-connections between "parallel" subcircuits become more active. This suggests that the normal dopaminergic system supports the segregation of the functional subcircuits of the basal ganglia. The finding of profound synchronization in the basal ganglia of MPTP-treated monkeys suggests that such elevated synchronization may also exist in human parkinsonian patients. It is an attractive hypothesis that the increase in recurrent inhibition of striatopallidal output activity by A_{2A} receptor antagonists might permit the restoration of segregated functional subcircuits in the basal ganglia and so normalize motor control (see Chapter 6).

E. ADENOSINE AND DOPAMINE RECEPTORS

$A_{2A}-D_2$ receptor interactions have been shown both within plasma membrane and intracellularly. Thus A_{2A} receptor stimulation affects the affinity of dopamine for D_2 receptors, stimulation of A_{2A} receptors counteracted a D_2 receptor mediated Ca^{2+} influx in A_{2A}/D_2 cotransfected cells, and A_{2A} agonists counteract the D_2 receptor mediated tonic inhibition of *c-fos* expression. A number of other studies showed that adenosine A_{2A} receptors exert opposing effects on D_2 receptor mediated effects, including signal transduction, gene expression, neurotransmitter release, and behavioral responses (Ferre *et al.*, 1997). From these results, together with similar opposing effects between adenosine A_1 and dopamine D_1, Ferre *et al.* (1997) have proposed that the $A_{2A}-D_2$ intramembrane receptor-receptor interaction, and a downstream interaction at the level of intracellular signal transduction, may provide the main molecular and cellular mechanism underlying many of the effects of adenosine agonists and antagonists (Ferre *et al.*, 1997).

However, there is increasing evidence that A_{2A} receptors can operate independently of D_2 receptors. Thus presynaptic A_{2A} receptors modulate recurrent feedback inhibition of striatal GABAergic spiny projection neurons (as described earlier), and inhibit GABA release from striatal synaptosomes in the absence of dopamine. In addition, in D_2 knockout mice, which show a parkinsonian-like locomotor phenotype (Baik *et al.*, 1995), blockade of adenosine A_{2A} receptors by KW-6002 reestablishes their locomotor activity and coordination of movement and lowers the level of striatal enkephalin expression to levels seen in normal mice. This means that A_{2A} receptors can regulate, in the absence of D_2 receptors, locomotor activity, coordination of movement, and gene expression (see Chapter 9). As expected, adenosine A_{2A} receptor knockout mice do not respond to the A_{2A} agonist CGS21680 and show reduced expression of enkephalin in the striatum (Ledent *et al.*, 1997).

When the nigrostriatal projection is preserved, both intramembrane A_{2A}/D_2 receptor interactions and independent A_{2A} and/or D_2 receptor actions will occur in striatopallidal neurons which express both of these receptors. However, when dopamine is depleted (e.g., in Parkinson's disease patients, MPTP-exposed monkeys, and D_2 knockout mice), the antiparkinsonian actions of adenosine A_{2A} receptor antagonists would be mediated directly, rather than by relief of an antagonistic interaction with endogenous dopamine. Thus, from the viewpoint of developing novel therapies for Parkinson's diseases, the direct effects of the A_{2A} receptor (i.e., effects in the absence of D_2 receptor stimulation) are the most important when considering the potential of A_{2A} receptor antagonists.

F. L-DOPA-INDUCED DYSKINESIAS AND A_{2A} RECEPTORS

The high prevalence of L-Dopa-induced dyskinesias in Parkinson's disease has led to marked interest in the underlying pathophysiological mechanisms. Dyskinesias such as chorea and ballism appear as a consequence of functional inactivation or lesion of the subthalamic nucleus (STN), leading to reduced neuronal activity in both the external segment of the globus pallidus (GP_e) and internal segment of the globus pallidus (GP_i) (see Fig. 1). It was proposed that hemichorea/ballism and dyskinesia induced by L-Dopa share a common pathophysiological mechanism, both resulting as a consequence of diminished activity of the STN-GP_i indirect pathway. However, the origin of L-Dopa-induced dyskinesias may not be so simple, since they are a relatively heterogeneous group of phenomena, with various manifestations occurring at different times after L-Dopa intake ("peak of dose," diphasic, and "off" period). The experimental MPTP monkey model treated with L-Dopa may only be a model for the "peak-dose" dyskinesias. According to the established model of basal ganglia pathophysiology, L-Dopa-induced dyskinesias arise when the activity in the STN or GP_i falls below a given level as a consequence of excessive inhibition from the GP_e. The abnormal pattern of neuronal activity transmitted from the GP_i to the thalamus and then to the motor cortical areas would introduce "noise" signals in the system, leading to involuntary activation of fragments of movements which intrude into the normal motor system (Obeso et al., 1997). Given the postulated mechanism of KW-6002, it is unlikely that excessive inhibition of the GP_i occurs with this agent. As discussed earlier, A_{2A} receptor antagonists might be expected to normalize motor control from the hypokinetic state. Indeed, in contrast to L-Dopa induced hyperactivity in MPTP-treated marmosets, locomotor activity of these animals treated with KW-6002 was increased at most to the level observed in normal animals, and dyskinesias were not seen (Chapters 11 and 12). In addition, locomotion improved by KW-6002 was discontinuous and similar to that seen in normal animals in terms of the behavior patterns, whereas L-Dopa or dopamine D_2 agonist produces a profound hyperactivity that greatly exceeds the activity of normal monkey (Chapter 11; Kanda et al., 1998). It is therefore proposed that, although KW-6002 enhances GP_e activity by disinhibition of the striatal recurrent collateral feedback inhibition mechanism, it is unable to cause excessive inhibition of the striatopallidal neurons and therefore induces no dyskinesia. Chase et al. have proposed overstimulation of glutamate receptor in the striatum as a mechanism for fluctuations in motor response to long-term L-Dopa treatment (Chase et al., 1996). The subunit composition and/or phosphorylation state of NMDA receptors expressed on dendritic spines of striatal medium spiny neurons changes in ways that compromise motor performance (Chase, 1998). It remains to be seen whether or not A_{2A} receptors are involved in such internal signaling mechanisms.

L-Dopa has long been the gold standard of therapy for Parkinson's disease but its long-term shortcomings are motor response complications such as dyskinesias, end-of-dose deterioration or wearing-off, and fluctuating control of motor symptoms (on–off fluctuation). Alternative therapeutic approaches are clearly needed that improve motor control without motor response complications. In this respect adenosine antagonists directed at A_{2A} receptors might be very efficient in reestablishing the normal physiological properties of striatal neurons in parkinsonian patients. Adenosine A_{2A} receptor antagonists thus provide a possible new approach to the treatment of Parkinson's disease.

REFERENCES

Albin, R. L., Young, A. B., and Penny, J. B. (1989). The functional anatomy of basal ganglia disorders. *Trends Neurosci.* 12, 366–375.
Alexander, G. E., and Grutcher, M. D. (1990). Functional architecture of basal ganglia circuits: Neural substrates of parallel processing. *Trends Neurosci.* 13, 266–271.
Baik, J.-H., Picetti, R., Saiardi, A., Thiriet, G., Dierich, A., Depulis, A., Le Meur, M., and Borrelli, E. (1995). Parkinsonian-like locomotor impairment in mice lacking dopamine D_2 receptors. *Nature* 377, 424–428.
Bergman, H., Feingold, A., Nini, A., Raz, A., Slovin, H., Abeles, M., and Vaadia, E. (1998). Physiological aspects of information processing in the basal ganglia of normal and parkinsonian primates. *Trends Neurosci.* 21, 32–38.
Brundege, J. M., and Dunwiddie, T. V. (1996). Modulation of excitatory synaptic transmission by adenosine released from single hippocampal pyramidal neurons. *J. Neurosci.* 16, 5603–5612.
Brundege, J. M., and Dunwiddie, T. V. (1997). Role of adenosine as a modulator of synaptic activity in the central nervous system. *Adv. Pharmacol.* 39, 353–391.
Burnstock, G. (1986). The changing face of autonomic neurotransmission. *Acta Physiol. Scand.* 126, 67–91.
Chase, T. N. (1998). Novel approaches to the palliation of Parkinson's disease. *Mov. Dis.* 13, M39.
Chase, T. N., Engber, T. M. and Mouradian, M. M. (1996). Contribution of dopaminergic and glutamatergic mechanism to the pathogenesis of motor-response complications in Parkinson's disease. *Adv. Neurol.* 69, 497–501.
Chen, G., and Van den Pol, A. N. (1997). Adenosine modulation of calcium currents and presynaptic inhibition of GABA release in suprachiasmatic and arcuate nucleus neurons. *J. Neurophysiol.* 77, 3035–3047.
Craig, G. C., and White, T. D. (1992). Low-level N-methyl-D-aspartate receptor activation provides a purinergic inhibitory threshold against further N-methyl-aspartate-mediated neurotransmission in the cortex. *J. Pharmacol. Exp. Ther.* 260, 1278–1284.
Craig, G. C., and White, T. D. (1993). N-methyl-D-aspartate and non-N-methyl-D-aspartate-evoked adenosine release from rat cortical slices: Distinct purinergic sources and mechanisms of release. *J. Neurochem.* 60, 1073–1080.
DeLong, M. R. (1990). Primate model of movement disorders of basal ganglia origin. *Trends Neurosci.* 13, 281–285.
Drury, A. N., and Szent-Györgyi, A. (1929). The physiological activity of adenosine compounds with especial reference to their action upon the mammalian heart. *J. Physiol. (London)* 68, 213–237.
Dunwiddie, T. V., Dialo, L., and Proctor, W. R. (1997). *J. Neurosci.* 17, 7673–7682.
Ferre, S., Fredholm, B. B., Morelli, M., Popoli, P., and Fuxe, K. (1997). Adenosine–dopamine

receptor–receptor interactions as an integrative mechanism in the basal ganglia. *Trends Neurosci.* **20**, 482–487.

Ferre, S., O'Connor, W. T., Fuxe, K., and Ungerstedt, U. (1993). The striopallidal neuron: A main locus for adenosine–dopamine interaction in the brain. *J. Neurosci.* **13**, 5402–5406.

Fredholm, B. B., Abbracchio, M. P., Burnstock, G., Daly, J. W., Harden, T. K., Jacobson, K. A., Leff, P., and Williams, M. (1994). Nomenclature and classification of purinoceptors. *Pharmacol. Rev.* **46**, 143–156.

Fredholm, B. B., and Svenningsson, P. (1998). Striatal adenosine A_{2A} receptors: Where are they? What do they do? *Trends Pharmacol. Sci.* **19**, 46–47.

Gereau, R. W., and Conn, P. J. (1994). Potentiation of cAMP responses by metabotropic glutamate receptors depresses excitatory synaptic transmission by a kinase-independent mechanism. *Neuron* **12**, 1121–1129.

Grover, L. M., and Teyler, T. J. (1993). Role of adenosine in heterosynaptic, posttetanic depression in area CA1 of hippocampus. *Neurosci. Lett.* **154**, 39–42.

Gubitz, A. K., Widdowson, L., Kurokawa, M., Kirkpatrick, K. A., and Richardson, P. J. (1996). Dual signalling by the adenosine A_{2A} receptor involves activation of both N- and P-type calcium channels by different G proteins and protein kinases in the same striatal nerve terminals *J. Neurochem.* **67**, 374–381.

Jaeger, D., Kita, H., and Wilson, C. J. (1994). Surround inhibition among projection neurons is weak or nonexistent in the rat neostriatum. *J. Neurophysiol.* **72**, 2555–2558.

James, S., and Richardson, P. J. (1993). Production of adenosine from extracellular ATP at the striatal cholinergic synapse. *J Neurochem.* **60**, 219–227.

Kanda, T., Jackson, M. J., Smith, L. A., Pearce, R. K. B., Nakamura, J., Kase, H., Kuwana, Y., and Jenner, P. (1998). Adenosine A_{2A} antagonist: A novel antiparkinsonian agent that does not provoke dyskinesia in parkinsonian monkeys. *Ann. Neurol.* **43**, 507–513.

Kirk, I. P., and Richardson, P. J. (1995). Inhibition of striatal GABA release by the adenosine A_{2A} receptor is not mediated by increases in cyclic AMP. *J. Neurochem.* **64**, 2801–2809.

Kita, H. (1996). Two pathways between the cortex and the basal ganglia output nuclei and the globus pallidus. *in* "The Basal Ganglia V" (Ohye *et al.*, Eds.), pp. 77–94. Plenum, New York.

Kurokawa, M., Kirk, I. P., Kirkpatrick, K. A., Kase, H., and Richardson, P. J. (1994). Inhibition by KF17837 of adenosine A_{2A} receptor-mediated modulation of striatal GABA and Ach release. *Br. J. Pharmacol.* **113**, 43–48.

Ledent, C., Vaugeois, J.-M., Schiffmann, S. N., Pedrazzini, T., El Yacoubi, M., Vanderhaeghen, J.-J., Costentin, J., Heath, J. K., Vassart, G., and Parmentier, M. (1997). Agressiveness, hypoalgesia and high blood pressure in mice lacking the adenosine A_{2A} receptor. *Nature* **388**, 674–678.

Manzoni, O. J., Manabe, T., and Nicoll, R. A. (1994). Release of adenosine by activation of NMDA receptors in the hippocampus. *Science* **265**, 2098–2101.

Mayfield, R. D., Suzuki, F. and Zahniser, N. R. (1993). Adenosine A_{2A} receptor modulation of electrically evoked endogenous GABA release from slices of rat globus pallidus. *J. Neurochem.* **60**, 2334–2337.

Mayfield, R. D., Larson, G., Orana, A., and Zahniser, N. R. (1996). Opposing actions of adenosine A_{2A} and dopamine D_2 receptor activation on GABA release in the basal ganglia: Evidence for an A_{2A}/D_2 receptor interaction in globus pallidus. *Synapse* **22**, 132–138.

Michell, J. B., Lupica, C. R., and Duwiddie, T. V. (1993). Activity dependent release of endogenous adenosine modulates synaptic responses in the rat hippocampus. *J. Neurosci.* **13**, 3439–3447.

Mori, A., Shindou, T., Ichimura, M., Nonaka, H., and Kase, H. (1996). The role of adenosine A_{2A} receptors in regulating GABAergic synaptic transmission in striatal medium spiny neurons. *J. Neurosci.* **16**, 605–611.

Nomoto, M., Shimizu, T., Iwata, S.-I., Kaseda, S., Mitsuda, M., and Fukuda, T. (1998). The metabolism of adenosine increased in the striatum of parkinsonism in common marmosets induced by 1-methyl-4-phenyl-1,2,3,6-tetrahydropyridine. *Adv. Neurol.* (in press).

Nonaka, H., Ichimura, M., Takeda, M., Nonak, Y., Shimada, J., Suzuki, F., Yamaguchi, K., and Kase, H. (1994a). KF17837 ((*E*)-8-(3,4-dimethoxystyryl)-1,3-dipropyl-7-methylxanthine), a potent and selective adenosine A$_2$ receptor antagonist. *Eur. J. Pharmacol.* **267**, 335–341.

Nonaka, H., Mori, A., Ichimura, M., Shindou, T., Yanagawa, K., Shimada, J., Kase, H. (1994b). Binding of [^{3}H]KF17837S, a selective adenosine A$_2$ receptor antagonist, to rat brain membranes. Mol. Pharmacol. **46**, 817-822.

Obeso, J. A., Rodriguez, M. C., and DeLong, M. R. (1997). Basal ganglia pathophysiology— A critical review. *in* "Advances in Neurology" (J. A. Obeso, N. R. DeLong, C. Ohye, and C. D. Marsden, Eds.), Vol. 74, pp. 3–8. Lippincott-Raven Publishers, Philadelphia.

Olah, M. E., and Stiles, G. L. (1995). Adenosine receptor subtype: Characterization and therapeutic regulation. *Annu. Rev. Pharmacol. Toxicol.* **35**, 581–606.

Ongini, E., and Fredholm, B. B. (1996). Pharmacology of adenosine A$_{2A}$ receptors. *Trends Pharmacol. Sci.* **17**, 362–372.

Park, T. J., Chung, S. K., Han, M. K., Kim, U. H. and Kim, K. T. (1998). Inhibition of voltage-sensitive calcium channels by the A$_{2A}$ adenosine receptor in PC12 cells. *J. Neurochem.* **71**, 1251–1260.

Park, T. J., Song, S. K,. and Kim, K. T. (1997). A$_{2A}$ adenosine receptors inhibit ATP-induced Ca^{2+} influx in PC12 cells by involving protein kinase A. *J. Neurochem.* **68**, 2177–2185.

Richardson, P. J., and Brown, S. J. (1987). ATP release from affinity-purified rat cholinergic nerve terminals. *J. Neurochem.* **48**, 622–630.

Richardson, P. J., Kase, H., and Jenner, P. G. (1997). Adenosine A$_{2A}$ receptor antagonists as new agents for the treatment of Parkinson's disease. *Trends Pharmacol. Sci.* **18**, 338–344.

Richardson, P. J., Kase, H., and Jenner, P. G. (1998). Richardson *et al.* Reply. *Trends Pharmacol. Sci.* **19**, 47–48.

Robertson, S. J., and Edwards, F. A. (1998). ATP and glutamate are released from separate neurones in the rat medial habenula nucleus: Frequency dependence and adenosine-mediated inhibition of release. *J. Physiol. (London).* **508**, 691–701.

Rosenberg, P. A., Knowles,. R., Knowles, K. P., and Li, Y. (1994). Beta-adrenergic receptor-mediated regulation of extracellular adenosine in cerebral cortex in culture. *J. Neurosci.* **14**, 2953–2965.

Rosenberg, P. A., and Li, Y. (1995). Adenylyl cyclase activation underlies intracellular cyclic AMP accumulation, cyclic AMP transport, and extracellular adenosine accumulation evoked by beta-adrenergic receptor stimulation in mixed cultures of neurons and astrocytes derived from rat cerebral cortex. *Brain Res.* **692**, 227–232.

Rosin, D. L., Botkin, S. M., and Linden, J. (1997). Ultrastructural localization of adenosine A$_{2A}$ receptor immunoreactivity in rat striatum. *Soc. Neurosci. Abstr.* **23**, 588.5.

Silinsky, E. M. (1975). On the association between transmitter secretion and the release of adenine nucleotides from mammalian motor nerve terminals. *J. Physiol. (London)* **247**, 145–162.

Smith, Y., Bevan, M. D., Shink, E., and Bolam, J. P. (1998). Microcircuitry of the direct and indirect pathways of the basal ganglia. *Neuroscience* **86**, 353–387.

Stern, E. A., Jaeger, D., and Wilson, C. J. (1998). Membrane potential synchrony of simultaneously recorded striatal spiny neurons *in vivo*. *Nature* **394**, 475–478.

Ziganshin, A. U., Hoyle, C. H., and Burnstock, G. (1994). Ecto-enzymes and metabolism of extracellular ATP. *Drug Dev. Res.* **32**, 134–146.

Zimmermann, H. (1992). 5-Nucleotidase: Molecular structure and functional aspects. *Biochem. J.* **285**, 345–365.

CHAPTER 2

Localization of Adenosine Receptors in Brain and Periphery

SARAH J. AUGOOD

Neurology Research, Massachusetts General Hospital and Harvard Medical School, Boston, Massachusetts

PIERS C. EMSON

Department of Neurobiology, The Babraham Institute, Cambridge, United Kingdom

DAVID G. STANDAERT

Neurology Research, Massachusetts General Hospital and Harvard Medical School, Boston, Massachusetts

I. ADENOSINE

Adenosine is released from metabolically active cells and is generated extracellularly by degradation of adenosine triphosphate (ATP). It is a potent biological molecule and modulates the activity of numerous neuronal and non-neuronal cell types within both the peripheral nervous system (PNS) and the central nervous system (CNS). Within the PNS, adenosine acts to modulate the activity of platelets, neutrophils [62], mast cells, and vascular smooth muscle cells. Within the brain, extracellular levels of adensoine in unrestrained rats are around 50–300 nM [3], rising significantly during periods of increased nerve activity. Under pathological conditions, high concentrations of adenosine are released by neurons, leading to the suggestion that adenosine may play a pivotal role in protecting cells from stress-induced damage, especially ischemic damage [11,50]. Consistent with this hypothesis, micromolar administration of selective adenosine receptor agonists, such as 5′-(N-ethylcarboxamido)-adenosine (NECA) and CGS-21680, can induce the production of nerve growth factor mRNA and protein by rat cortical microglia *in vitro* [19] and be mitogenic in human umbilical venous endothelial cell cultures [56].

The actions of adenosine within both the PNS and the CNS are mediated via interaction with a family of G-protein coupled adenosine receptors. The first proposal that adenosine receptors could be subdivided was made by van Calker in 1979 [4], based on the observation that adenosine could either inhibit or stimulate adenylyl cyclase activity *in vitro*. These opposing effects were suggested to be mediated via A_1 (inhibition) or A_2 (stimulation) adenosine receptors. Four family members have now been identified by molecular cloning and these have been termed A_1, A_{2A}, A_{2B}, and A_3 adenosine receptors. In this chapter, we review the literature concerning the anatomical localization of all four adenosine receptor subtypes. A brief review of the localization and putative functions of each adenosine receptor subtype is given, focusing primarily on their cellular localization within the mammalian CNS.

II. RECEPTOR SUBTYPES

A. ADENOSINE A_1 RECEPTORS

The adenosine A_1 receptor has now been cloned from a number of species (see Table I), including rat [33,46] and human [61]. In humans, the complete gene consists of at least six exons and five introns, although only a single intron interrupts the coding sequence [44]. The complete nucleotide sequence of the rat cDNA has an open reading frame encoding a protein of approximately 326 amino acids, with a theoretical molecular mass of 37 KDa. In contrast to the other members of the adenosine receptor family, two distinct transcripts are detected in rat and human tissue by Northern blot analysis [33] (see Table 2). These are expressed in a tissue-specific manner [44] and contain distinct exons transcribed from two separate promoters [45]. Study of human tissue by polymerase chain reaction (RT-PCR) revealed transcripts containing exons 4, 5, and 6 in all tissues examined (frontal cortex, basal ganglia, thalamus, cerebellum, fat, heart, skeletal muscle, aorta, liver, and spleen), whereas an alternative transcript containing exons 3, 5, and 6 (but not exon 4) was seen only in frontal cortex, cerebellum, and kidney but not in fat, skeletal muscle, or heart [44]. In rat, the distribution of mRNA encoding the A_1 receptor has been studied extensively by RT-PCR, Northern blot analysis, and *in situ* hybridization [10,27,33,46]. Consistent with the expression of A_1 receptor transcripts in human tissue, two receptor transcripts (5.6 kb and 3.1 kb) are detected in rat tissues [33]. Despite the widespread distribution of both receptor transcripts within many CNS and PNS tissues, there appears to be a differential enrichment of the two mRNAs within different tissues: the higher molecular weight transcript (5.6 kb) being predominant within the CNS and the lower molecular weight transcript (3.1 kb) dominating within the PNS [33]. The one exception appears to be the eye where only the 5.6-kb transcript has been detected [33], expressed exclusively by retinal ganglion cells [27]. Within brain, A_1 transcripts are enriched within the olfactory bulb, cerebral cortex, hippocampal formation, mesencephalon, striatum, and cerebellum [10,33,46]. *In situ* hybridization studies have essentially confirmed and extended the distribution of mRNA revealed by Northern blot analysis. Additional structures found to be enriched in mRNA include the thalamus, medial geniculate nucleus, ventral tegmental nucleus, brain stem, and spinal cord. Furthermore, discrete patterns of neuronal labeling are observed and a specific mRNA signal is observed localized to pyramidal neurons in the hippocampal formation, granule cells in the cerebellum [33], and large putative cholinergic cells within the striatum [10]. Within the PNS, an abundance of adenosine A_1 receptor mRNA is detected (by Northern blot analysis) in the spleen, stomach, and eye with a less intense signal seen in the testis, adipose tissue, heart, kidney, liver, and bladder [10,33,46]. Whether A_1 receptor mRNA is expressed in the pituitary is controversial.

Adenosine A_1 receptor binding sites have been localized in rat and human brain tissue by *in vitro* autoradiography using [^{3}H]-N^6-cyclohexyladenosine (CHA) as the A_1-specific high-affinity ligand [1,14,17,18]. As predicted from previous biochemical studies, a widespread distribution of [^{3}H]-CHA binding was observed with the highest density of binding sites obseved in the molecular and polymorphic layers of the hippocampus and dentate gyrus, the molecular layer of the cerebellum, and within the temporal gyrus. Moderate densities are observed within several basal ganglia structures including the caudate nucleus and putamen, substantia nigra pars reticulata, and within the spinal cord (substantia gelatinosa). Specific labeling of most white matter areas as well as certain hypothalamic structures is neglible. Within the periphery, high-affinity [^{3}H]-CHA binding sites are associated with spermatocytes within the seminiferous tubule epithelium [36]. More recently, site-directed mutagenesis studies have identified particular amino acids in transmembrane domains 1–4 that are believed to be important for the binding of A_1 receptor-subtype specific ligands [49].

As the rat A_1 receptor was one of the first adenosine receptors to be cloned, A_1-specific antisera are now available. Using an affinity-purified antipeptide A_1-specific antibody directed against a conserved sequence in both the rat and human A_1 receptors, Rivkees and colleagues [48] mapped, in detail, the distribution of A_1-like immunoreactivity in the rat brain. As predicted from *in situ* hybridization studies and ligand binding studies, A_1-like immunoreactivity was found localized to specific neuronal populations and cellular processes. Brain structures exhibiting a strong immunopositive signal include the hippocampal formation, cerebellum, cerebral cortex, and several thalamic nuclei and cranial nerves. Specifically, intense somatic and axonal labeling was associated with pyramidal neurons in most regions of the cerebral cortex and hippocampal formation and basket cells in the cerebellum (granule cells were moderately immunopositive). Within basal ganglia structures, A_1-immunopositive cells were observed in the striatum (38% of neurons), globus pallidus (43%), subthalamic nucleus, and ventral tegmental area, although the precise chemical phenotype of these immunopositive cells has not been determined. Additional brain structures enriched in A_1-immunoreactivity include the corpus callosum [60], several thalamic nuclei, the superior and inferior colliculi, the habenular, and the facial, trigeminal, and hypoglossal nuclei. One unexpected finding of this study was the enrichment of A_1-like immunoreactivity within specific hypothalamic structures as Goodman and Snyder [18] reported a relative dearth of A_1 binding sites here. To date, the distribution of A_1-immunoreactivity in human brain has not been reported, although one would predict a similar pattern of staining as autoradiography studies using [^{3}H]-CHA as the specific A_1 receptor ligand show numerous parallels between the distribution in rat [23] and human [17] brain. That is, an enrichment of A_1 binding sites is observed in the human cerebral cortex, striatum, hippocampus, thalamus, and cerebellum.

Concerning the functional roles of adenosine A_1 receptors in the mammalian nervous system, it is now known that A_1 receptors can interact with a variety of signal transduction pathways to inhibit/modulate renin secretion and renal vasoconstriction and acid secretion in the gastrointestinal tract (see [7]), and to have cardioprotective effects by promoting survival of cardiac myocytes. In vitro, stimulation of cell surface A_1 receptors on DDT_1MF-2 smooth muscle cells causes a rapid clustering of receptor molecules, resulting in receptor internalization and densensitization [6]. Together, these data suggest that A_1 receptors may play an important role in modulating cellular activity via high-affinity receptor densensitization. Within the CNS, several mechanisms contributing to the cytoprotective role of adenosine have been proposed, including the depression of neuronal firing rate and neuronal metabolism by A_1 receptor activation. Biochemical data suggest that, in vitro, oxidative stress increases A_1 receptor expression by activating nuclear factor kB regulatory sites on the A_1 receptor gene [37], promoting the cytoprotective role of adenosine. Whether a parallel mechanism exists in vivo during times of ischemic insult, for example, awaits clarification. Within the CNS, however, A_1 receptors have been involved in modulating neurotransmitter release and inhibiting synaptic transmission; one putative mechanism involves interaction with axonal A_1 receptors [8,60]. An involvement of A_1 receptors in the psychiatric disorder of bipolar affective disorder has recently been proposed, although this preliminary finding could not be replicated in a larger study [9].

B. ADENOSINE A_{2A} RECEPTORS

The human A_{2A} receptor is encoded by a single gene containing one intron in the open reading frame located on chromosome 22 [41]. Northern blot analysis of CNS and peripheral tissue reveal the mRNA encoding this receptor to be a single band of about 2.5 kb, consistent with its predicted size [2,16]. Site-directed mutagenesis studies coupled with functional biochemical work have demonstrated that certain amino acids in the first transmembrane domain [20] and in the second extracellular loop are important for A_{2A} ligand binding [26]. Furthermore, *in vitro* activation of the G-protein G_s is predominantly dictated by the NH_2-terminal segment of the third intracellular loop [39].

The distribution of mRNA encoding the rat and human A_{2A} receptor has been studied in detail using RT-PCR, Northern blot analysis, and sensitive *in situ* hybridization methodologies (see Table 2). In contrast to the widespread distribution of A_1 receptor transcripts within the CNS, the distribution of A_{2A} receptor transcripts seems to be more restricted [2,16,54,55], although Dixon and colleagues [10] report a more widespread distribution by RT-PCR than is detected by *in situ* hybridization and Northern blot analysis. Sensitive *in situ* techniques report an enrichment of A_{2A} receptor mRNA in the caudate nucleus and putamen (striatum), nucleus accumbens, islands of Calleja, and olfactory tubercle [2,16,54]. A study of human postmortem tissues reveals a similar enrichment of A_{2A} transcripts within the striatum [55]. A weak signal is detected, however, in other CNS tissues (amygdala, occipital cortex, substantia nigra, and cerebellum) by Northern blot analysis and in peripheral tissues, including heart, lung, small intestine, and kidney [41]. Within the CNS, the chemical phenotype of A_{2A} mRNA-expressing neurons has been investigated in detail. Within the striatum, approximately 50% of neurons within both the rat [2,16,54] and human [55] brain express A_{2A} receptor transcripts. Of these A_{2A} mRNA-positive neurons, the vast majority are GABAergic projection neurons coexpressing the neuropeptide enkephalin [2,35,55]. Consistent with this cellular data, an enrichment of A_{2A} binding sites [^{3}H]-CGS-21680 are detected almost exclusively within the striatum and within target structures of striatal GABA/enkephalin neurons, namely the GPe [23,34]. There exists, however, some debate surrounding the expression of this receptor by the small population (<15% of striatal neurons) of aspiny striatal cholinergic interneurons [25]. The majority of double-label *in situ* hybridization studies have failed to detect $A_{2A}R$ expression in either rat or postmortem human tissue [2,35,55], although this finding has been contested by PCR [10]. Concerning the precise cellular localization of A_{2A} receptor protein in the CNS, no detailed ultrastructural studies are currently available although they are eagerly awaited.

To gain a deeper understanding of the putative function(s) of this receptor in vivo A_{2A} receptor-deficient mice have been generated [28]. These homozygous mice are viable and develop normally, suggesting that the A_{2A} receptor function may not be critical during neurogenesis. However, these A_{2A} receptor-deficient mice display behaviors reflecting increased anxiety and hyperaggression (in males). The neural basis of these behaviors is uncertain because developmental compensatory mechanisms involving other adenosine receptors are possible. However, the observation that A_{2A} receptors are localized within limbic structures is noteworthy indicating that, in the intact animal, endogenous adenosine acting on A_{2A} receptors may have antianxiolytic properties [52]. As within most transgenic animal studies, the issue of background genotype requires careful consideration

Of the four adenosine receptor subtypes, the A_{2A} receptor is the focus of intense research within the neurological field, particularly in relation to the hypoactive and hyperactive movement disorders of Parkinson's disease [47] and Huntington's disease, respectively, where the efficacy and chronic use of drug therapies are limited. A study by Kanda and colleagues [24] have reported that oral administration of KW-6002, a selective A_{2A} receptor antagonist, to hypoactive parkinsonian MPTP-treated marmosets results in a modest and sustained increase in motor activity without the onset of abnormal dyskinetic movements. Furthermore, oral administration of KW-6002 during the 21-day trial was well tolerated. This indeed is an interesting development and strengthens the hypothesis that adenosine A_{2A} receptors may be an important therapeutic target for future development.

C. ADENOSINE A_{2B} RECEPTORS

The rat adenosine A_{2B} receptor gene encodes a 332 amino acid protein [58]. Analogous to the A_1 and A_{2A} receptor genes, the coding region of the A_{2B} receptor gene is interrupted by a single intron corresponding to the second intracellular loop of the proposed seven transmembrane domain topography [22]. In contrast to the other members of the adenosine receptor family, a human A_{2B} pseudogene has also been identified and localized to chromosome 1q32 [22]. This pseudogene exhibits approximately 80% sequence homology to the A_{2B} protein and contains multiple deletions, point mutations, frame shifts, and in-frame stops, indicating that resulting translated proteins(s) would not be functional. Whether such a pseudogene exists in the genome of other mammalian species is not yet known.

Little is known about the localization of the A_{2B} receptor subtype in brain because sensitive in situ hybridization studies have failed to detect a positive mRNA signal at the cellular level [10,58], although a positive signal has been detected in the hypophyseal pars tuberalis [58]. The cellular phenotype of A_{2B} receptor expression in brain, therefore, has not been determined, although it may be expressed by rat astrocytes [40]. Examination of the tissue distribution of A_{2B} mRNA by RT-PCR, however, reveals a more widespread distribution with an A_{2B}-specific PCR product being detected in numerous structures in the forebrain, midbrain, and cerebellar tissue (see Table 2)[10]. Indeed, the human A_{2B} receptor gene was isolated from a human hippocampal library [42] consistent with the expression of this gene in brain tissue. Within the periphery, a restricted distribution is observed by both RT-PCR [10] and by Northern blot analysis [58]. An intense mRNA signal is detected in the large intestine, caecum, urinary bladder, lung, mast cells, and ciliary processes within the eye [10, 27, 58].

By use of an affinity-purified antipeptide antibody raised in chicken [43], immunopositive structures have been localized in human peripheral organs. Of note, Western blot analysis of human and rat tissue revealed a marked species heterogeneity with regard to the multiplicity and apparent size of the A_{2B}-immunopositive bands. In human and rat thymus and colon and human small intestine samples, a 50–55-KDa immunopositive band is detected, whereas in the rat small intestine, an additional 35-KDa band is observed. Using an immunohistochemical technique A_{2B}-immunopositive staining was detected in the epithelial cells of the crypts in the human colon, in addition to the syncytiotrophoblast cells of the placental villi, and in the basal zone of mouse choriallantoic placenta [43].

Concerning the putative functional roles of this adenosine receptor subtype, biochemical studies have demonstrated that this receptor protein can couple positively to adenylyl cyclase in rat primary astrocytes [40] and in human intestinal epithelia [59], in addition to inhibiting the growth of human aortic smooth muscle cells [13] and collagen and total protein synthesis in cardiac fibroblasts [12]. In addition to the putative clinical benefit of A_{2B} receptor-specific drugs in treating cardiac and diarrheal diseases [59], interest has focused on the role of this receptor subtype in the treatment of asthma [15] by virtue of mast cell activation. Indeed, enprofylline, an antiasthmatic drug, is the most selective, although not potent, A_{2B} receptor antagonist known to date.

D. Adenosine A_3 Receptors

The adenosine A_3 receptor is the more recent receptor in this gene family to be isolated and cloned. The proposed membrane topography (hydrophobicity analysis) of the deduced amino acid sequence predicts that the protein has seven hydrophobic domains consistent with this receptor protein being a

TABLE I   Cloning of Adenosine Receptors

Subtype	Organism	Source	Protein	Accession no.	Chromosome
A_1	Human	heart	327 a.a.[a]	AB004662	1q31–32.1
	Rat	brain	326 a.a.	M64299	n/a
	Cow	brain	326 a.a.	M86261	n/a
	Mouse	- - -	- - -	AF133099*	n/a
	Guinea pig (Hartley)	brain	326 a.a.	U04279	n/a
	Chicken (gallus gallus)	adipose	324 a.a.	U28380	n/a
	Rabbit	kidney	328 a.a.	L01700	n/a
A_{2A}	Human	lymphocytes	412 a.a.	U40771	22q11.2
	Rat	brain	410 a.a.	L08102	n/a
	Mouse	genomic	410 a.a.	Y13346	n/a
	Guinea pig	leukocyte	409 a.a	D63674	n/a
	Dog	thyroid	412 a.a.	X14052	n/a
A_{2B}	Human	brain	332 a.a.	M97759	17p11.2–p12
	Rat	brain	332 a.a.	M91466	n/a
	Mouse	colon	- - -	Al647254*	n/a
A_3	Human	Brain	318 a.a.	L22607	1p13.3
	Sheep	pars tuberalis	317 a.a.	S65334	n/a
	Rat	- - -	320 a.a.	M94152	n/a
	Mouse	- - -	319 a.a.	AF069778	3
	Rabbit	lung	319 a.a.	U90718.1	n/a
	Dog	mastocytoma	314 a.a.	U54792	n/a
	Chicken	brain	333 a.a.	AF115332	n/a

* = Partial sequence;   n/a = not mapped yet (June 99)   [a]a. a., amino acid.

member of the family of membrane-bound G-protein coupled receptors. The full-length cDNA encodes a 317–333 amino acid protein (see Table I), with an estimated molecular mass of 37 kDa. In contrast to the other member of the adenosine receptor family, there is a marked divergence in sequence among the different species so far isolated, in particular between the rat A_3 receptor sequence and the human and sheep homologues (see [31]). Direct comparison of sequence identity reveal that the rat A_3 receptor shares less than 85% sequence homology with the sheep and human A_3 receptor sequences. As there is more than 90% conservation of sequence identity between the rat and human for the other three adenosine receptors, the possibility of additional A_3 receptor subtypes has been suggested. This species-dependent diversity in sequence information is further reflected by the varying patterns of receptor expression that have been reported. In the rat, Northern blot analysis of several peripheral and CNS tissues reports an enrichment of A_3 receptor mRNA almost exclusively within the testis [64]. However, a widespread distribution of A_3 receptor mRNA has been reported using sensitive RT-PCR technology [10]. Of note, moderate amounts of mRNA are reported in all brain areas studied, including the striatum, hypothalamus, hippocampus, and cerebellum, as well as in numerous peripheral tissues, including the spleen, lung, uterus, and testis. A very weak signal was reported in the heart and eye. However, examination of tissue sections processed for *in situ* hybridization, to reveal the cellular sites of A_3 receptor mRNA expression, revealed a specific hybridization signal only within spermatocytes and spermatids in the testis. No signal was detected within the CNS or within other peripheral tissues [10], including the eye [27]. Whether these apparent differences in tissue distribution observed by RT-PCR and by *in situ* hybridization reflect differences in the sensitivity of the two techniques employed or are suggestive of multiple A_3 receptor subtypes [38] awaits further study. In the sheep, however, it is the lung and spleen, not the testis, that are reported to be enriched in A_3 receptor mRNA as are the pineal gland and pars tuberalis in the brain. No specific signal has been detected in heart tissue [30]. Similarly in human tissue, an enrichment of A_3 receptors is reported by some researchers [51] in the lung and liver with relatively lower levels in the brain. The detailed cellular localization of A_3 receptors within the human brain has yet to be reported. The introduction of relatively specific A_3 receptor ligands (see [21]), in addition to the availability of specific antisera directed against the A_3 receptor, will certainly clarify the situation and add greatly to our knowledge of the cellular localization of this receptor protein.

Undoubtedly, the relatively low levels of A_3 receptor detected have hampered the molecular anatomical studies; however, within the mammalian nervous system, numerous physiological roles have been ascribed to this enigmatic receptor, including a role in inflammation and nociception [53], via release of histamine and serotonin from activated mast cells; cardioprotection [29,57], via activation of cardiac ventricular cells; and apoptosis [63]. However, A_3 receptor, activation is reported to have both cytoprotective and cytotoxic effects, depending on the species, tissue, and agonist concentration studied. In general, nanomolar concentrations of selective agonists appear to be cytoprotective, whereas micromolar concentrations can evoke apoptosis and cell death [5]. For example, administration of IB-MECA and Cl-IB-MECA (A_3 agonists) can protect chick cardiac myocytes in culture from hypoxia/ischemia-induced cell death in a dose-dependent manner [29,57], this cytoprotective effect being blocked by the novel A_3 receptor antagonist,

MRS1191. Furthermore, administration of the novel antagonists MRS1191 and L-249313 (500 nM) can induce toxicity in human leukemia (HL-60) and lymphoma (U-937) cells in culture [63], suggesting that tonic activation of A_3 receptors *in situ* may be cytoprotective. Whereas administration of micromolar concentrations (>10 μM) of CI-IB-MECA, an A_3 selective agonist, to these human cell lines [63] and of 2-chloro-adenosine (3–10 μM), a nonselective adenosine receptor agonist, to rat glia cells in culture can induce DNA fragmentation [5,38], recognized markers of apoptotic cell death. This apoptotic process could be antagonized by 3 μM staurosporine supporting the involvement of protein kinase C activation in this pathway.

With regard to the putative role of A_3 receptors within the CNS, it is intriguing to note that the affinity of these receptors for adenosine is low in the micromolar range, suggesting that, *in vivo* at least, these receptors may be critically important during times of stress when pathological concentrations of adenosine are present within the brain, sufficient to activate these receptors. Whether the result of receptor activation is to promote neuronal cell survival by destruction of macrophages and activated microglia awaits further study. Macek and colleagues [32] reported that A_3 receptor activation may impair metabotropic glutamate receptor functioning, suggesting an indirect effect of adenosine on glutamatergic signaling. Furthermore, since A_3 receptor activation has been shown to promote mast cell degranulation within the periphery and release of histamines, the clinical potential of selective A_3 receptor antagonists may be significant for the treatment of asthma and other allergic and inflammatory disorders [21].

TABLE II   Localization of Adenosine Receptors:

	A_1	A_{2A}	A_{2B}	A_3
RT-PCR (see ref. 10)	CNS and PNS	CNS and PNS	CNS and PNS	CNS and PNS
Northern blot analysis	5.6 Kb + 3.1 Kb CNS and PNS	2.5 kb forebrain >> PNS	2.2 Kb PNS >> CNS	1.8 Kb PNS only
In situ hybridization (mRNA)	widespread in CNS: enriched in CBM, hippo + cortex.	restricted in CNS: forebrain >> PNS	PNS >> CNS colon, eye, large intestine, bladder	testis only
Immunochemical (protein)	widespread in CNS: enriched in CBM, hippo + cortex.	blood vessels, neurons + neuropil. forebrain and PNS	intestine + colon	specific antisera?
Ligand binding in CNS	[3H]CHA: widespread in brain	[3H]CGS-21680: forebrain only	specific ligand?	specific ligand?

Summary of the distribution of adenosine receptor subtypes in rats and human tissues using different techniques.

III. SUMMARY

In this chapter, we provide an overview of the macroscopic and cellular localization of four adenosine receptor subtypes within the mammalian nervous system (see Table II) and attempt to highlight the potential functional roles of these receptors within both the CNS and the PNS. Indeed, it is clear that adenosine plays a pivotal physiological role in mammals, its effects mediated via interaction with adenosine A_1, A_{2A}, A_{2B}, and/or A_3 receptors.

REFERENCES

1. Alexander, S., and Reddington, M., The cellular localization of adenosine receptors in rat neostriatum. *Neurosci, 28* (1989) 645–651.
2. Augood, S. J., and Emson, P. C., Adenosine A_{2A} receptor mRNA is expressed by enkephalin cells but not by somatostatin cells in rat striatum: a co-expression study, *Brain Res, Mol Brain Res 22* (1994) 204–210.
3. Ballarin, M., Fredholm, B., Ambrosio, S., and Mahy, N., Extracellular levels of adenosine and its metabolites in the striatum of awake rats: inhibition of uptake and metabolism. *Acta Physiol Scand, 142* (1991) 97–103.
4. van Calker, D., Muller, M., and Hamprecht, B., Adenosine regulates via two different types of receptors: the accumulation of cyclic AMP in cultured brain cells. *J. Neurochem, 33* (1979) 999–1005.
5. Ceruti, S., Barbiere, D., Franchesi, C., Giammaroli, A., Rainaldi, G., Malorni, W., Kim, H., Lubitz, D. V., Jacobson, K., Cattabeni, F., and Abbracchio, M., Effects of adenosine A_3 receptor agonists on astrocytes: induction of cell protection at low and cell death at high concentrations. *Drug Dev Res, 3* (1996) 117.
6. Ciruela, F., Saura, C., Canela, E., Mallol, J., Lluis, C., and Franco, R., Ligand-induced phosphorylation, clustering, and densitization of A_1 adenosine receptors. *Mol Pharmacol, 52* (1997) 788–797.
7. Collis, M., and Hourani, S., Adenosine receptor subtypes. *Trends in Pharmacological Sciences, 14* (1993) 360–365.
8. Cunha, R., Sebastiao, A., and Ribeiro, J., Inhibition by ATP of hippocampal synaptic transmission requires localized extracellular catabolism by ecto-nucleotidases into adenosine and channeling to adenosine A_1 receptors. *J Neurosci, 18* (1998) 1987–1995.
9. Deckert, J., Nothen, M., Albus, M., Franzek, E., Rietschel, M., Ren, H., Stiles, G., Knapp, M., Weiglt, B., Maier, W., Beckmann, H., and Propping, P., Adenosine A_1 receptor and bipolar affective disorder: systematic screening of the gene and association studies. *Am J Med Genetics 81* (1998) 18–23.
10. Dixon, A., Gubitz, A., Sirinathsinghji, D., Richardson, P., and Freeman, T., Tissue distribution of adenosine receptor mRNAs in the rat. *Br J Pharmacol, 118* (1996) 1461–1468.
11. Dragunow M., Adenosine: the brain's natural anticonvulsant? *Trends in Pharmacological Sciences, 7* (1986) 128–130.
12. Dubey, R., Gillespie, D., and Jackson, E., Adenosine inhibits collagen and protein synthesis in cardiac fibroblasts: a role of A_{2B} receptors. *Hypertension, 31* (1998) 943–948.
13. Dubey, R., Gillespie, D., Mi, Z., and Jackson, E., Adenosine inhibits growth of human aortic smooth muscle cells via A_{2B} receptors. *Hypertension, 31* (1998) 516–521.
14. Fastbom, J., Pazos, A., Probst, A., and Palacios, J., Adenosine A_1 receptors in the human brain: a quantitative autoradiographic study. *Neurosci, 22* (1987) 827–839.

15. Feoktistov, I., Polosa, R., Holgate, S., and Biaggioni, I., Adenosine A_{2B} receptors: a novel therapeutic target in asthma? *Trends in Pharmacological Sciences, 19* (1998) 148–153.

16. Fink, J., Weaver, D., Rivkees, S., Peterfreund, R., Pollack, A., Adler, E., and Reppert, S., Molecular cloning of the rat A_2 adenosine receptor: selective co-expression with D_2 dopamine receptors in rat striatum. *Mol Brain Res, 14* (1992) 186–195.

17. Glass, M., Faull, R., and Dragunow, M., Localisation of the adenosine uptake site in the human brain: a comparison with the distribution of adenosine A_1 receptors. *Brain Res, 710* (1996) 79–91.

18. Goodman, R., and Snyder, S., Autoradiographic localization of adenosine receptors in rat brain using [^{3}H]cyclohexyladenosine. *J Neurosci, 2* (1982) 1230–1241.

19. Heese, K., Fiebich, B., Bauer, J., and Otten, U., Nerve growth factor (NGF) expression in rat microglia is induced by adenosine A_{2A}-receptors. *Neurosci Lett, 231* (1997) 83–86.

20. Ijzerman, A.P., Von Frijtag Drabbe Kunzel, J.K., Kim, J., Jiang, Q., and Jacobson, K.A., Site-directed mutagenesis of the human adenosine A_{2A} receptor. Critical involvement of Glu13 in agonist recognition. *Eur J Pharmacol, 310* (1996) 269–272.

21. Jacobson, K., Adenosine A_3 receptors: novel ligands and paradoxical effects. *Trends in Pharmacological Sciences, 19* (1998) 184–191.

22. Jacobson, M., Johnson, R., Luneau, C., and Salvatore, C., Cloning and chromosomal localization of the human A_{2B} adenosine receptor gene (ADORA2B) and its pseudogene. *Genomics, 27* (1995) 374–376.

23. Jarvis, M., and Williams, M., Direct autoradiographic localization of adenosine A_2 receptors in the rat brain using the A_2-selective agonist, [3H]CGS21680. *Eur J Pharmacol, 168* (1989) 243–246.

24. Kanda, T., Jackson, M., Smith, L., Pearce, R., Nakamura, J., Kase, H., Kuwana, Y., and Jenner, P., Adenosine A_{2A} antagonists: a novel antiparkinsonian agent that does not provoke dyskinesia in parkinsonian monkeys. *Ann Neurol, 43* (1998) 507–513.

25. Kawaguchi, Y., Wilson, C. J., Augood, S. J., and Emson, P .C., Striatal interneurones: chemical, physiological and morphological characterization [published erratum appears in *Trends Neurosci, 19*(4) (1996) 143. *Trends Neurosci, 18* (1995) 527–535.

26. Kim, J., Jiang, Q., Glashofer, M., Yehle, S., Wess, J., and Jacobson, K. A., Glutamate residues in the second extracellular loop of the human A_{2A} adenosine receptor are required for ligand recognition. *Mol Pharmacol, 49* (1996) 683–691.

27. Kvanta, A., Sergard, S., Sejersen, S., Kull, B., and Fredholm, B., Localization of adenosine receptor messenger RNAs in the rat eye. *Exp Eye Res, 65* (1997) 595–602.

28. Ledent, C., Vaugeois, J.-M., Schiffmann, S., Pedrazzini, T., Yacoubi, M., Vanderhaeghen, J.-J., Costentin, M., Heath, J., Vassart, G., and Parmentier, M., Aggressiveness, hypoalgesia and high blood pressure in mice lacking the adenosine A_{2A} receptor. *Nature, 388* (1997) 674–678.

29. Liang, B., and Jacobson, K., A physiological role of the adenosine A_3 receptor: sustained cardioprotection. *Proc Natl Acad Sci USA, 95* (1998) 6995–6999.

30. Linden, J., Taylor, E., Robeva, A., Tucker, A., Stehle, J., Rivkees, S., Fink, J., and Reppert, S., Molecular cloning and functional expression of a sheep A_3 adenosine receptor with widespread tissue distribution. *Mol Pharmacol, 44* (1993) 524–532.

31. Lubitz, D.V., Adenosine A_3 receptor and brain: a culprit, a hero, or merely yet another receptor. *Ann N Y Acad Sci, 825* (1997) 49–67.

32. Macek, T., Schaffhauser, H., and Conn, P. Protein kinase C and A_3 adenosine receptor activation inhibit presynaptic metabotropic glutamate (mGluR) function and uncouple mGluRs from GTP-binding proteins. *J Neurosci, 18* (1998) 6138–6146.

33. Mahan, L.C., McVittie, L.D., Smyk-Randall, E., Nakata, H., Monsma, F.J. Jr., Gerfen, C., and Sibley, D., Cloning and expression of an A_1 adenosine receptor from rat brain. *Mol Pharmacol, 40* (1991) 1–7.

34. Martinez-Mir, M., Probst, A., and Palacios, J., Adenosine A_2 receptors: selective localization in the human basal ganglia and alterations with disease. *Neurosci, 42* (1991) 697–706.

35. Moratalla, R., Sacerdote, M., Martin, D., Cuellar, B., Chen, J.-F., and Standaert, D., Localization of adenosine A_{2A} receptor mRNA in neurochemically identified striatal neurons in the human compared to the rat. Soc Neurosci, 28th meeting (1998).

36. Murphy, K., Goodman, R., and Snyder, S., Adenosine receptor localization in rat testes: biochemical and autoradiographic evidence for association with spermatocytes. *Endocrinol, 113* (1983) 1299–1305.

37. Nie, Z., Mei, Y., Rybak, F., Marcuzzi, A., Ren, H., Stiles, G., and Ramkumar, V., Oxidative stress increases adenosine receptor expression by activating nuclear factor kB. *Mol Pharmacol, 53* (1998) 663–669.

38. Ogata, T., and Schubert, P., Programmed cell death in rat microglia is controlled by extracellular adenosine. *Neurosci Lett, 218* (1996) 91–94.

39. Olah, M.E., Identification of A_{2A} adenosine receptor domains involved in selective coupling to G_s. Analysis of chimeric A_1/A_{2A} adenosine receptors. *J Biol Chem, 272* (1997) 337–344.

40. Peakman, M., and Hill, S., Adenosine A_{2B}-receptor-mediated cyclic AMP accumulation in primary rat astrocytes. *Br J Pharmacol, 111* (1994) 191–198.

41. Peterfreund, R. A., MacCollin, M., Gusella, J., and Fink, J. S., Characterization and expression of the human A_{2A} adenosine receptor gene. *J Neurochem, 66* (1996) 362–368.

42. Pierce, K., Furlong, T., Selbie, L., and Shine, J., Molecular cloning and expression of an adenosine A_{2B} receptor from human brain. *Biochem Biophys Res Commun, 187* (1992) 86–93.

43. Puffinbarger, N., Hansen, K., Resta, R., Laurent, A., Knudsen, T., Madara, J., and Thompson, L., Production and characterization of multiple antigenic peptide antibodies to the adenosine A_{2B} receptor. *Mol Pharmacol, 47* (1995) 1126–1132.

44. Ren, H., and Stiles, G., Characterization of the human A_1 adenosine receptor gene. Evidence for alternative splicing. *J Biol Chem, 269* (1994) 3104–3110.

45. Ren, H., and Stiles, G., Separate promoters in the human A_1 adenosine receptor gene direct the synthesis of distinct messenger RNAs that regulate receptor abundance. *Mol Pharmacol, 48* (1995) 957–980.

46. Reppert, S., Weaver, D., Stehle, J., and Rivkees, S., Molecular cloning and characterization of a rat A_1-adenosine receptor that is widely expressed in brain and spinal cord. *Mol Endocrinol, 5* (1991) 1037–1048.

47. Richardson, P., Kase, H., and Jenner, P., Adenosine A_{2A} receptor antagonists as new agents for the treatment of Parkinson's disease. *Trends Pharmacol Sci, 18* (1997) 338–344.

48. Rivkees, S., Price, S., and Zhou, F., Immunohistochemical detection of A_1 adenosine receptors in rat brain with emphasis on localization in the hippocampal formation, cerebral cortex, cerebellum and basal ganglia. *Brain Res, 677* (1995) 193–203.

49. Rivkees, S. A., Lasbury, M. E., and Barbhaiya, H., Identification of domains of the human A_1 adenosine receptor that are important for binding receptor subtype-selective ligands using chimeric A_1/A_{2A} adenosine receptors, *J Biol Chem, 270* (1995) 20485–20490.

50. Rudolphi, K., Schubert, P., Parkinson, F., and Fredholm, B., Neuroprotective role of adenosine in cerebral ischaemia *Trends in Pharmacological Sciences., 13* (1992) 439–445.

51. Salvatore, C., Jacobson, M., Taylor, H., Linden, J., and Johnson, R., Molecular cloning and characterization of the human A_3 adenosine receptor. *Proc Natl Acad Sci USA, 90* (1993) 10365–10369.

52. Salzman, C., Miyawaki, E., Bars, P. I., and Kerrihard, T., Neurobiological basis of anxiety and its treatment. *Harvard Rev Psychiatry, 1* (1993) 197–206.

53. Sawynok, J., Adenosine receptor activation and nociception. *Eur J Pharmacol, 347* (1998) 1–11.

54. Schiffmann, S., Jacobs, O., and Vanderhaeghen, J.-J. Striatal restricted adenosine A_2 receptor (RDC8) is expressed by enkephalin but not substance P neurons: an *in situ* hybridization histochemistry study. *J Neurochem, 57* (1991) 1062–1067.

55. Schiffmann, S. N., Libert, F., Vassart, G., and Vanderhaeghen, J.-J., Distribution of adenosine A_2 receptor mRNA in the human brain. *Neurosci Lett, 130* (1991) 177–181.

56. Sexl, V., Mancusi, G., Holler, C., Gloria, M. E., Schutz, W., and Freissmuth, M., Stimulation of the mitogen-activated protein kinase via the A_{2A}-adenosine receptor in primary human endothelial cells. *J Biol Chem, 272* (1997) 5792–5799.

57. Stambaugh, K., Jacobson, K., Jiang, J., and Liang, B., A novel cardioprotective function of adenosine A_1 and A_3 receptors during prolonged simulated ischemia. *Am J Physiol, 273* (1997) H501–H505.

58. Stehle, J., Rivkees, S., Lee, J., Weaver, D., Deeds, J., and Reppert, S., Molecular cloning and expression of the cDNA for a novel A_2-adenosine receptor subtype. *Mol Endocrinol, 6* (1992) 384–393.

59. Strohmeier, G., Reppert, S., Lencer, W., and Madara J., The A_{2B} adenosine receptor mediates cAMP responses to adenosine receptor agonists in human intestinal epithelia. *J Biol Chem, 270* (1995) 2387–2394.

60. Swanson, T., Krahl, S., Liu, Drazba, J., and Rivkees, S., Evidence for physiologically active axonal adenosine receptors in the rat corpus callosum. *Brain Res, 784* (1998) 188–198.

61. Townsend-Nicholson, A., and Shine, J., Molecular cloning and characterization of a human brain A_1 adenosine receptor cDNA. *Mol Brain Res, 16* (1992) 365–370.

62. Walker, B. A., Rocchini, C., Boone, R. H. Ip, S., and Jacobson, M. A., Adenosine A_{2A} receptor activation delays apoptosis in human neutrophils. *J Immunol, 158* (1997) 2926–29231.

63. Yao, Y., Sei, Y., Abbracchio, M., Jiang, J., Kim, Y., and Jacobson, K., Adenosine A_3 receptor agonists protect HL-60 and U-937 cells from apoptosis induced by A_3 antagonists. *Biochem Biophys Res Commun, 232* (1997) 317–322.

64. Zhou, Q.-Y., Li, C., Olah, M., Johnson, R., Stiles, G., and Civelli, O., Molecular cloning and characterization of an adenosine receptor: the A_3 adenosine receptor. *Proc Natl Acad Sci USA, 89* (1992) 7432–7436.

Medicinal Chemistry of Adenosine Receptors in Brain and Periphery

JUNICHI SHIMADA AND FUMIO SUZUKI

Drug Discovery Research Laboratories, Pharmaceutical Research Institute, Kyowa, Hakko Kogyo Co., Ltd., Nagaizumi-cho, Sunto-gun, Shizuoka, Japan

I. INTRODUCTION

Adenosine modulates a variety of biological functions, both in the central nervous system (CNS) and peripheral tissues (Pelleg and Porter, 1990). Most of these effects appear to be mediated via specific cell surface receptors. On the basis of both pharmacological and biochemical studies, these receptors have been divided into four subtypes—termed adenosine A_1, A_{2A}, A_{2B}, and A_3 receptors—which belong to the superfamily of receptors coupled to G-proteins (Fredholm *et al.*, 1994). The different receptor subtypes regulate the intracellular signaling system in various ways. The A_1 and A_3 receptors inhibit adenylate cyclase and activate phospholipase C. The A_1 receptor may also stimulate phosphoinositide metabolism and potassium flux as well as inhibit calcium flux. In addition, the A_{2A} and A_{2B} receptors both stimulate adenylate cyclase. The most thoroughly investigated subtypes are the high-affinity A_1 and A_{2A} receptors, both of which are activated by adenosine in low, nanomolar, or at least submicromolar concentrations, depending on the cell system investigated. All the adenosine receptors are present in brain, with the adenosine A_1 and A_{2A} receptor subtypes being differentially distributed. A_{2A} receptors are found predominantly in the striatum, whereas A_1 receptors predominate in hippocampus and cortex.

Theophylline and other xanthine derivatives are widely used therapeutically, particularly as broncholytics, but also as mild diuretics, cardiac stimulants, and as CNS stimulatory agents. Xanthines exert pharmacological effects primarily through blockade of adenosine receptors (Fredholm, 1980). However, they are nonselective antagonists and having weak affinities for both A_1 and A_2 receptors. Considerable effort (van Galen et al.,1992) have been invested in a search of selective antagonists to elucidate the physiological role of adenosine. These efforts were made mainly by modifying the structure of theophylline.

II. A_1 ADENOSINE RECEPTOR ANTAGONISTS

A. STRUCTURE–ACTIVITY RELATIONSHIPS

Studies on structure–activity relationships of xanthines revealed that alkyl substitution, such as a propyl group at the 1- and 3-positions, markedly increased affinity for A_1 and A_{2A} receptors (Bruns et al., 1983; Martinson et al., 1987). The rank order of potency for both subtypes was methyl < ethyl < n-propyl ≦ iso-butyl. Substitution in the 1-position is very important for high A_1 affinity, whereas substitution in the 3-position is not an absolute requirement for high affinity (Müller et al., 1993). Overall, for high A_1 affinity, propyl substitution at both the 1- and 3-positions are an optimum alkyl substituent combination. The most significant enhancements in affinity and subtype selectivity come with substitution at the 8-position of xanthine (Katsushima et al., 1990; Shamim et al., 1988). Introduction of an aryl or cycloalkyl substituent in the 8-position increased the affinity to a high degree and led to selective and potent A_1 antagonists. The sp^3 carbon-containing cycloalkyl ring has a more favorable interactions with a hydrophobic pocket of the A_1 receptor than the sp^2 carbons in an aryl ring. Bulky nonaromatic substituents in the xanthine 8-position, such as cyclopentyl (DPCPX) (Bruns et al., 1987a; Lohse et al., 1987), dicyclopropylmethyl (KF15372) (Shimada et al., 1991), and endo-norbornyl (Shimada et al.,1992b), are particularly favorable for high A_1 affinity and selectivity. N^6-Cycloalkyl or N^6-bicycloalkyladenosines, such as N^6-cyclopentyladenosine (CPA) or N^6-endo-norbornyladenosine, are known to be selective A_1 agonists (Paton et al., 1986; Trivedi et al., 1989). Furthermore, the 8-substituent of xanthine exhibits stereoselectivity in a manner that parallels the N^6 substituent of agonists, as shown by the receptor binding affinity of 8-RS-, -8R-, and -8S-phenylisopropylxanthi-

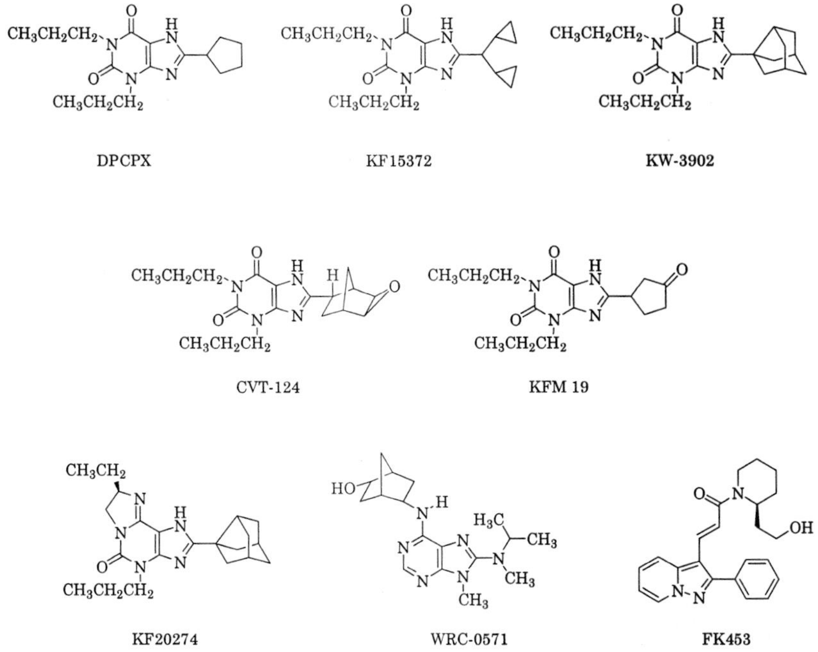

FIGURE 1 Chemical structures of A_1 adenosine antagonist.

nen (Peet *et al.*, 1993). Thus the 8-substituent of xanthine appears to bind to the same region of the A_1 receptor.

The conformation of the cyclopentyl group is not restricted at room temperature. Conformation was fixed using tricycloalkane systems, which contain quaternary carbons in the 1'-position of the substituent. This modification causes a remarkable enhancement of affinity for the A_1 receptor. The resulting 1,3-dipropyl-8-(3-noradamantyl)xanthine (KW-3902) (Shimada *et al.*, 1992b) is a selective and highly potent A_1 receptor antagonist. Because corresponding N^6-substituted agonist (Nair and Fasbender, 1993) has a lower affinity for the A_1 receptor, a quaternary carbon at the 1'-position of N^6-substituents (substitution at the S-4 subregion) is not tolerated in agonists.

An unsubstituted N—H group in the 7-position of xanthines is important as a hydrogen bond donor for binding to the A_1 receptor (Dooley *et al.*, 1996). 8-Substituted 8-azaxanthine derivatives, which contain a nitrogen atom (—N=) but no —NH— group in the 7-position, show low affinity for adenosine receptors (Franchetti *et al.*, 1994). 7-Substitution decreases the affinity of 1,3,8-substituted xanthines for adenosine A_1 receptors (Shamim *et al.*, 1989).

TABLE I A_1 and A_{2A} Receptor Binding of Nonselective and A_1-Selective Antagonists

| | K_i (nM) | | K_i ratio | |
Compound	$A_1{}^a$	$A_{2A}{}^b$	A_{2A}/A_1	References
Theophylline	8,470	25,300	3.0	Bruns et al., 1986
Caffeine	29,100	48,100	1.7	Bruns et al., 1986
DPCPX	0.46	340	740	Bruns et al., 1987a
KF15372	0.99	430	430	Suzuki et al., 1993
KW-3902	0.19	380	2,000	Shimada et al., 1992b
CVT-124	0.67	1,250	1,900	Pfister et al., 1997
KFM 19	10.5^c	1512^d	140	Schingnitz et al., 1991
KF20274	0.56	290	520	Suzuki et al., 1993
WRC-0571	1.7^e	105^e	60	Martin et al., 1996
FK 453	17^f	$11,300^f$	660	Terai et al., 1995

[a] Inhibition of radioligand binding to membranes from rat brain, otherwise noted.
[b] Inhibition of radioligand binding to membranes from rat striatum, otherwise noted.
[c] Inhibition of binding to membranes from rhesus monkey cortex.
[d] Inhibition of binding to membranes from rhesus monkey striatum.
[e] Inhibition of binding membranes from HEK-293 cells stably transfected with recombinant human adenosine receptors.
[f] IC_{50} value.

The most intensively investigated class of adenosine A_1 antagonists besides the xanthines are adenine derivatives. These compounds are derived from the physiological agonist adenosine, but they lack the ribose moiety that is necessary for receptor activation. Structure—activity relationships of a series of 9-methyl adenine derivatives were similar to that of N^6-substituted adenosine A_1 agonists (Ukena et al., 1987). Amongst these adenine derivatives is endo-(5-hydroxynorbotnyl)-8-(N-methyl-N-isopropylamino)-9-methyladenine (WRC-0572) (Martin et al., 1996), which is a potent A_1-selective adenosine receptor antagonist.

The chemical structures and adenosine receptor binding affinity of representative adenosine A_1 antagonists are shown in Figure 1 and Table I, respectively.

B. Pharmacology of A_1 Receptor Antagonists

1. Kidney

The diuretic effects of xanthines, such as caffeine and theophylline, were described since before the late 1800s. The pharmacological basis of these diuretic actions has been proposed to be adenosine receptor antagonism (Osswald *et al.*, 1978). In fact, exogenous adenosine produces antidiuretic and antinatriuretic effects in many species, and these effects are competitively antagonized by theophylline and mimicked by several adenosine analogues (Collis *et al.*, 1986). The diuretic and natriuretic activities of a variety of adenosine antagonists suggest that blockade of A_1 receptors is more important than that of A_{2A} receptors and that endogenous adenosine directly enhances tubular sodium reabsorption in the kidney. In fact, potent A_1-selective antagonists, such as DPCPX (Knight *et al.*, 1993) and KW-3902 (Kobayashi *et al.*, 1993; Mizumoto *et al.*, 1993) are potent diuretic and natriuretic agents in rat and dog with little effect on potassium excretion. Moreover, A_1-selective antagonists did not affect renal blood flow or glomerular filtration rate (GFR) (Mizumoto and Karasawa, 1993). A_1-selective adenosine receptor antagonists belonging to different structural classes, including xanthine [(*S*)-dipropyl-8-[2-(5,6-epoxynorbonyl)]xanthine (CVT-124)] (Pfister *et al.*, 1997) and nonxanthine [*R*-[(*E*)-3-(2-phenylpyrazolo[1,5-*a*]pyridin-3-yl)acryloyl]-2-piperidine ethanol (FK-453)] derivatives (Terai *et al.*, 1995), which have been reported to show similar diuretic and natriuretic actions. In contrast, adenosine A_{2A} antagonists exhibited no diuretic effect (Suzuki *et al.*, 1992a).

Adenosine also plays a role in mediating the hemodynamic changes (decreasing GFR) in acute renal failure. Studies of structure–activity relationships of 8-substituted xanthines have demonstrated that the adenosine, acting on the A_1 receptor, is an important mediator in acute renal failure (Suzuki *et al.*, 1992a; Yao *et al.*, 1994). Furthermore, KW-3902 shows protective effects against acute renal failure induced by cytostatics, such as cisplatin, X-ray, or radio contrast media (Arakawa *et al.*, 1996; Nagashima *et al.*, 1995).

2. Central Nervous System

A_1 receptors in hippocampus are densely concentrated in the CA1 and CA3 regions (Onodera and Kogure, 1988). In general, the presynaptic A_1 receptors cause an inhibition of the release of neurotransmitters and the postsynaptic A_1 receptors cause a decrease in excitability (Dunwiddie and Fredholm, 1989). Previous work revealed that A_1 receptors also play a role in the development of long-term potentiation (LTP), particularly in the CA1 region (Arai *et al.*, 1990; Tanaka *et al.*, 1990). LTP is one of the most striking examples of synaptic plasticity, which is postulated to underly learning and memory. From these results, A_1 antagonists might be expected to enhance the release of various neurotransmitters, such as acetylcholine to depolarize postsynaptic neurons and to increase LTP (Suzuki, 1992).

Systematic administration of A_1 receptor agonists, such as N^6-((*R*)-phenyl-isopropyl)adenosine ((*R*)-PIA) or CPA, but not *N*-ethyladenosin-5′-uronamide

(NECA; A_1 and A_{2A} agonist), dose-dependently impaired passive avoidance behavior (Normile and Barraco, 1991; Shiozaki et al., 1990). These findings suggest that selective activation of a central population of A_1 receptors, presumably in the hippocampus, impairs retention of a passive avoidance, possibly via an influence on hippocampal excitability. In fact, A_1-selective antagonist, such as KF15372, showed antiamnesic activity in (R)-PIA- and scopolamine-induced amnesia, whereas A_{2A}-selective antagonists had no effects (Suzuki et al., 1993). KF15372 also improves learning performance in nucleus basalis magnocellularis (NBM)-lesioned rats (Shiozaki et al., 1993). These results suggest that adenosine A_1 antagonists may have therapeutic potential for the treatment of cognitive deficits in humans.

Water-soluble adenosine A_1 antagonists with antiamnesic activity, such as (R)-7,8-dihydro-8-ethyl-2-(3-noradamantyl)-4-propyl-1H-imidazo[2,1-i]purin-5(4H)-one (KF20274) (Suzuki et al., 1992b) or 1,3-dipropyl-8-(3'-oxocyclopentyl)xanthine (KFM-19) (Schingnitz et al., 1991), have also been reported.

III. A_{2A} ADENOSINE RECEPTOR ANTAGONISTS

A. STRUCTURE–ACTIVITY RELATIONSHIP

Whereas many selective ligands A_1 receptors have been synthesized, it is only recently that A_{2A}-selective agonists and antagonists have been found (Baraldi et al., 1995). Some caffeine derivatives, such as 3,7-dimethyl-1-propargylxanthine or 1,3-dipropyl-7-methylxanthine, have been reported to possess a moderate degree of A_{2A} selectivity (Daly et al., 1986; Ukena et al., 1986). Surprisingly, 8-cycloalkyl substituents (cyclopentyl and cyclohexyl) increase the affinity of caffeine and 1,3-dipropyl-7-methylxanthine for the A_{2A} receptor (Shamim et al., 1989). Introduction of some parasubstituted phenyl groups such as 4-[N-[2-(dimethylamino)ethyl]-N-methyl]aminosulfonyl)phenyl (PD-115199) (Bruns et al., 1987b) or 4-[[(2-aminoethyl)aminocarbonyl]methoxy]phenyl (XAC) (Jacobson et al., 1987), into the 8-position potently enhanced affinity for A_1 and A_{2A} receptors. This observation suggests that a receptor pocket different from that recognized by 8-cycloalkyl substituents exists in A_1 and A_{2A} receptors.

(E)-Styryl substitution at the 8-position increased affinity for the A_{2A} receptor approximately 100-fold compared with the parent compound (1,3-dipropyl-7-methylxanthine) and resulted in high A_{2A} selectivity (69-fold) (Shimada et al., 1992a). 2-Phenylethyl or (E)-cinnamyl substitution does not cause increased affinity for the A_{2A} receptor. Incorporation of a methyl group into the vinylene group caused reduction in affinity for both A_1 and A_{2A} receptors. Thus, the vinylene group between the xanthine and the phenyl group appears to play an important role for the receptor interactions.

It is interesting that 7-methylation of 8-substituted xanthines generally resulted in a reduced affinity for both A_1 and A_{2A} receptors. However, if the 8-substituent was a styryl residue, the effect of 7-methylation is differed. A_1 affinity was still reduced, but A_{2A} affinity was unchanged or increased in 8-styrylxanthine derivatives. The reduced A_1 affinity can be explained by the importance of having a hydrogen bond donor at the 7-position of the xanthine nuclei for the binding to adenosine A_1 receptors (Dooley et al., 1996). In contrast, the enhanced A_{2A} affinity of 8-styrylxanthines by 7-methylation may be explained by steric factors. The methyl group may sterically interact with the styryl group to force the latter into a favorable conformation for interaction with the adenosine A_{2A} receptor. Similar to 8-styrylxanthines, 7-methyl substitution does not alter the affinity for A_{2A} receptors in 8-(2-phenylethyl) and (E)-cinnamyl xanthines. In contrast to this observation, introduction of a methyl group into the 7-position of 8-(2-cyclopentylethyl)- or 8-cyclopentyl-substituted xanthine results in decreased affinity for the A_{2A} receptor. Consequently, the electrostatic effects of the 2-phenylethyl or cinnamyl group appears to be more favorable for an interaction with the A_{2A} receptor than those of a cyclopentyl group.

Introduction of methoxy substituents into the phenyl group of (E)-l,3-dipropyl-7-methyl-8-styrylxanthine enhanced the A_{2A} selectivity in general. Two or three substitution of the phenyl moiety with methoxy or methyl groups at 2,3,4-, 3,4,5-, and 3,4-positions is especially favored and resulted in the synthesis of the first potent, truly A_{2A}-selective xanthine, (E)-1,3-dipropyl-8-(3,4-dimethoxystyryl)-7-methylxanthine (KF17837) (Shimada et al., 1992a). 2,4,5-Trisubstitution remarkably reduced affinity for the adenosine A_{2A} receptor (Shimada et al., 1997). The A_{2A} selectivity of the compounds could also be enhanced by monosubstitution of the phenyl ring with a halogen atom, preferably in the metaposition (Jacobson et al., 1993a). Replacement of the styryl phenyl group by heterocycles, such as thienyl, furyl, and pyridyl, also led to adenosine A_{2A} antagonists, but these compounds were inferior to the styryl-substituted xanthines with regard to selectivity and/or potency (Giudice et al., 1996). Aza-analogues of 8-styryl-xanthine, in which the ethenyl bridge is replaced by an imine, amide, or azo function, show relatively high A_{2A} affinity (Müller et al., 1997a). Ring-constrained styryl analogues, containing an 8-(2-benzofuran) group, are antagonists showing only weak binding to adenosine receptors (Shimada et al., 1992b).

Alkyl substitution at the 1-position of 8-styrylxanthine is a critical determinant of affinity for the A_{2A} receptor. No apparent differences in the

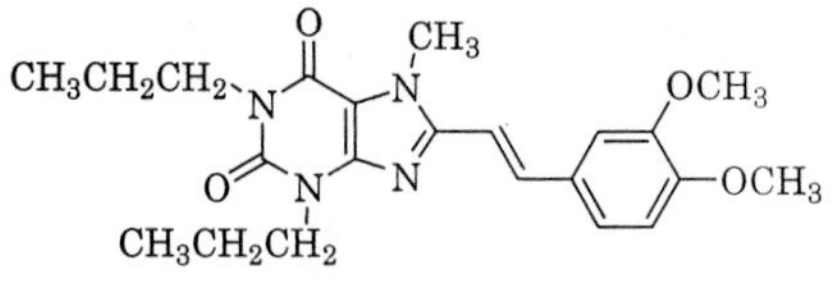

KF17837

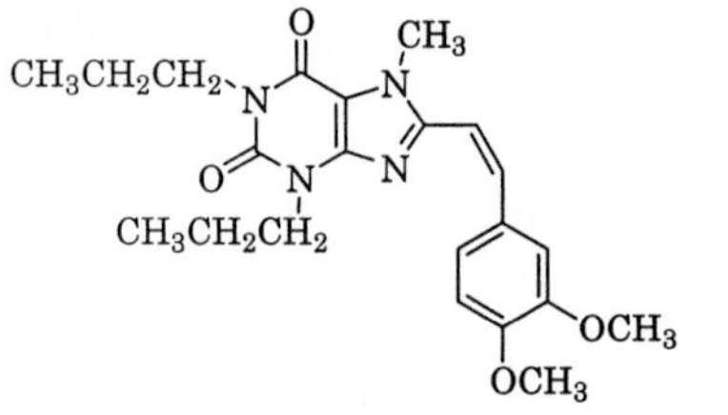

(*Z*)- KF17837 = GK4-1866

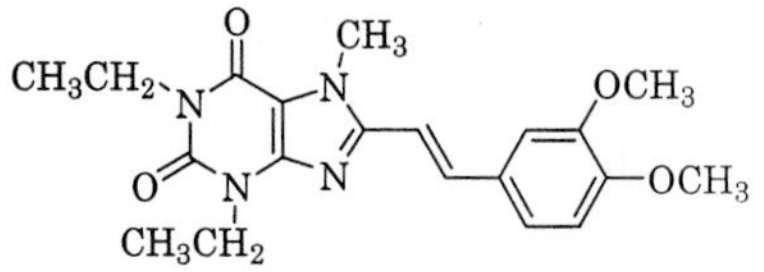

KW-6002

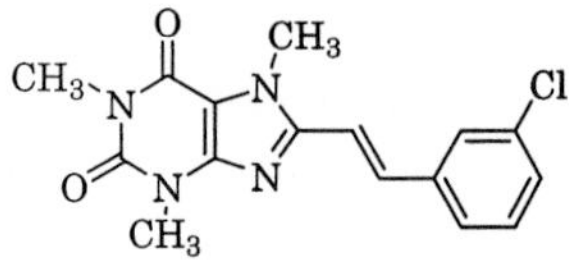

CSC

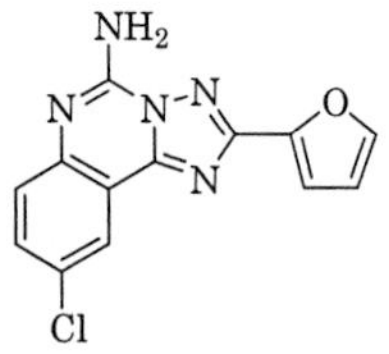

CGS15943

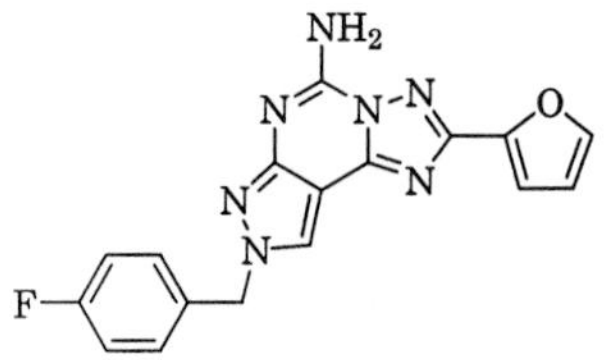

8FB-PTP

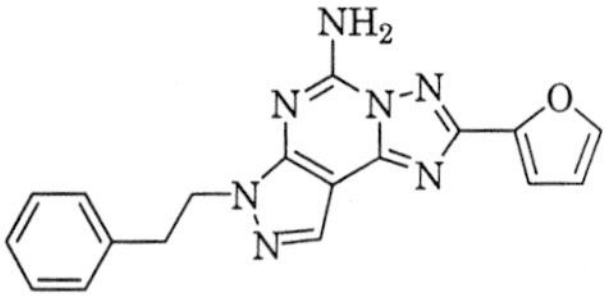

SCH58261

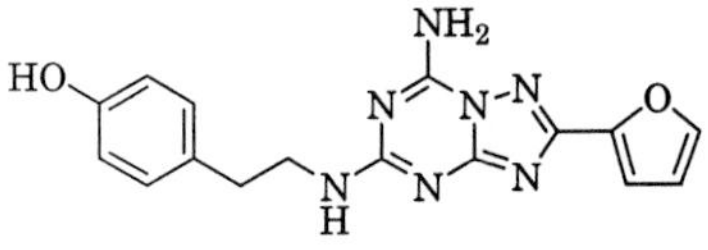

ZM241385

FIGURE 2 Chemical structures of A_{2A} adenosine antagonist.

affinity for the A_{2A} receptor were observed between 1,3-dialkyl-7-methyl-8-styrylxanthines, but 1,3-dipropyl or 1,3-diethyl substitution enhanced A_{2A} affinity. The 1,3-diethyl analogue (KW-6002) (Shimada *et al.*, 1997) of KF17837 showed almost the same potency and selectivity as KF17837. 1,3-Dimethyl or 1,3-diallyl substitution at the 1- and 3-positions reduced affinity for the A_1 receptor, resulting in higher A_{2A} selectivity. An extension of our work led to the development of 8-(3-chlorostyryl)caffeine (CSC) (Jacobson *et al.*, 1993a, 1993b; Mathot *et al.*, 1995), a selective A_{2A} antagonist, with lower potency compared with KF17837. Introduction of a propargyl moiety at

TABLE II A_1 and A_{2A} Receptor Binding of A_{2A}-Selective Antagonists

Compound	K_i (nM)		K_i ratio	References
	$A_1{}^a$	$A_{2A}{}^b$	A_1/A_{2A}	
KF17837	62	1.0	62	Nonaka et al., 1993
KF17837S[c]	390	7.8	50	Shimada et al., 1992a
GK4-1866[d]	>10,000	860	>12	Nonaka et al., 1993
KW-6002	150	2.2	68	Shimada et al., 1997
KW-6002S[c]	580	13	45	Shimada et al., 1997
CSC	28,200	54	520	Jacobson et al., 1993a
CGS 15943	20.5	3.3	6.2	Williams et al., 1987
3-FB-PTP	3.3	1.2	2.8	Zocchi et al., 1996
SCH 58261	121	2.3	53	Baraldi et al., 1996
ZM 241385	2,040[e]	0.30[e]	6,800	Poucher et al., 1995

[a]Inhibition of radioligand binding to membranes from rat brain.
[b]Inhibition of radioligand binding to membranes from rat striatum.
[c]$E-Z$ equilibrium mixture.
[d]Z-isomer of KF17837.
[e]IC_{50} value.

the 1-position of styrylxanthine is reported to enhance A_{2A} affinity (Müller et al., 1997b).

A number of nonxanthine heterocyclic derivatives were found to be potent but nonselective for A_{2A} receptors. Example of such compounds are the triazoloquinazoline, CGS15943 (Williams et al., 1987), and the triazoloqinoxaline, CP66713 (Sarges et al., 1990). A series of CGS15943 derivatives in which the m-chlorophenyl group was replaced by a heterocycle ring, such as pyrazole or imidazole, have been described in the literature. From these modification, some potent and selective A_{2A} antagonists arose, namely 3-FB-PTP (Dionisotti et al., 1994) and SCH58261 (Baraldi et al., 1996; Zocchi et al., 1996). A related class of compounds consisting of a bicyclic instead of a tricyclic ring system (e.g., ZM241385) has also been developed (Poucher et al., 1995; Keddie et al., 1996).

Chemical structures and adenosine binding affinity of representative adenosine A_{2A} antagonists are shown in Figure 2 and Table II, respectively.

B. PHOTOISOMERIZATION OF 8-STYRYLXANTHINES

Studies have shown that photoisomerization of an ethylenic double bond (Waldeck, 1991) and light-induced isomerization of the 8-styrylcaffeine derivative (Philip and Szulczewski, 1973) are general phenomena. When methanolic solutions of KF17837 were prepared and exposed to a fluorescent lamp for varying periods of time (Nonaka et al., 1993), the sequential ultraviolet (UV) spectrum of this solution changed very rapidly, whereas no change was observed in the dark. When the reaction mixture was analyzed by high-performance liquid chromatography (HPLC), it was found to contain KF17837 and a new product (Z-isomer of KF17837: GK4-1866). Because dimethyl sulfoxide (DMSO) has been used in the receptor binding assay for dissolving KF17837, we examined the photoliability of KF17837 and the Z-isomer in this solvent (fluorescent lamp, 1000x). Rates of photoisomerization were greatly dependent on the initial concentration of substrate; photoisomerization being slow ($t_{1/2}$ = 27 h) at high concentrations (e.g., 10 mM) and crystalline KF17837 was stable under photoillumination. Consequently, photoisomerization was not a problem during synthesis of KF17837. However, at low concentration (e.g., 0.1 mM), photoisomerization was very fast ($t_{1/2}$ = 0.5 h) and an equilibrium mixture (82% Z-18% E) was formed. This finding was confirmed by similarly exposing the Z-isomer (0.1 mM) to light, which resulted in the same equilibrium mixture. The change in HPLC peak areas due to the E- or Z-isomer as a function of time was governed by pseudo-first-order analysis according to Eq. 1.

$$\log|CP - CP_\infty| = -(k_{obs}/2.303)t + \text{const} \tag{1}$$

CP and CP∞ are the percentages of the E-isomer present at time t and at infinity where an equilibrium mixture was obtained, respectively, and k_{obs} is the pseudo-first-order rate constant for the isomerization. The k_{obs} values (0.1 mM) obtained from the decrease in the E-isomer (the increase in the Z-isomer) and from the increase in the E-isomer (the decrease in the Z-isomer) were 1.8 and 2.4 h^{-1}, respectively, and agreed approximately with each other. An identical process of isomerization was observed when methanol was used as solvent.

This fast photoisomerization could obviously lead to anomolous experimental results. Thus, it is probable that the binding data for KF17837 in the first report (Shimada et al., 1992a) was derived from experiments using the E–Z equilibrium mixture (KF17837S) and that differences in apparent affinities determined in different laboratories (Jacobson et al., 1993a) were due to differences in the degree of photoisomerization of KF17837.

The potency of the E- and Z-isomers and their equilibrium mixture for adenosine A$_1$ and A$_{2A}$ receptors was determined by standard radioligand binding procedures (Nonaka et al., 1993; Nonaka et al., 1994). All procedures in the binding assay were performed in the dark to avoid photoisomerization. The E-isomer (KF17837) possessed high affinity for the A$_{2A}$ receptor (K_i = 1.0 nM) and resulted in high A$_{2A}$ selectivity (62-fold). In contrast, the

Z-isomer showed low affinity for both A_1 and A_{2A} receptor (A_1, $K_i > 10$ μM; A_{2A}, $K_i = 860$ nM). The active principle of the $E-Z$ equilibrium mixture (KF17837S) is therefore the E-isomer, KF17837. Most published radioligand binding data of styryl xanthines contain data from stable $E-Z$ equilibrium mixtures rather than pure (E)-isomers. The $E-Z$ ratio present is between 2 : 8 and 3 : 7 in 8-(methoxy substituted styryl) derivatives but will depend on the substitution of the phenyl group of the styryl moiety (Shimada *et al.*, 1997).

C. Pharmacology of A_{2A} Receptor Antagonists

1. In Vivo Characterization

8-styryl-1,3-dialkyl-7-methylxanthines have been identified as a selective A_{2A} receptor antagonist. Before evaluating their pharmacological activity in the CNS, we confirmed their *in vivo* A_{2A} antagonism on the cardiovascular system. NECA, nonselective adenosine agonist, caused a dose-dependent decrease in heart rate and blood pressure in anesthetized rats (Fredholm *et al.*, 1987). KF17837 produced a rightward shift of the NECA dose–response curves, and the shift was larger for blood pressure than that of heart rate at the oral dose of 10 mg/kg (Shimada *et al.*, 1992a). In contrast, theophylline, a nonselective antagonist, produced equivalent rightward shifts in both dose–response curves. Adenosine is reported to reduce heart rate via A_1 receptor and blood pressure via A_{2A} receptors (Mathot *et al.*, 1996). Thus, KF17837 was identified as a selective adenosine A_{2A} antagonist *in vivo*. The diethyl analogue (KW-6002) almost abolished the hypotensive response to NECA at a dose of 1 mg/kg, which did not affect the bradycardic responses. This potent activity is explained by differences in oral absorption of the two compounds since the bioavailability of KF17837 and KW-6002 at a dose of 30 mg/kg in rat was 3.6% and 20.6%, respectively. No photoisomerization of 8-styrylxanthines was observed in 0.3% Tween 80 suspensions which were used for oral administration, presumably due to its low water solubility (<1 μg/mL). The results indicate that KF17837 and KW-6002 can be used to evaluate the role of adenosine A_{2A} receptors in the action of adenosine *in vivo* (Jackson *et al.*, 1993).

2. Central Nervous System

A_1-selective agonists, such as CHA, R-PIA, and the nonselective agonist NECA, are potent locomotor depressants in rodents. However, the ability of adenosine agonists to depress locomotor activity was found to correlate with their activity at A_{2A} adenosine receptors and not A_1 adenosine receptors (Durcan and Morgan, 1989). The discrete distribution of A_{2A} receptors (striatum, nucleus accumbens, and olfactory tubercle) suggests a specific functional role for A_{2A} receptors in basal ganglia and associated nuclei (Jarvis and Williams, 1989; Martinez-Mir et al., 1991; Parkinson and Fredholm, 1990). Methylxanthines, such as theophylline and caffeine, are known to enhance locomotor activity, and their stimulant effects are related, at least in part, to their ability to block adenosine receptors (Snyder et al., 1981). However, these methylxanthines are nonselective antagonists and have weak affinity for both A_1 and A_{2A} receptors. Therefore, the role of receptor subtypes in the behavioral effects associated with methylxanthines has been unclear because of the lack of selective adenosine A_{2A} antagonists.

Evidence has been accumulated to show that adenosine A_{2A} receptors have a profound influence on motor function (Ongini and Fredholm, 1996). For example, the intracerebroventricular injection of adenosine A_{2A}-selective agonist, 2-[p-(2-carboxyethyl)phenethylamino]-5'-N-ethylcarboxamidoadenosine (CGS 21680) induces catalepsy, and this response is antagonized by treatment with A_{2A} an antagonist (KF17837) (Kanda et al., 1994). In contrast, the cataleptic response is not affected by an A_1 antagonist (KFM-19). KF17837 also ameliorated the cataleptic response produced by the dopamine D_2 antagonist (haloperidol). In the striatum, adenosine A_{2A} receptors are selectively located on GABA/enkephalin-containing neurons bearing D_2 receptors, which constitute the indirect output pathway projecting to the external segment of globus pallidus (Schiffmann et al., 1991). A_{2A} receptors appear to modulate the striatal output activity through the regulation of GABA and acetylcholine release (Kurokawa et al., 1994; Mori et al., 1996; see Chapters 6 and 7).

To establish the precise relationships of adenosine A_{2A} antagonism with motor control, structure–activity relationships for anticataleptic activity (inhibitory activity on haloperidol-induced catalepsy in mice) of 8-styrylxanthines was studied (Shimada et al., 1997). Two or three substitution of the phenyl moiety with methoxy or methyl at 2,3,4-, 3,4,5- and 3,4-position favored in vivo activity. Derivatives with mono substitution or a simple phenyl group showed weak activity. Surprisingly, diethyl substitution at the 1- and 3-position dramatically potentiated the activity without exception presumably due to increased oral bioavailability. For example, the ED_{50} values of KF17837 and KW-6002 were 2.7 and 0.03 mg/kg, po, respectively, giving KW-6002 a potency that is approximately 90 times that of KF17837.

IV. CONCLUSION

Adenosine is neuromodulator with wide-ranging effects throughout the human body. Because of the potent bioactivity of adenosine, intensive research for novel therapeutic applications that exploit the adenosine signal transmission pathways has been conducted. Two promising areas where A_1 antagonists may be therapeutic are cognitive deficit and acute renal failure. Several A_1-selective compounds such as KW-3902 are under clinical trial at this time as renal protectants. Although many ligands selective for A_1 receptors have been synthesized, it is only recently that A_{2A}-selective antagonists have been reported. Important progress has been made with the synthesis of new compounds, such as 8-styrylxanthines, and new nonxanthine heterocycles. The most probable therapeutic application of these agents appears to be in the CNS area and, specifically, for the treatment of basal ganglia disorders, such as Parkinson's disease. Among these agents, KW-6002 was identified as an adenosine A_{2A}-selective antagonist with potent anticataleptic activity. Theophylline, the nonselective adenosine antagonist, has been shown to improve motor scores and the mental state of parkinsonian patients (Mally and Stone, 1994). Selective adenosine A_{2A} antagonists such as KW-6002 should provide new possibilities for the treatment of Parkinson's disease (Kanda et al., 1998; Richardson et al., 1997).

REFERENCES

Arai, A., Kessler, M., and Lynch, G. (1990). The effect of adenosine on the development of long-term potentiation. *Neurosci Lett* 119, 41–44.

Arakawa, K., Suzuki, H., Naitoh, M., Matsumoto, A., Hayashi, K., Matsuda, H., Ichihara, A., Kubota, E., and Saruta, T. (1996). Role of adenosine in the renal responses to contrast medium. *Kidney Int* 49, 1199–1206.

Baraldi, P.G., Cacciari, B., Spalluto, G., Borioni, A., Viziano, M., Dionisotti, S., and Ongini, E. (1995). Current developments of A_{2A} adenosine receptor antagonists. *Curr Med Chem* 2, 707–722.

Baraldi, P.G., Cacciari, B., Spalluto, G., Villatoro, M.J.P.I., Zocchi, C., Dionisotti, S., and Ongini, E. (1996). Pyrazolo[4,3-*e*]-1,2,4-triazolo[1,5-*c*]pyrimidine derivatives: potent and selective A_{2A} adenosine antagonists. *J Med Chem* 39, 1164–1171.

Bruns, R.F., Daly, J.W., and Snyder, S.H. (1983). Adenosine receptor binding: structure–activity analysis generates extremely potent xanthine antagonists. *Proc Natl Acad Sci USA* 80, 2077–2080.

Bruns, R.F., Fergus, J.H., Badger, E.W., Bristol, J.A., Santay, L.A., Hartman, J.D., Hays, S.J., and Huang, C.C. (1987a). Binding of the A_1-selective adenosine antagonist 8-cyclopentyl-1,3-dipropylxanthine to rat brain membranes. *Naunyn-Schmiedeberg's Arch Pharmacol* 335, 59–63.

Bruns, R.F., Fergus, J.H., Badger, E.W., Bristol, J.A., Santay, L.A., and Hays, S.J. (1987b). PD 115,199: an antagonist ligand for adenosine A_2 receptors. *Naunyn-Schmiedeberg's Arch Pharmacol* 335, 64–69.

Bruns, R.F., Lu, G.H., and Pugsley, T.A. (1986). Characterization of the A_2 adenosine receptor labeled by [^{3}H]NECA in rat striatal membranes. *Mol Pharmacol* 29, 331–346.

Collis, M.G., Baxter, G.S., and Keddie, J.R. (1986). The adenosine receptor antagonist, 8-phenyltheophylline, causes diuresis and saliuresis in the rat. *J Pharm Pharmacol* 38, 850–852.

Daly, J.W., Padgett, W.L., and Shamim, M.T. (1986). Analogues of caffeine and theophylline: effect of structural alterations on affinity at adenosine receptors. *J Med Chem* 29, 1305–1308.

Dionisotti, S., Conti, A., Sandoli, D., Zocchi, C., Gatta, F., and Ongini, E. (1994). Effects of the new A_2 adenosine receptor antagonist 8FB-PTP, an 8-substituted pyrazolo-triazolo-pyridine, on *in vivo*. *Br J Pharmacol* 112, 659–665.

Dooley, M.J., Kono, M., and Suzuki, F. (1996). Theoretical structure–activity studies of adenosine A_1 ligands: requirements for receptor affinity. *Bioorg Med Chem* 4, 923–924.

Dunwiddie, T.W., and Fredholm, B.B. (1989). Adenosine A_1 receptors inhibit adenylate cyclase activity and neurotransmitter release and hyperpolarize pyramidal neuron in rat hippocampus. *J Pharmacol Exp Ther* 249, 31–37.

Durcan, M.J., and Morgan, P.F. (1989). Evidence for adenosine A_2 receptor involvement in the hypomobility effects of adenosine analogues in mice. *Eur J Pharmacol* 168, 285–290.

Franchetti, P., Messini, L., Cappellacci, L., Grifantini, M., Lucacchini, A., Martini, C., and Senatore, G. (1994). 8-Azaxanthine derivatives as antagonists of adenosine receptors. *J Med Chem* 37, 2970–2975.

Fredholm, B.B. (1980). Are methylxanthine effects due to antagonism of endogenous adenosine? *Trends Pharmacol Sci* 1, 129–132.

Fredholm, B.B., Jacobson, K.A., Jonzon, B., Kirk, K.L., Li, Y.O., and Daly, J.W. (1987). Evidence that a novel 8-phenyl-substituted xanthine derivative is a cardioselective adenosine receptor antagonist *in vivo*. *J Cardiovasc Pharmacol* 9, 396–400.

Fredholm, B.B., Abbracchio, M.P., Burnstock, G., Daly, J.W., Harden, T.K., Jacobson, K.A., Leff, P., and Williams, M. (1994). Nomenclature and classification of purinoceptors. *Pharmacol Rev* 46, 143–156.

Giudice, M.R.D., Borioni, A., Mustazza, C., Gatta, F., Dionisotti, S., Zocchi, C., and Ongini, E. (1996). (*E*)-1-(Heterocyclyl or cyclohexyl)-2-[1,3,7-trisubstituted(xanthin-8-yl)]ethenes as A_{2A} adenosine receptor antagonists. *Eur J Med Chem* 31, 59–63.

Jackson, E.K., Herzer, W.A., and Suzuki, F. (1993). KF17837 is an A_2 adenosine receptor antagonist *in vivo*. *J Pharmacol Exp Ther* 267, 1304–1310.

Jacobson, K.A., Gallo-Rodriguez, C., Melman, N., Fischer, B., Maillard, M., van Bergen, A., van Galen, P.J.M., and Karton, Y. (1993a). Structure–activity relationships of 8-styrylxanthines as A_2-selective adenosine antagonists. *J Med Chem* 36, 1333–1342.

Jacobson, K.A., Kirk, K.L., Padgett, W.L., and Daly, J.W. (1987). A functionalized congener approach to adenosine receptor antagonists: amino acid conjugates of 1,3-dopropylxanthine. *Mol Pharmacol* 29, 126–133.

Jacobson, K.A., Nikodijevic, O., Padgett, W.L., Gallo-Rodriguez, C., Maillard, M., and Daly, J.W. (1993b). 8-(3-Chlorostyryl)caffeine (CSC) is a selective A_2-adenosine antagonist *in vitro* and *in vivo*. *FEBS Lett* 323, 141–144.

Jarvis, M.F., and Williams, M. (1989). Direct autoradiographic localization of adenosine A_2 receptors in the rat brain using the A_2-selective agonist [^{3}H]CGS 21680. *Eur J Pharmacol* 168, 243–246.

Kanda, T., Jackson, M.J., Smith, L.A., Pearce, R.K.B., Nakamura, J., Kase, H., Kuwana, Y., and Jenner, P. (1998). Adenosine A_{2A} antagonist: a novel antiparkinsonian agent that does not provoke dyskinesia in parkinsonian monkeys. *Ann Neurology* 43, 507–513.

Kanda, T., Shiozaki, S., Shimada, J., Suzuki, F., and Nakamura, J. (1994). KF 17837: a novel selective adenosine A_{2A} receptor antagonist with anticataleptic activity. *Eur J Pharmacol* 256, 263–268.

Katsushima, T., Nieves, L., and Wells, J.N. (1990). Structure–activity relationships of 8-cycloalkyl-1,3-dipropylxanthines as antagonists of adenosine receptors. *J Med Chem* 33, 1906–1910.

Keddie, J.R., Poucher, S.M., Shaw, G.R., Brooks, R., and Collis, M.G. (1996). *In vivo* characterization of ZM 241385, a selective adenosine A_{2A} receptor antagonist. *Eur J Pharmacol* 301, 107–113.

Knight, R.J., Browmer, C.J., and Yates, M.S. (1993). The diuretic action of 8-cyclopentyl-1,3-dipropylxanthine, a selective A_1 adenosine receptor antagonist. *Br J Pharmacol* 109, 271–277.

Kobayashi, T., Mizumoto, H., and Karasawa, A. (1993). Diuretic effects of KW-3902 (8-(no-radamantan-3-yl)-1,3-dipropylxanthine), a novel adenosine A_1 receptor antagonist, in conscious dogs. *Biol Pharm Bull* 16, 1231–1235.

Kurokawa, M., Kirk, I.P., Kirkpatrick, K.A., Kase, H., and Richardson, P.J. (1994). Inhibition by KF17837 of adenosine A_{2A} receptor-mediated modulation of striatal GABA and Ach release. *Br J Pharmacol* 113, 43–48.

Lohse, M.J., Klotz, K.-N., Lindenborn-Fotinos, J., Reddington, M., Schwabe, U., and Olsson, R.A. (1987). 8-Cyclopentyl-1,3-dipopylxanthine (DPCPX)—a selective high affinity antagonist radioligand for A_1 adenosine receptors. *Naunyn-Schmiedeberg's Arch Pharmacol* 336, 204–210.

Mally, J., and Stone, T.W. (1994). The effect of theophylline on parkinsonian symptoms. *J Pharm Pharmacol* 46, 515–517.

Martin, P.L., Wysocki, R.J., Jr., Barrett, R.J., May, J.M., and Linden, J. (1996). Characterization of 8-(N-methylisopropyl)amino-N^6-(5'-endohydroxy-endonorbornyl)-9-methyladenine (WRC-0571), a highly potent and selective, nonxanthine antagonist of A_1 adenosine receptors. *J Pharmacol Exp Ther* 276, 490–499.

Martinez-Mir, M.I., Probst, A., and Palacios, J.M. (1991). Adenosine A_2 receptors: selective location in the human basal ganglia and alterations with disease. *Neurosci* 42, 697–706.

Martinson, E.A., Johnson, R. A., and Wells, J.N. (1987). Potent adenosine receptor antagonists that are selective for the A_1 receptor subtype. *Mol Pharmacol* 31, 247–252.

Mathot, R.A.A., Gubbens-Stibbe, J.M., Soudjin, W., and Jacobson, K.A. (1995). Quantification of the *in vivo* potency of the adenosine A_2 receptor antagonist 8-(3-chlorostyryl)caffeine. *J Pharmacol Exp Ther* 275, 245–253.

Mathot, R.A.A., Soudjin, W., Breimer, D.D., Ijzerman, A.P., and Danhof, M. (1996). Pharmacokinetic–haemodynamic relationships of 2-chloroadenosine at adenosine A_1 and A_{2A} receptors *in vivo*. *Br J Pharmacol* 118, 369–377.

Mizumoto, H., and Karasawa, A. (1993). Renal tubular site of action of KW-3902, a novel adenosine A_1-receptor antagonist, in anesthetized rats. *Jpn J Pharmacol* 61, 251–253.

Mizumoto, H., Karasawa, A., and Kubo, K. (1993). Diuretic and renal protective effects of 8-(no-radamantan-3-yl)-1,3-dipropylxanthine (KW-3902), a novel adenosine A_1-receptor antagonist, via pertussis toxin insensitive mechanism. *J Pharmacol Exp Ther* 266, 200–206.

Mori, A., Shindou, T., Ichimura, M., Nonaka, H., and Kase, H. (1996). The role of adenosine A_{2A} receptors in regulating GABAergic synaptic transmission in striatal medium spiny neurons. *J Neurosci* 16, 605–611.

Müller, C.E., Geis, U., Hipp, J., Schobert, U., Frobenius, W., Pawlowski, M., Suzuki, F., and Sandoval-Ramírez, J. (1997b). Synthesis and structure–activity relationships of 3,7-dimethyl-1-propargylxanthine derivatives, A_{2A}-selective adenosine receptor antagonists. *J Med Chem* 40 4396–4405.

Müller, C.E., Shi, D., Manning, M., Jr., and Daly, J.W. (1993). Synthesis of paraxanthine analogs (1,7-disubstituted xanthines) and other xanthines unsubstituted at the 3-position: structure–activity relationships at adenosine receptors. *J Med Chem* 36, 3341–3349.

Müller, C.E., Sauer, R., Geis, U., Frobenius, W., Talik, P., and Pawlowski, M. (1997a). Aza-analog of 8-styrylxanthines as A_{2A}-adenosine receptor antagonist. *Arch Pharm Med Chem* 330, 181–189.

Nagashima, K., Kusaka, H., and Karasawa, A. (1995). Protective effects of KW-3902, an adenosine A_1-receptor antagonist, against cisplatin-induced acute renal failure in rats. *Jpn J Pharmacol* 67, 349–357.

Nair, V., and Fasbender, A.J. (1993). C-2 functionalized N^6-cyclosubstituted adenosines: highly selective agonists for the adenosine A_1 receptor. *Tetrahedron* **49**, 2169–2184.

Nonaka, H., Ichimura, M., Takeda, M., Nonaka, Y., Shimada, J., Suzuki, F., Yamaguchi, K., and Kase, H. (1994). KF 17837 ((*E*)-8-(3,4-dimethoxystyryl)-1,3-dipropyl-7-methylxanthine), a potent and selective adenosine A_2 receptor antagonist. *Eur J Pharmacol* **267**, 335–341.

Nonaka, Y., Shimada, J., Nonaka, H., Koike, N., Aoki, N., Kobayashi, H., Kase, H., Yamaguchi, K., and Suzuki, F. (1993). Photoisomerization of a potent and selective adenosine A_2 antagonist, (*E*)-1,3-pipropyl-8-(3,4-dimethoxystyryl)-7-methylxanthine. *J Med Chem* **36**, 3731–3733.

Normile, H.J., and Barraco, R.A. (1991). N^6-cyclopentyladenosine impairs passive avoidance retention by selective action at A_1 receptors. *Brain Res Bull* **27**, 101–104.

Ongini, E., and Fredholm, B.B. (1996). Pharmacology of adenosine A_{2A} receptors. *Trends Pharmacol Sci* **17**, 364–372.

Onodera, H., and Kogure, K. (1988). Differential localization of adenosine A_1 receptors in the rat hippocampus: quantitative autoradiographic study. *Brain Res* **458**, 212–217.

Osswald, H., Spielman, W.S., and Knox, F.G. (1978). Mechanism of adenosine-mediated decreases in glomerular filtration rate in dogs. *Circ Res* **43**, 465–469.

Parkinson, F.E., and Fredholm, B.B. (1990). Autoradiographic evidence for G-protein coupled A_2-receptors in rat neostriatum using [^{3}H]CGS 21680 as a ligand. *Naunyn-Schmiedeberg's Arch Pharmacol* **342**, 85–89.

Paton, D.M., Olsson, R.A., and Thompson, R.T. (1986). Nature of the N^6 region of the adenosine receptor in guinea-pig ileum and rat vas deferens. *Naunyn-Schmiedeberg's Arch Pharmacol* **333**, 313–322.

Peet, N.P., Lentz, N.L., Dudley, M.W., Ogden, A.M.L., McCarty, D.R., and Racke, M.M. (1993). Xanthines with C^8 chiral substituents as potent and selective adenosine A_1 antagonists. *J Med Chem* **36**, 4015–4020.

Pelleg, A., and Porter, R.S. (1990). The pharmacology of adenosine. *Pharmacother* **10**, 157–174.

Pfister, J.R., Belardinelli, L., Lee, G., Lum, T.L., Milner, P., Stanley, W.C., Linden, J., Baker, S.P., and Schreiner, G. (1997). Synthesis and biological evaluation of the enantiomers of the potent and selective A_1-adenosine antagonist 1,3-dipropyl-8-[2-(5,6-epoxynorbonyl)]xanthine. *J Med Chem* **40**, 1773–1778.

Philip, J., and Szulczewski, D.H. (1973). Photo-induced isomerization of 8-(3,4,5-trimethoxystyryl)caffeine as possible route of drug decomposition. *J Pharm Sci* **62**, 1885–1886.

Poucher, S.M., Keddie, J.R., Singh, P., Stoggall, S.M., Caulkett, P.W.R., Jones, G., and Collis, M.G. (1995). The *in vitro* pharmacology of ZM 241385, a potent, nonxanthine, A_{2A} selective adenosine receptor antagonist. *Br J Pharmacol* **115**, 1096–1102.

Richardson, P.J., Kase, H., and Jenner, P.G. (1997). Adenosine A_{2A} receptor antagonists as new agents for the treatment of Parkinson's disease. *Trends Pharmacol Sci* **18**, 338–344.

Sarges, R., Howard, H.R., Browne, R.G., Lebel, L.A., Seymour, P.A., and Koe, B.K. (1990). 4-Amino[1,2,4]triazolo[4,3-*a*]quinoxalines. A novel class of potent adenosine receptor antagonists and potential rapid-onset antidepressants. *J Med Chem* **33**, 2240–2254.

Schiffmann, S.N., Jacobs, O., and Vanderhaeghen, J.-J. (1991). Striatal restricted adenosine A_2 receptor (RDC8) is expressed by enkephalin but not by substance P neurons: an *in situ* hybridization histochemistry study. *J Neurochem* **57**, 1062–1067.

Schingnitz, C., Küfner-Mühl, U., Ensinger, H., Lehr, E., and Kuhn, F.J. (1991). Selective A_1 antagonists for treatment of cognitive deficits. *Nucleosides Nucleotides* **10**, 1067–1076.

Shamim, M.T., Ukena, D., Padgett, W.L., and Daly, J.W. (1989). Effects of 8-phenyl and 8-cycloalkyl substituents on the activity of mono-, di-, and trisubstituted alkylxanthines with substitution at the 1-, 3-, and 7-positions. *J Med Chem* **32**, 1231–1237.

Shamim, M.T., Ukena, D., Padgett, W.L., Hong, O., and Daly, J.W. (1988). 8-Aryl- and 8-cy-cloalkyl-1,3-dipropylxanthines: further potent and selective antagonists for A_1-adenosine receptors. *J Med Chem* 31, 613–617.

Shimada, J., Suzuki, F., Nonaka, H., Karasawa, A., Mizumoto, H., Ohno, T., Kubo, K., and Ishii, A. (1991). 8-(Dicyclopropylmethyl)-1,3-dipropylxanthine: a potent and selective adenosine A_1 antagonist with renal protective and diuretic activities. *J Med Chem* 34, 466–469.

Shimada, J., Suzuki, F., Nonaka, H., Ishii, A., and Ichikawa, S. (1992a). (*E*)-1,3-Dialkyl-7-methyl-8-(3,4,5-trimethoxystyryl)xanthines: potent and selective adenosine A_2 antagonists. *J Med Chem* 35, 2342–2345.

Shimada, J., Suzuki, F., Nonaka, H., and Ishii, A. (1992b). 8-Polycycloalkyl-1,3-dipropylxan-thines as potent and selective antagonists for A_1 adenosine receptors. *J Med Chem* 35, 924–930.

Shimada, J., Koike, N., Nonaka, H., Shiozaki, S., Yanagawa, K., Kanda, T., Kobayashi, H., Ichimura, M., Nakamura, J., Kase, H., and Suzuki, F. (1997). Adenosine A_{2A} antagonists with potent anti-cataleptic activity. *Bio Med Chem Lett* 7, 2349–2352.

Shiozaki, S., Ishii, A., Shuto, K., and Suzuki, F. (1990). Effects of N^6-(L-phenylisopropyl)adeno-sine on the passive avoidance in mice. *Jpn J Pharmacol* 52 (Suppl. II), 107P.

Shiozaki, S., Nonaka, H., Shimada, J., Suzuki, F., Nakamura, J., and Ishii, A. (1993). Behavioral pharmacological studies of KF15372, a selective adenosine A_1 antagonist. *Jpn J Pharmacol* 55 (Suppl. I), 188P.

Snyder, S.H., Katims, J.J., Annau, Z., Bruns, R.F., and Daly, J.W. (1981). Adenosine receptors and behavioral actions of methylxanthines. *Proc Natl Acad Sci USA* 75, 3260–3264.

Suzuki, F. (1992). Adenosine A_1 antagonists: a new therapeutic approach to cognitive deficits and acute renal failure. *Drug News Perspect* 5, 587–591.

Suzuki, F., Shimada, J., Mizumoto, H., Karasawa, A., Kubo, K., Nonaka, H., Ishii, A., and Kawakita, T. (1992a). Adenosine A_1 antagonists. 2. Structure–activity relationships on di-uretic activities and protective effects against acute renal failure. *J Med Chem* 35, 3066–3075.

Suzuki, F., Shimada, J., Nonaka, H., Ishii, A., Shiozaki, S., Ichikawa, S., and Ono, E. (1992b). 7,8-Dihydro-8-ethyl-2-(3-noradamantyl)-4-propyl-1*H*-imidazo[2,1-i]purin-5(4*H*)-one: a potent and water-soluble adenosine A_1 antagonist. *J Med Chem* 35, 3578–3581.

Suzuki, F., Shimada, J., Shiozaki, S., Ichikawa, S., Ishii, A., Nakamura, J., Nonaka, H., Kobayashi, H., and Fuse, E. (1993). Adenosine A_1 antagonists. 3. Structure–activity relationships on amelioration against scopolamine- or N^6-((R)-phenylisopropyl)adenosine-induced cognitive disturbance. *J Med Chem* 36, 2508–2518.

Tanaka, Y., Sakurai, M., Goto, M., and Hayashi, S. (1990). Effect of xanthine derivatives on hip-pocampal long-term potentiation. *Brain Res* 522, 63–68.

Terai, T., Kita, Y., Kusunoki, T., Shimazaki, T., Ando, T., Horiai, H., Akanane, A., Shiokawa, Y., and Yoshida, K. (1995). A novel non-xanthine adenosine A_1 receptor antagonist. *Eur J Phar-macol* 279, 217–225.

Trivedi, B.K., Bridges, A.J., Patt, W.C., Priebe, S.R., and Bruns, R.F. (1989). N^6-Bicycloalkyl-adenosines with unusually high potency and selectivity for the adenosine A_1 receptor. *J Med Chem* 32, 8–11.

Ukena, D., Padgett, W.L., Hong, O., Daly, J.W., Daly, D.T., and Olsson, R.A. (1987). N^6-Substi-tuted 9-methyladenines: a new class of adenosine receptor antagonists. *FEBS Lett* 215, 203–208.

Ukena, D., Shamim, M.T., Padgett, W., and Daly, J.W. (1986). Analogs of caffeine: antagonists with selectivity for A_2 adenosine receptors. *Life Sci* 39, 743–750.

Van Galen, P.J.M., Stiles, G.L., Michaels, G., and Jacobson, K.A. (1992). Adenosine A_1 and A_2 re-ceptors: structure–function relationships. *Med Res Rev* 12, 423–471.

Waldeck, D.H. (1991). Photoisomerization dynamics of stilbenes. *Chem Rev* 91, 415–436.

48   J. Shimada and F. Suzuki

Williams, M., Francis, J., Ghai, G., Psychoyos, S., Stone, G. A., and Cash, W.D. (1987). Biochemical characterization of the triazoloquinazoline, CGS15943, a novel nonxanthine adenosine antagonist. *J Pharm Exp Ther* **241**, 414–420.

Yao, K., Kusaka, H., Sano, J., Sato, K., and Karasawa, A. (1994). Diuretic effects of KW-3902, a novel adenosine A_1-receptor antagonist, in various models of acute renal failure in rats. *Jpn J Pharmacol* **64**, 281–288.

Zocchi, C., Ongini, E., Conti, A., Monopoli, A., Negretti, A., Baraldi, P.G., and Dionisotti, S. (1996). The non-xanthine heterocyclic compound SCH 58261 is a new potent and selective A_{2A} adenosine receptor antagonist. *J Pharmacol Exp Ther* **276**, 398–404.

CHAPTER 4

Overview of the Physiology and Pharmacology of Adenosine in the Peripheral System

AKIRA KARASAWA

Pharmaceutical Research and Development Center, Kyowa Hakko Kogyo Co., Ltd., Tokyo, Japan

Adenosine elicits a variety of physiological and pharmacological actions in many tissues and organs, and most of its actions are mediated via specific receptors on the cell surface (Daly, 1982; Williams, 1987; Belardinelli *et al.*, 1989; Daval *et al.*, 1996). Adenosine interacts with at least four different receptor subtypes, namely, A_1, A_{2A}, A_{2B}, and A_3 receptors (Collis and Hourani, 1993; Fredholm *et al.*, 1994). In some disease states, local or systemic adenosine levels are elevated and thus adenosine seems to be involved in the development of various diseases (Zhang and Lautt, 1992; Driver *et al.*, 1993; Funaya *et al.*, 1997). These elevations of endogenous adenosine levels represent adaptive counterregulatory mechanisms attempting to maintain homeostasis, pathogenic consequences that may aggravate the disease, or both. In fact, endogenous or exogenous adenosine as well as its specific agonists could retard the development of some diseases such as myocardial ischemia and inflammation, whereas excessive adenosine administration can also elicit various adverse events (Macallum *et al.*, 1991).

TABLE I Physiological Responses to Adenosine and Its Receptor Subtypes Involved

Physiological response	Receptor subtype[a]
Central nervous system	
Sedation	A_1
Decrease of locomotor activity	A_{2A}
Anticonvulsant action	A_1
Inhibition of allodinia	A_1
Peripheral nervous system	
Inhibition of sympathetic nerves	A_1
Inhibition of parasympathetic nerves	A_1
Stimulation of chemoreceptor	A_2
Stimulation of parasympathetic nerves	A_{2A}
Modulation of sensory nerves	A_1, A_2, A_3
Cardiovascular system	
Vasodilation (vascular smooth muscle)	A_1, A_{2A}, A_{2B}, A_3
Release of EDRF from endothelium	A_{2B}
Vasoconstriction (vascular smooth muscle)	A_1
Negative chronotropic action	A_1
Negative inotropic action	A_1
Negative dromotropic action	A_1
Preconditioning	A_1, A_3
Inhibition of platelet aggregation	A_{2A}
Respiratory and pulmonary system	
Bronchodilation	A_2
Bronchoconstriction	A_1
Renal system	
Antidiuresis (tubular sodium reabsorption)	A_1
Constriction of afferent arteriole	A_1
Dilation of efferent arteriole	A_{2A}
Contraction of mesangial cell	A_1
Tubuloglomerular feedback response	A_1
Inhibition/stimulation of renin release	A_1/A_{2A}
Erythropoietin production	A_{2A}
Gastrointestinal system	
Inhibition of transmitter release	A_1
Potentiation of transmitter release	A_{2A}
Inhibition of gastric acid output	A_1
Stimulation of intestinal secretion	A_2
Inhibition of stimulated intestinal secretion	?
Hormonal and exocrine system	
Inhibition of lipolysis	A_1
Increase/decrease of insulin sensitivity	$A_1/?$
Inhibition of pancreatic insulin secretion	A_1
Stimulation of pancreatic glucagon secretion	A_2
Potentiation of pancreatic exocrine secretion	A_1, A_2
Stimulation of gluconeogenesis	A_2

(continues)

TABLE I (*continued*)

Physiological response	Receptor subtype[a]
Immune System	
Inhibition of neutrophil superoxide generation	A_{2A}
Inhibition of expression of cell adhesion molecule	A_{2A}
Inhibition of cytokine synthesis	A_2, A_3
Enhancement of cytokine synthesis	?
Degranulation of mast cell	A_2
Promotion of neutrophil chemotaxis	A_2
Inhibition of eosinophil migration	A_3
Immunosuppression	A_{2A}

[a] ?: receptor subtype not specified; A: A_{2A} or A_{2B} not clear.

Based on the understanding of the adenosine physiology and the availability of specific agonists, antagonists, and various kinds of modulators, the pharmacological manipulation of adenosine or its actions has become possible and is expected to serve in the development of various therapeutic applications (Daly, 1982; Stone *et al.*, 1995). However, if therapeutic application of adenosine-related drugs (e.g., adenosine A_{2a} receptor antagonists as an anti-parkinsonian agent) is attempted, both the pharmacological aspects of the drug target and potential side effects have to be determined. This chapter focuses on the physiological effects of adenosine in the peripheral system and on its pharmacological manipulation. The current knowledge of various physiological effects of adenosine and its receptor subtypes involved is summarized in Table I.

I. METABOLISM, RECEPTORS, AND MODULATION OF ADENOSINE

Adenosine is formed via two metabolic pathways (Fig. 1). One is the route from the high-energy phosphate ATP, by degradation or metabolism, to adenosine via ADP and AMP. This route is accelerated by conditions in which ATP synthesis is inhibited, e.g., hypoxia or ischemia. The hydrolysis of AMP is catalyzed by 5'-nucleotidase, which is present both intracellularly (cytosolic form) and extracellularly (membrane-bound form). Another route to adenosine formation is by hydrolysis of ATP, via *S*-adenosylmethionine (SAH) to *S*-adenosylhomocysteine, in an oxygen-insensitive fashion. It is reported that, in the kidney, SAH hydrolysis contributes about 30% of the total adenosine formation under normoxic conditions, whereas during hypoxia most of the adenosine is formed in the cell derived from dephosphorylation of AMP (Kloor *et al.*, 1996).

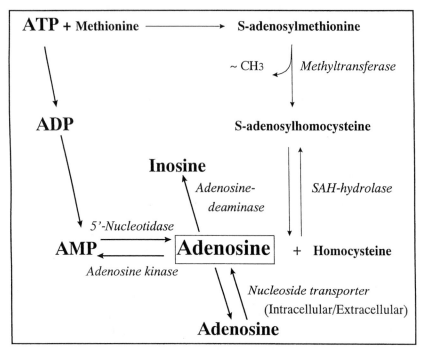

FIGURE 1. Pathways of adenosine formation and metabolism in the cell. SAH: *S*-adenosylhomocysteine.

Adenosine diffuses through plasma membranes via specific transporters. Thorn and Jarvis (1996) recently reviewed the various forms of adenosine transporters. Two broad types of adenosine transporter exist: facilitated carriers and active processes driven by the transmembrane sodium gradient. Facilitated-diffusion adenosine carriers are either sensitive (es) or insensitive (ei) to the transport inhibitor nitrobenzylthioinosine (NBMPR). Recently, molecular cloning of the various adenosine transporters has successfully been completed (Wang *et al.*, 1997; Yao *et al.*, 1997; Crawford *et al.*, 1998). Cells, including erythrocytes and endothelial cells, can take up adenosine with high affinity from the interstitial space, especially via the es-type adenosine transporters.

Adenosine, once formed, is metabolized by adenosine kinase (AK) or adenosine deaminase (ADA): AK phosphorylates adenosine to AMP whereas ADA, located both intracellularly and extracellularly, deaminates adenosine to produce inosine. Among many cell types, the endothelium plays a crucial role in the uptake and metabolism of adenosine. The half-life of adenosine in the extracellular space and in the bloodstream is very short (in the range of $3-10$ s). Thus the regulation of the extracellular adenosine concentration is a highly dynamic process with a high turnover rate. The basal levels of adenosine in the interstitium vary among the various tissues and are generally in the range between 10^{-8} and 10^{-7} M (Headrick, 1996; Siragy and Linden, 1996). In the ischemic condition, the interstitial adenosine level increases due to the decrease in energy charge. The cell surface receptors are assumed to be stimulated depending on the extracellular concentration of adenosine in the interstitium (Martin *et al.*, 1997).

The purine receptors are divided into two groups, P_1 and P_2. This division has been based on the potency order of agonists: ATP > ADP > AMP > adenosine and adenosine > AMP > ADP > ATP for the P_2- and the P_1-purinergic receptors, respectively. Accordingly, adenosine, if present extracellularly, almost exclusively acts on the P_1-purinergic receptors. The P_1 receptors are subdivided into A_1, A_{2A}, A_{2B}, and A_3 receptors (Collis and Hourani, 1993), for which structural information is now available (Stehle *et al.*, 1992; Van Galen *et al.*, 1992; Zhou *et al.*, 1992). Whereas the A_{2A} and A_{2B} receptors interact with G_s to stimulate adenylate cyclase activity and elevate cyclic AMP levels (see Chapter 5), the A_1 and A_3 receptors couple productively with members of the G_i/G_o family. Each receptor exhibits the seven transmembrane-spanning topography characteristics of almost all G protein coupled receptors (Palmer and Stiles, 1995). A_1 receptors can act through multiple effectors, including adenylate cyclase, potassium channels, calcium channels, phospholipase A_2 or C, and guanylyl cyclase (Olsson and Pearson, 1990; see Chapter 5). The receptor-selective ligands are addressed in Chapter 3.

On the basis of our understanding of the metabolic pathways of adenosine, several kinds of adenosine potentiators have been developed and their potential usefulness as therapeutic agents has been explored. These adenosine potentiators include adenosine deaminase inhibitors, adenosine (nucleoside) transport inhibitors, and adenosine kinase inhibitors, all of which are expected to increase local or systemic adenosine concentrations and to enhance the beneficial actions of endogenous adenosine. ADA inhibitors such as deoxycoformycin, which have been used as anticancer agents, could increase the tissue concentration of adenosine. The inhibition of ADA activity has been reported to protect against the extension of myocardial infarction (Martin *et al.*, 1997) and the nephropathy induced by puromycin aminonucleoside (Nosaka *et al.*, 1997). Adenosine transport inhibitors may also enhance local generation of adenosine. The conventional vasodilators dipyridamole and dilazep are known to inhibit the es-type adenosine transporters, though they are not specific. R75231 is reported to be a specific inhibitor of the es-type adenosine transporter (Baer *et al.*, 1991). Though the potential cardioprotective effect of inhibitors of the es-type transporter has been described, the most appropriate clinical indications for the es-type transport inhibitors await further investigations. At this point, inhibitors of adenosine transporters other than the es type are still not available and thus the physiological functions involving each adenosine transporter have not been fully elucidated. AK inhibitors can also potentiate the local generation of adenosine; one such inhibitor (GP-1-515) has been suggested to be a potential anti-inflammatory agent (Cronstein et al., 1995; Firestein et al., 1995).

II. PERIPHERAL NERVOUS SYSTEM

Adenosine is a potent and ubiquitous modulator of neurotransmitter release in both the central and peripheral nervous systems. In the periphery, adenosine is known to modulate the transmission of many types of nerves, including the sympathetic, parasympathetic, sensory, and motor nerves.

It is well known that adenosine presynaptically inhibits adrenergic neurotransmission in many tissues and organs. In various vascular preparations, adenosine, via A_1 receptors, inhibits noradrenaline release and sympathetic neurotransmission (Hedqvist and Fredholm, 1976; Brown and Collis, 1983). In the dog in vivo, intravenous infusion of adenosine attenuated the femoral vasoconstrictor response to sympathetic nerve stimulation, and the inhibitory action of adenosine was antagonized by theophylline (Hom and Lokhandwala, 1981a). Recently, Tamaoki et al. (1997) investigated the possible involvement of the endothelium in the modulation by adenosine of vascular sympathetic neurotransmission. In the isolated canine pulmonary artery, adenosine and its agonists inhibited the release of noradrenaline. The adenosine transport inhibitor dipyridamole and the ADA inhibitor deoxycoformycin enhanced the inhibition by adenosine in the presence of the endothelium but not in the absence of the endothelium. This observation suggests an involvement of the endothelium, either via uptake or metabolism of adenosine, in sympathetic neurotransmission in the vasculature. Adenosine also inhibits noradrenaline release from sympathetic nerve endings in the heart (Hom and Lokhandwala, 1981b; Richardt et al., 1987). This inhibition by adenosine of noradrenaline release seems to be one of the mechanisms of the cardioprotective action of adenosine in the ischemic myocardium (Cook and Karmazyn, 1996). Moreover, in other organs such as the kidney and the vas deferens, adenosine has also been reported to inhibit sympathetic neurotransmission (Muller and Paton, 1979; Ekas et al., 1981). Collectively, it seems to be a general feature that adenosine, via activation of A_1 receptors, exhibits an inhibitory modulation of sympathetic neurotransmission.

As compared with the sympathetic nervous system, the action of adenosine on the parasympathetic nervous system has not extensively been investigated.

In the guinea pig ileum longitudinal muscle, the adenosine antagonist 8-(p-sulfophenyl)theophylline was shown to increase the release of acetylcholine (Gustafsson, 1984). In the guinea pig ileum, adenosine or its agonists, either via activation of A_1 or A_{2A} receptors, inhibit or activate, respectively, the twitch contractions induced by transmural stimulation of the cholinergic nerve (Tomaru et al., 1995). These observations indicate that, at least in the guinea pig ileum, there exist adenosine receptors, probably of the A_1 type and A_{2A} type, negatively and positively modulating the release of acetylcholine at the presynaptic site. In contrast, in the guinea pig bronchi, adenosine seems to only minimally affect cholinergic neurotransmission (Kamikawa and Shimo, 1989).

Adenosine also affects neurotransmission of the sensory nerves in various tissues. In the rat mesenteric arterial bed, analogues of adenosine were reported to inhibit the vasodilator response to electrical stimulation of capsaicin-sensitive sensory-motor nerves (Rubino et al., 1993). The selective A_1 receptor agonist N^6-cyclopentyladenosine potently inhibited the neurotransmission whereas the A_{2A} agonist CGS 21680 did not affect it, suggesting that the A_1-adenosine receptor mediates the inhibition of sensory nerve transmission. In the guinea pig atria subjected to the transmural stimulation of sensory nerves, adenosine was shown to inhibit neurotransmission, resulting in the inhibition of the positive inotropic effect mediated by the sensory nerve (Rubino et al., 1990). The same study also showed that the cardiac response to the nerve stimulation was enhanced by 8-phenyltheophylline and was reduced by dipyridamole, suggesting a modulatory role of endogenous adenosine in the neurotransmission of the cardiac sensory nerve.

Motor nerve neurotransmission is also regulated by adenosine. In the phrenic nerve–hemidiaphragm preparation from rats, adenosine and related agonists affected electrically evoked acetylcholine release; both inhibitory A_1 receptors and excitatory A_{2A} receptors were suggested to be functioning in this preparation (Correia-de-Sa and Riberio, 1996).

III. CARDIOVASCULAR SYSTEM

In a variety of vascular preparations, adenosine induces vasodilator responses via activation of A_2 receptors (Li and Fredholm, 1985; Mathie et al., 1991; Utterback et al., 1994; Rongen et al., 1997). The vasodilation, when induced systemically, causes hypotension. Recently, Belardinelli et al. (1998), using the specific A_{2A} receptor antagonist SCH58261, clarified that the A_{2A} receptor was involved in coronary vasodilation in the isolated guinea pig perfused heart. On the other hand, the stimulation of A_1 receptors may also mediate vascular relaxation in the porcine coronary artery, via the activation of glyburidesensitive potassium channels (Merkel *et al.*, 1992), though the vasodilation mediated by A_2 receptors seems to be more important than that mediated by A_1 receptors. Moreover, adenosine, via stimulation of A_1 receptors, inhibits sympathetic neurotransmission, resulting in the reduced tonus of the vasculature (Hedqvist and Fredholm, 1976; Brown and Collis, 1983). Collectively, stimulation of adenosine receptors is assumed to cause vasodilation, rather than vasoconstriction, in most of the vasculature. Adenosine, however, exceptionally causes vasoconstriction in the renal preglomerular arteriole (Osswald *et al.*, 1997) and in the pulmonary vasculature (Wiklund *et al.*, 1987; Biaggioni *et al.*, 1989), via the stimulation of A_1 receptors.

In the heart, adenosine exhibits a variety of effects on cardiac function via the activation of A_1 receptors (Fredholm and Sollevi, 1986; Belardinelli and Pelleg, 1990; Rongen *et al.*, 1997). First, adenosine suppresses impulse formation in the sinus node, leading to bradycardia (i.e., a negative chronotropic action). However, *in vivo,* the effect of adenosine on heart rate is rather complex, since it also causes vasodilation, resulting in the activation of sympathetic nerve reflex, and chemoreceptor stimulation. Second, adenosine, acting on the proximal portion of the atrioventricular junction, prolongs atrioventricular conduction time (i.e., a negative dromotropic action). Third, adenosine depresses cardiac contractility of both the atrial and ventricular myocardium (i.e., a negative inotropic action) when the contractility is increased by β-adrenoceptor agonists. All these actions of adenosine are mediated by the activation of A_1 receptors (Belardinelli *et al.*, 1989). Adenosine is clinically indicated for the treatment of supraventricular tachycardias that incorporate the sinus node and atrioventricular node as part of the arrhythmic circuit or for unmasking atrial tachyarrythmias or ventricular preexcitation (Wilbur and Marchlinski, 1997). Adenosine is also effective against some unique atrial and ventricular tachycardias. These antiarrhythmic effects of adenosine are mainly ascribed to its negative chronotropic and dromotropic actions resulting from the A_1 receptor activation, though the involvement of A_2 receptors cannot be excluded.

One of the most well-studied features of adenosine is its cardioprotective action. Adenosine has been shown to protect the jeopardized ischemic myocardium in a variety of animal models of myocardial infarction (Cook and Karmazyn, 1996; Granger, 1997). There may be a variety of mechanisms involved in the cardioprotective effect of adenosine. First, the cardioprotective effect of adenosine seems to be at least partly due to its A_1 receptor-mediated cardiac depressant action, which leads to the decrease in myocardial energy consumption. Second, a coronary vasodilator action, which results in increased oxygen supply to the heart, seems to play a role, especially in coronary microembolization (Hori *et al.*, 1989). Third, preconditioning mediated via adenosine could also be involved in the cardioprotection. In fact, adenosine is a probable mediator for the establishment of cardiac preconditioning (Baxter,

1997), which is a defense mechanism preparing for successive episodes of cardiac ischemia. Both A_3 receptors, which cause protein kinase C activation, and A_1 receptors are likely to be involved in this phenomenon (Thornton et al., 1992; Armstrong and Ganote, 1994; Kitakaze et al., 1997). Fourth, anti-inflammatory effects of adenosine, as will be addressed later, could also contribute to the protection against the extension of myocardial infarction, especially during the reperfusion period when neutrophil activation occurs. Finally, the inhibition of P-selectin expression may also contribute to the cardioprotective action of adenosine, since this is reported to play a role in the extension of myocardial infarction (Weyrich et al., 1993). The increase in extracellular adenosine formation during hypoxia and ischemia is assumed to be "a natural defence substance against the consequence of ischemia" (Rongen et al., 1997). Moreover, ecto-5'-nucleotidase is reported to be induced by the brief ischemic insult in the myocardium, possibly via the activation of protein kinase C (Kitakaze et al., 1997). This induction of ecto-5'-nucleotidase is likely to contribute to the efficient formation of adenosine and consequently to the effective achievement of the cardioprotective action of adenosine in the ischemic myocardium.

Based on the various cardioprotective actions of adenosine, pharmacological manipulation of endogenous adenosine could exert either beneficial effects or adverse effects on the ischemic heart. In dogs subjected to coronary occlusion and reperfusion, intravenous infusion of adenosine was demonstrated to attenuate the infarct size when the cardiac function and the transmural blood flow were well preserved (Pitarys et al., 1991). Moreover, adenosine potentiation by AICA-riboside, nucleoside transport inhibitors, or ADA inhibitors was reported to be cardioprotective in animal models of cardiac infarction (Gruber et al., 1989; Masuda et al., 1991; Martin et al., 1997). In contrast, blockade of adenosine receptors was shown to enhance the extension of acute myocardial infarction (Zhao et al., 1994). From analysis of the effects of specific adenosine receptor antagonists, activation of A_1 and A_2 receptors was demonstrated to be cardioprotective during the ischemic period and the reperfusion period, respectively, in a canine model of myocardial ischemia and reperfusion. The influence of adenosine receptor blockade during the chronic phase of myocardial ischemia or infarction remains to be established, though; in the acute phase of ischemia, adenosine blockade is assumed to aggravate the ischemic myocardium.

Adenosine may also regulate arterial smooth muscle cell growth and proliferation, which are key events in atherogenesis. In aortic smooth muscle cells isolated from both normal and streptozotocin-induced diabetic rats, adenosine was shown to inhibit the growth rate, and the cells from diabetic rats were more sensitive to adenosine (Pares-Herbute et al., 1996). Moreover, adenosine is reported to inhibit serum-induced growth of cardiac fibroblasts from rats (Dubey *et al.*, 1997). Adenosine thus might play a role as an endogenous anti-atherogenic and anti-fibrotic substance.

Platelet aggregation is inhibited by adenosine via activation of A_{2A} receptors and cyclic AMP formation in platelets (Cristalli *et al.*, 1994). In the adenosine A_{2A} receptor knockout mouse, the anti-aggregatory effect of the adenosine agonist NECA was shown to be diminished (Ledent *et al.*, 1997). Moreover, a recent study by Minamino *et al.* (1998) demonstrated that adenosine, via activation of A_2 receptors, inhibited the expression of P-selectin on platelets and subsequent platelet–neutrophil adhesion, resulting in the reduced formation of coronary thromboemboli in dogs during coronary hypoperfusion. Thus adenosine, either directly or indirectly, inhibits platelet aggregation, leading to the prevention of various forms of thrombosis. The adenosine transport inhibitor dipyridamole is reported to potentiate the ADP-induced platelet aggregation (Di Minno *et al.*, 1980).

Various forms of systemic shock may also involve adenosine. In an animal model of hemorrhagic shock, venous adenosine levels were shown to increase (Zhang and Lautt, 1992). The modulation of adenosine or its action may therefore be useful for the treatment of various systemic shock states. The administration of adenosine and an A_1 receptor antagonist protected against the systemic shock caused by splanchnic artery occlusion and reperfusion in rats (Karasawa *et al.*, 1992). Additionally, patients with shock due to gram-negative sepsis suffer from systemic inflammatory responses and elevated proinflammatory cytokine levels (Dinarello *et al.*, 1993), both of which can be mitigated by adenosine or its agonists (Cronstein *et al.*, 1985; Sajjadi *et al.*, 1996; Eigler *et al.*, 1997). Accordingly, Firestein *et al.* (1994) reported that an AK inhibitor protected against septic shock. From these observations, adenosine is assumed to be a modulator for the pathophysiology of systemic shock, either via its hemodynamic actions or its anti-inflammatory actions.

IV. RENAL EFFECTS

In the kidney, adenosine exhibits a variety of physiological actions including effects on hemodynamics, tubular function, and the release of renin (Spielman and Arend, 1991; Osswald *et al.*, 1997). Adenosine constricts preglomerular (afferent) arterioles and dilates postglomerular (efferent) arterioles via activation of adenosine A_1 and A_{2A} receptors, respectively. Adenosine also induces mesangial cell contraction via the stimulation of A_1 receptors (Oliver *et al.*, 1989). These site-specific actions of adenosine result in a decrease in glomerular capillary pressure (Haas and Osswald, 1981). Adenosine, acting on the renal tubule, also has an antidiuretic action. Coulson *et al.* (1991) reported that, in the proximal tubule, adenosine stimulates phosphate and glucose transport in the opossum kidney epithelial cell line, suggesting that adenosine, presumably via a decrease in cyclic AMP, stimulates the availability of Na phosphate and Na glucose cotransporters, thus promoting reabsorption of Na and water in the renal tubule. This is consistent with the prominent diuretic action of adenosine A_1 receptor antagonists (Mizumoto and Karasawa, 1993; Mizumoto et al., 1993). A_1 receptor antagonists have also been shown to decrease Na-dependent phosphate transport in a proximal tubular cell line and to inhibit the cotransporter of $NaHCO_3$ in the isolated proximal tubule (Takeda et al., 1993; Cai et al., 1995). The A_1 receptor mediated inhibition of renin release (Arend et al., 1984) results in reduced angiotensin II production and aldosterone release. In contrast, activation of A_2-adenosine receptors was shown to stimulate renin secretion in rat cortical slices (Churchill and Churchill, 1985). In dogs, infusion of the adenosine A_{2A} agonist CGS-21680A into the renal artery increased plasma renin activity and renal blood flow with minimal effects on urinary volume or urinary Na excretion (Levens et al., 1991).

The tubuloglomerular feedback (TGF) mechanism refers to a series of events whereby changes in the NaCl concentration in the tubular fluid at the end of the thick ascending limb of Henle's loop are sensed by the macula densa, which then elicits afferent arteriolar vasoconstriction, leading to an antidiuretic action. Schnermann et al. (1990) showed that the blockade of the adenosine A_1 receptor inhibited the TGF and that adenosine, acting on A_1 receptors, is a mediator of TGF. Thus the diuretic action of A_1 receptor antagonists may at least partly be due to the inhibition of TGF.

Adenosine may play a role in the pathogenesis of some forms of acute renal failure. Osswald et al. (1977, 1997) observed that postocclusive renal vasoconstriction was accompanied by an increase in renal adenosine content and was blocked by an adenosine receptor antagonist. These authors concluded that adenosine, accumulated during the ischemic period, can induce postocclusive vasoconstriction in the kidney, which may then lead to further, excessive renal ischemia, which could be harmful to the failed kidney. In fact, the renal failure sometimes observed following the injection of contrast medium involves renal ischemia and accompanies an increased level of adenosine in the kidney (Rudnick et al., 1996). In accordance with these observations, adenosine A_1 receptor antagonists have been shown to ameliorate acute renal failure following various nephrotoxic insults, including cis-platinum, contrast medium, and gentamycin (Yao et al., 1994b; Nagashima et al., 1995; Arakawa et al., 1996). Moreover, adenosine A_1 receptor antagonists, not conventional diuretics, cause diuretic effects even in animals with acute renal failure (Yao et al., 1994a). Such adenosine A_1 antagonists thus seem to be promising candidate drugs for the treatment of acute renal failure.

In contrast, potentiation of the actions of adenosine may be effective against diabetic nephropathy and glomerular nephritis. It is reported that, in rats with streptozotocin-induced diabetic mellitus, dipyridamole, presumably by inhibition of adenosine transport and the resultant increased interstitial adenosine concentration, inhibited the development of proteinuria (Vallon and Osswald, 1994). In patients with diabetic nephropathy, a combined treatment with aspirin–dipyridamole for 6 weeks significantly reduced the total 24-h urinary protein excretion (Hopper et al., 1989). In addition, dipyridamole is reported to attenuate the development of nephritis and retard proteinuria (Okada et al., 1981; Woo, 1996). The beneficial effect of dipyridamole seems to be not only due to its antiplatelet action but its effect on renal hemodynamics, leading to the reduced intraglomerular pressure, as is the case with angiotensin I converting enzyme inhibitors.

Renal erythropoietin production is increased by the stimulation of A_2-adenosine receptors with NECA in the tubular epithelial cell line, and the augmented erythropoietin production is paralleled by increased intracellular cyclic AMP (Fisher and Nakajima, 1992). In rats in vivo, adenosine agonists such as NECA and CGS-21680A dose-dependently stimulated production of erythropoietin (Nagashima and Karasawa, 1996). Moreover, the same study demonstrated that elevated urinary excretion of adenosine is accompanied by anemia following partial withdrawal of blood and that the increase of erythropoietin following anemic hypoxia was inhibited by an adenosine A_{2A} receptor antagonist. These results suggest that adenosine, presumably by stimulation of A_{2A} receptors, increases erythropoietin production in response to hypoxia or anemia. Thus adenosine is assumed to be a mediator which, by sensing systemic anemia in the kidney, maintains the homeostasis of hematocrit.

V. RESPIRATORY AND PULMONARY SYSTEM

In conscious humans and animals, adenosine stimulates carotid and aortic chemoreceptors (McQueen and Ribeno, 1981; Biaggioni et al., 1987), resulting in the stimulation of respiration and ventilation. The receptor subtype involved has not been determined.

Adenosine is likely to be involved in the pathophysiology of asthma, an inflammatory disease of airways associated with bronchial hyperresponsiveness and variable airflow obstruction (Church and Holgate, 1986; Polosa and Holgate, 1997). In fact, increased amounts of adenosine in the bronchial lavage fluid have been demonstrated in subjects with asthma (Driver et al., 1993). Adenosine could play roles in the pathogenesis of asthma either as a proinflammatory substance or as a bronchoconstrictor. Aside from these two main pathogenic mechanisms, adenosine and its triphosphate nucleotide ATP were found to induce chloride secretion in the nasal epithelium (Knowles *et al.*, 1991), which might also be involved in the pathophysiology of asthma.

Adenosine, released perhaps from mast cells, platelets, or epithelia, may modulate airway inflammation by promoting neutrophil chemotaxis. Adenosine also increases histamine release from immunologically activated human lung mast cells and circulating basophils by stimulation of specific cell surface receptors (Hughes *et al.*, 1984; Rose *et al.*, 1988). In rat mast cells, adenosine is reported to potentiate the histamine release induced by anti-IGE or concanavarin, in a manner antagonized by theophylline (Marquardt *et al.*, 1978). Moreover, Feoktistov and Biaggioni (1995) have recently shown that adenosine elicits secretion of IL-8, a potent chemoattractant, from human mast cells by the stimulation of A_{2B} receptors, suggesting that mast cell derived cytokines might be involved in the persistent airway inflammatory responses.

Adenosine provokes concentration-related bronchoconstriction when administered by inhalation to asthmatic patients but not to normal volunteers (Cushley *et al.*, 1983). It seems that adenosine indirectly, rather than directly, constricts airway smooth muscles through activation of specific receptors on intermediary inflammatory cells or on afferent nerve endings. Adenosine has been shown to enhance histamine release and prostanoid generation from human lung mast cells (Hughes *et al.*, 1984; Peachell *et al.*, 1988). Thus, histamine and bronchoconstricting prostanoids (e.g., prostaglandin D_2, thromboxane A_2), released from mast cells, seem to be involved in the bronchoconstriction of patients with asthma. Activation of neural pathways may also contribute to the contraction of airway smooth muscles. A reflex cholinergic mechanism is suggested in the bronchoconstriction, since an anticholinergic agent, administered by inhalation, attenuated the airway effect of adenosine in subjects with stable asthma (Polosa *et al.*, 1991). In addition, the involvement of sensory nerves has been suggested (Manzini and Ballati, 1990). Recently, Meade *et al.* (1996) showed that, in BED rats, adenosine increased pulmonary resistance by stimulating neuropeptide-containing nerves prior to mast cell activation, suggesting that the release of contractile neuropeptides from sensory nerve endings is important for bronchoconstriction following adenosine challenge. In contrast, in normal guinea pig bronchi, adenosine inhibited tachykininergic contraction in a manner antagonized by aminophylline (Kamikawa and Shimo, 1989).

It has been reported that adenosine-induced bronchoconstriction was reduced by antisense oligonucleotides, which reduced the number of adenosine A_1 receptors in the lung of an animal model with allergic asthma (Nyce and Metzger, 1997; Richardson, 1997). Theophylline is one of the most widely used anti-asthmatic agents. Though its effect has previously been ascribed to inhibition of phosphodiesterase activity, its antagonistic action at adenosine receptors is now believed to be involved in the therapeutic efficacy of this drug. In fact, theophylline inhibits neutrophil chemotactic factor release associated with adenosine challenge in patients with asthma (Driver *et al.*, 1991), and this drug also inhibits adenosine-induced bronchoconstriction (Cushley *et al.*, 1984). The clinical investigation of subtype-specific adenosine antagonists for the treatment of asthma is therefore warranted.

VI. GASTROINTESTINAL SYSTEM

In the gastrointestinal tract, adenosine has been shown to modulate neuro-transmission (Gustafsson, 1984; Broad *et al.*, 1992; Christofi and Wood, 1993). Adenosine is known to inhibit the release of major contractile neuro-transmitters such as acetylcholine and neurokinins. In the guinea pig ileum, adenosine inhibited neurotransmitter release by suppressing the presynaptic influx of calcium ions during depolarization of cholinergic terminals (Shi-nozuka *et al*, 1985). Accordingly, adenosine A_1 receptor agonists inhibit the giant migrating contractions induced in rats by glycerol enema (Tomaru *et al.*, 1993). In addition, the adenosine agonist NECA has been shown to inhibit peristalsis in the rat ileum, though its precise mechanism is obscure (Coupar and Hancock, 1994). On the other hand, an adenosine A_1 receptor antagonist was found to increase defecation (Tomaru *et al.*, 1994). It seems that in-hibitory A_1 and stimulatory A_{2A} receptors exist in cholinergic nerves of the in-testine (Tomaru *et al.*, 1995). Indeed, an adenosine A_1 agonist inhibited, and an adenosine A_{2A} agonist potentiated, the twitch contraction of the isolated guinea pig ileum subjected to transmural nerve stimulation. The ability of adenosine A_1 receptor antagonists to induce gastrostimulatory action and defecation suggests that endogenous adenosine plays a physiological role in sustained inhibition of gastrointestinal motility via adenosine A_1 receptors.

Adenosine receptors are also present in the gastric fundus, where they inhibit gastric acid secretion in rats and dogs (Westerberg and Geiger, 1989; Gerber *et al.*, 1985). In canine parietal cells, moreover, adenosine A_1 receptor agonists decreased histamine-induced aminopyrine (AP) accumulation, an in-dex of gastric acid secretion, whereas 8-phenyltheophylline increased AP ac-cumulation (Gerber and Payne, 1988). The inhibitory effect of adenosine was specific to histamine and it did not affect either carbachol or dibutyryl cyclic AMP stimulated acid secretion.

On the other hand, the effect of adenosine on intestinal secretion is rather complex. Adenosine is reported to stimulate chloride (Cl^-) secretion in the rabbit ileum, as examined by determination of the short-circuit current, with simultaneous measurement of cyclic AMP content in the isolated ileum (Dobbins *et al.*, 1984). In accordance with this result, adenosine and its agonists, presumably via A_2 receptors, caused sustained Cl^- secretion across monolayers of T84, a human colonic epithelial cell line (Barrett *et al.*, 1990).

On the other hand, the adenosine agonist NECA is reported to reverse PGE_2-induced Cl^- secretion and inhibit VIP-induced Cl^- secretion in the jejunum (Couper and Hancock, 1994). A recent study by Tally *et al.* (1996) demonstrated that adenosine, via stimulation of A_{2B} receptors, increased Cl^- secretion in the ischemic intestine whereas, under normal conditions, extracellular levels of adenosine were maintained below the prosecretory threshold and thus adenosine limited the activation of Cl^- secretion. Adenosine thus seems to exert dual regulatory effects on intestinal secretion.

VII. INFLAMMATION AND IMMUNE SYSTEM

Adenosine, via stimulation of A_2 receptors, inhibits some, but not all, neutrophil functions; thus adenosine inhibits phagocytosis, the generation of toxic oxygen metabolites and adhesion, whereas adenosine does not inhibit degranulation nor chemotaxis (Cronstein *et al.*, 1985; Cronstein, 1994). In N-formylmethionylleucylphenylalanine (FMLP)-stimulated neutrophils, adenosine and its analogs suppress the generation of superoxide anion and hydrogen peroxide in a theophylline-sensitive manner. However, the effect of adenosine on neutrophil activation is dependent on the stimuli and the species examined (Cronstein *et al.*, 1987; Ward *et al.*, 1988). In human as well as rat neutrophils, adenosine enhanced superoxide anion generation in cells stimulated with immune complexes; in contrast, when FMLP was used as a stimulant, the oxygen radical generation of human neutrophils was suppressed, but that of rat neutrophils was enhanced. Irrespective of this complexity, most of the effects of adenosine on human neutrophils are inhibitory rather than stimulatory in nature.

In addition to neutrophils, adenosine affects other types of inflammatory cells such as macrophages and mast cells. In mouse peritoneal macrophages, exogenous adenosine stimulated superoxide secretion whereas the xanthine oxidase inhibitor alloprinol inhibited this superoxide secretion (Tritsche and Niswander, 1983). On the other hand, in mouse peritoneal macrophages, adenosine inhibited zymozan particle-stimulated β-glucuronidase secretion in a theophylline-resistant fashion (Riches *et al.*, 1985). In rat mast cells, adenosine potentiated the histamine release induced by anti-IGE, concanavalin A, or the calcium ionophore A23187 without influencing spontaneous release, and this effect was antagonized by theophylline (Marquardt *et al.*, 1978). In human eosinophils, adenosine inhibits the migration via A_3-receptors (Knight *et al.*, 1997).

The expression of various cell adhesion molecules is modulated by adenosine. Adenosine, via activation of A_2 receptors, directly inhibits CD11/CD18 (β_2-integrin adhesion molecule) expression on the surface of polymorphonuclear cells and subsequent superoxide generation (Cronstein *et al.*, 1985;

Wollner et al., 1993). In human endothelial cells, expression of the adhesion molecules E-selectin and vascular cell adhesion molecule-1 (VCAM-1) was also reduced by adenosine (Bouma et al., 1996). Adenosine interferes with neutrophil–endothelial adhesion by effects on both neutrophils and endothelial cells (Grisham et al., 1989; Cronstein et al., 1992). These results suggest that the vascular endothelium, in addition to the neutrophils, constitutes an important target for the anti-inflammatory actions of adenosine. Moreover, in dogs subjected to coronary hypoperfusion, endogenous adenosine inhibited the expression of P-selectin and subsequent thromboemboli (Minamoto et al., 1998). Thus adenosine inhibits leukocyte adherence to the endothelium and the following extravasation (Grisham et al., 1989; Cronstein et al., 1992; Jordan, 1997).

Recently, the modulatory effects of adenosine on the expression and secretion of various cytokines have been elucidated by a number of authors. Adenosine has been shown to inhibit TNF expression in macrophages and monocytes, possibly via the stimulation of adenosine A_2 or A_3 receptors (Sajjadi et al., 1996; Eigler et al., 1997). Adenosine was also found to inhibit the release of interleukin (IL)-6 and IL-8 from stimulated endothelial cells (Bouma et al., 1996). Moreover, adenosine is known to enhance the secretion of IL-10, an anti-inflammatory cytokine, from human monocytes (Le Moine et al., 1996). Thus all the known effects of adenosine on cytokines are anti-inflammatory.

Taken together, adenosine exhibits a prominent anti-inflammatory action via inhibitory effects on neutrophils and macrophages, inhibition of the expression of cell adhesion molecules, and the modulation of various cytokines in monocytes and endothelial cells. Interestingly, ecto-5'-nucleotidase is reported to be induced by proinflammatory cytokines such as IL-1 and TNF in human monocytes and rat mesangial cells (Murray et al., 1988; Savic et al., 1990). Thus, by the induction of 5'-nucleotidase and the subsequent increase in local generation of adenosine, the inflammatory response and the subsequent extravasation could be effectively mitigated in a negative-feedback manner. Endogenous adenosine therefore seems to be a counterregulator of the inflammatory responses.

In accordance with the anti-inflammatory properties of adenosine, adenosine agonists have been shown to ameliorate the carrageenan-induced pleural inflammatory response in rats in vivo (Schrier et al., 1990). Moreover, a strategy to augment adenosine action has also been attempted: an AK inhibitor, via the enhancement of endogenous adenosine, inhibits neutrophil–endothelium adhesion (Firestein et al., 1995) and exhibits an anti-inflammatory effect in a rat model of carrageenan-induced inflammation in air pouches in vivo (Cronstein et al., 1995). In addition, the antirheumatoid agent methotrexate, conventionally described as a dihydrofolate reductase inhibitor, has been shown to promote the release of adenosine, which seems to be at least partly responsible for the efficacy of this agent in the treatment of rheumatoid arthritis (Cronstein, 1997).

Adenosine is immunosuppressive and its effects on lymphocytes are very important (Girbert *et al.*, 1972; Hirschhorn, 1995). Accumulation of adenosine in the absence of ADA activity is lymphotoxic and results in severe combined immunodeficiency (e.g., inherited ADA deficiency). In accordance with this observation, adenosine modulates T-cell subset-specific antigen expression, facilitating T8 antigen expression and activating radioresistant suppressor activity (Moroz and Twig, 1985). The immunosuppressive action of adenosine is mediated via A_{2A} receptors (Huang *et al.*, 1997; Koshiba *et al.*, 1997).

VIII. ENDOCRINE AND EXOCRINE EFFECTS

Adenosine has various metabolic effects in many cells and tissues. In the pancreatic endocrine system, adenosine via activation of A_1 receptors inhibits insulin secretion from B cells, whereas it stimulates glucagon secretion from A cells via A_2 receptors (Chapal *et al.*, 1985; Hillaire-Buys *et al.*, 1987, 1994). Thus the action of adenosine on the pancreatic endocrine system tends to increase blood glucose levels. The peripheral metabolic effects of adenosine on various tissues or organs are more complex and dependent upon the types of cells or tissues. In adipocytes, adenosine generally facilitates the action of insulin on various processes, including glucose transport, oxidation, and lipolysis, where A_1 receptors are involved (Joost and Steinfelder, 1982; Heseltine *et al.*, 1995). In the myocardium, adenosine was also shown to potentiate insulin-stimulated glucose uptake, independent of changes in coronary blood flow in dogs (Law and Raymond, 1988). In the liver, adenosine has been shown to stimulate glycogen synthesis (de Sánchez *et al.*, 1972). These observations indicate that the sensitivity to insulin is increased in the adipocyte, myocardium, and the liver. In contrast, in skeletal muscle, the opposite effect of adenosine has been reported by Epsinal *et al.* (1983), who showed that depletion of adenosine, by the addition of ADA to the incubation medium surrounding stripped soleus muscle from rats, increased the sensitivity of the muscle to insulin. This inhibitory effect of adenosine on skeletal muscle insulin sensitivity was supported by the observation that the adenosine agonist 2-chloroadenosine decreased soleus muscle sensitivity to the glycolytic effect of insulin, whereas the adenosine antagonist 8-phenyltheophylline increased insulin sensitivity (Boudohoski *et al.*, 1984). Taking into account the nature of adenosine being generated locally in response to hypoxia, adenosine may play a role in increasing energy supply in jeopardized skeletal muscles during hypoxia (e.g., during excessive exercise) by increasing glycogen degradation.

Adenosine may also affect the pancreatic exocrine system. Exogenous adenosine has been shown to potentiate secretin-stimulated pancreatic secretion in the dog (Yamagishi *et al.*, 1985). Moreover, in isolated pancreatic lobules, the adenosine agonists R-PIA and NECA increased amylase secretion (Rodríguez-Nodal *et al.*, 1995). The increase of amylase secretion induced by adenosine was inhibited by either the A_1-selective antagonist PD116,948 or the A_2-selective antagonist PD115,199, suggesting that the action of adenosine is mediated by both A_1 and A_2 receptors. At this point, however, it is uncertain whether or not the effect of adenosine on the pancreatic exocrine system is of physiological or pathophysiological significance.

Several studies have examined the effects of adenosine on hormone secretion. In the isolated bovine adrenal zona fasciculata cells, adenosine stimulated or augmented basal, angiotensin II and cyclic AMP-stimulated steroidogenesis, whereas adenosine blockade with ADA or 8-phenyltheophylline enhanced ACTH-stimulated steroidogenesis (Koper *et al.*, 1988). These results suggest a dual regulation of adenosine in the secretion of corticosterone. On the other hand, the adenosine agonist R-PIA was shown to elevate plasma ACTH and corticosterone levels in the rat *in vivo* (LeBlanc and Soucy, 1994). In the *in vivo* situation, the peripheral vasodilating effect of this agonist may also be involved in the elevation of ACTH and corticosterone. In fact, systemic hypotension, which can be caused by adenosine agonists, is known to release corticotropin (ACTH)-releasing factor (Plotsky *et al.*, 1986), resulting in the stimulated release of ACTH and corticosterone. The adenosine receptor antagonist caffeine has also been reported to elevate ACTH and corticosterone levels in rats (Leblanc *et al.*, 1995), whereas in man, theophylline has been shown to produce a small and transient increase in cortisone secretion (Tulin-Silver *et al.*, 1981). The anxiogenic action of the antagonist, in addition to its direct action on the adrenocortical cells, seems to be involved in the increased level of corticosterone *in vivo*.

A central action of adenosine modulating the release of prolactin has also been reported (Dorfinger and Schonbrunn, 1985; Ondo *et al.*, 1989). In the clonal GH4C1 pituitary cell line, adenosine and the selective agonist R-PIA inhibited the release of prolactin and cyclic AMP accumulation in a theophylline-sensitive manner. In contrast to this *in vitro* action, adenosine, injected intraventricularly, caused dose-related rises in plasma prolactin levels without affecting plasma levels of leutinizing hormone or thyrotropin in rats, and this effect of adenosine was also antagonized by theophylline. Though the responses *in vitro* and *in vivo* differ, adenosine seems to play a role in the control of prolactin secretion. Further studies are required to clarify the details of this effect.

IX. CONCLUDING REMARKS

This chapter surveyed the current knowledge of the physiology and pharmacology of adenosine in the peripheral system. Adenosine is an endogenous substance generated by all living cells which, in normal physiological conditions and in some disease states, plays important roles in the modulation of many cell functions. Recent work in this diverse field has brought new insights into the basic science of adenosine action and the potential therapeutic applications of adenosine regulating agents. Such agents include receptor subtype-specific agonists and antagonists and modulators of the metabolic pathways involving adenosine. However, as little time has elapsed since the subtype-specific ligands and the modulators have become available, further investigations are required in both the basic and the applied aspects of adenosine research.

REFERENCES

Arakawa, K., Suzuki, H., Naito, M., Matsumoto, A., Hayashi, K., Matsuda, H., Ichihara, A., Kubota, E., and Saruta, T. (1996). Role of adenosine in the renal response to contrast medium. *Kidney Int.* **49**, 1199–1206.

Arend, L. J., Haramati, A., Thompson, C. I., and Spielman, W. S. (1984). Adenosine-induced decrease in renin release: Dissociation from hemodynamic effects. *Am. J. Physiol.* **247**, F447–F452.

Armstrong, S., and Ganote, C. E. (1994). Adenosine receptor specificity in preconditioning of isolated rabbit cardiomyocytes: Evidence of A_3 receptor involvement. *Cardiovasc. Res.* **28**, 1049–1056.

Baer, H. P., Seriner, V., Moorji, A., and Van Belle, H. (1991). *In vivo* effectiveness of several nucleoside transport inhibitors in mice and hamsters. *Naunyn-Schmiedeberg's Arch. Pharmacol.* **343**, 365–369.

Barrett, K. E., Cohn, J. A., Huott, P. A., Wasserman, S. I., and Dharmsathaphorn, K. (1990). Immune-related intestinal chloride secretion. II. Effect of adenosine on T84 cell line. *Am. J. Physiol.* **258**, C902–C912.

Baxter, G. F. (1997). Ischaemic preconditioning of myocardium. *Ann. Med.* **29**, 345–352.

Belardinelli, L., Linden, J., and Bern, R. M. (1989). The cardiac effects of adenosine. *Prog. Cardiovasc. Dis.* **32**, 73–97.

Belardinelli, L., and Pelleg, A. (1990). Cardiac electrophysiology and pharmacology of adenosine. *J. Cardiovasc. Electrophysiol.* **1**, 327–339.

Belardinelli, L., Shryock, J. C., Snowdy, S., Zhang, Y., Monopoli, A., Lozza, G., Ongini, E., Olsson, R. A., and Dennis, D. M. (1998). The A_{2A} adenosine receptor mediates coronary vasodilation. *J. Pharmacol. Exp. Ther.* **284**, 1066–1073.

Biaggioni, I., Olafsson, B., Robertson, P. M., Hollister, A. S., and Robertson, D. (1987). Cardiovascular and respiratory effects of adenosine in conscious man. Evidence for chemoreceptor activation. *Circ. Res.* **61**, 779–786.

Biaggioni, I., King, L. S., Enayat, N., Robertson, D., and Newman, J. H. (1989). Adenosine produces pulmonary vasoconstriction in sheep. Evidence for thromboxane A_2/prostaglandin endoperoxide-receptor activation. *Circ. Res.* **65**, 1516–1525.

Bouma, M. G., Van den Wildenberg, F. A. J. M., and Buurman, W. A. (1996). Adenosine inhibits cytokine release and expression of adhesion molecules by activated human endothelial cells. *Am. J. Physiol.* **270**, C522–C529.

Broad, R. M., McDonald, T. J., Brondin, E., and Cook, M. A. (1992). Adenosine A_1 receptors mediate inhibition of tachykinin release from enteric nerve ending. *Am. J. Physiol.* **262**, G525–G531.

Brown, C. M., and Collis, M. G. (1983). Adenosine A_1 receptor mediated inhibition of nerve stimulation-induced contractions of the rabbit portal vein. *Eur. J. Pharmacol.* **93**, 277–282.

Cai, H., Batuman, V., Puschett, D. B., and Puschett, J. B. (1995). Phosphate transport inhibition by KW-3902, an adenosine A1 receptor antagonist, is mediated by cyclic adenosine monophosphate. *Am. J. Kidney Dis.* **26**, 825–830.

Chapal, J., Loubatieres-Mariani, M. M., Petit, P., and Roye, M. (1985). Evidence for an A2-subtype adenosine receptor on pancreatic glucagon secreting cells. *Br. J. Pharmacol.* **86**, 565–569.

Christofi, F. L., and Wood, J. D. (1993). Presynaptic inhibition by adenosine A1 receptors on guinea pig small intestinal myenteric neurons. *Gastroenterology* **104**, 1420–1429.

Church, M. K., and Holgate, S. T. (1986). Adenosine and asthma. *Trends Pharmacol. Sci.* **7**, 49–50.

Churchill, P. C., and Churchill, M. C. (1985). A_1 and A_2 adenosine receptor activation inhibits and stimulates renin secretion of rat cortical slices. *J. Pharmacol. Exp. Ther.* **232**, 589–594.

Collis, M. G., and Hourani, M. O. (1993). Adenosine receptor subtypes. *Trends Pharmacol. Sci.* **14**, 360–366.

Cook, M. A., and Karmazyn, M. (1996). Cardioprotective actions of adenosine and adenosine analogues. *In* "Myocardial Ischemia: Mechanisms, Reperfusion, Protection" (M. Kamazyn, Ed.), pp. 325–344. Birkhaüser Verlag, Basel.

Correia-de-Sa, P., and Ribeiro, J. A. (1996). Adenosine uptake and deamination regulate tonic A2a receptor facilitation of evoked [^{3}H]acetylcholine release from the rat motor nerve terminals. *Neuroscience* **73**, 85–93.

Coulson, R., Johnson, R. A., Olsson, R. A., Cooper, D. R., and Scheinman, S. J. (1991). Adenosine stimulates phosphate and glucose transport in opossum kidney epithelial cells. *Am. J. Physiol.* **260**, F921–F928.

Couper, I. M., and Hancock, D. L. (1994). The adenosine agonist NECA inhibits intestinal secretion and peristalsis. *J. Pharm. Pharm.* **46**, 801–804.

Crawford, C. R., Patel, D. H., Naeve, C., and Belt, J. A. (1998). Cloning of the human equilibrative, nitrobenzylmercaptopurine riboside (NBMPR)-insensitive nucleoside transporter ei by functional expression in a transport-deficient cell line. *J. Biol. Chem.* **273**, 5288–5293.

Cristalli, G., Vittori, S., Thompson, R. D., Padgett, W. L., Shi, D., Daly, J. W., and Olsson, R. A. (1994). Inhibition of platelet aggregation by adenosine receptor agonists. *Naunyn-Schmiedeberg's. Arch. Pharmacol.* **349**, 644–650.

Cronstein, B. N., Rosenstein, E. D., Kramer, S. B., Weissmann, G., and Hirschhorn, R. (1985). Adenosine, a physiologic modulator of superoxide anion generation by human neutrophils. Adenosine acts via an A_2 receptor on human neutrophils. *J. Immunol.* **135**, 1366–1371.

Cronstein, B. N., Kubersky, S. M., Weissmann, G., and Hirschhorn, R. (1987). Engagement of adenosine receptors inhibits hydrogen peroxide (H_2O_2) release by activated human neutrophils. *Clin. Immunol. Immunopathol.* **42**, 76–85.

Cronstein, B. N., Levin, R. I., Philips, M. Hirschhorn, R., Abramason, S. B., and Weossman, G. (1992). Neutrophil adherence to endothelium is enhanced via adenosine A_1 receptors and inhibited via adenosine A_2 receptors. *J. Immunol.* **148**, 2201–2206.

Cronstein, B. N. (1994). Adenosine, an endogenous anti-inflammatory agent. *J. Appl. Physiol.* **76**, 5–13.

Cronstein, B. N., Naime, D., and Firestein, G. (1995). The anti-inflammatory effects of an adenosine kinase inhibitor are mediated by adenosine. *Arthritis Rheum.* 38, 1040–1045.

Cronstein, B. N. (1997). The mechanism of methtrexate. *Rheum. Dis. Clin. North Am.* 23, 739–755.

Cushley, M. J., Tattersfield, A. E., and Holgate, S. T. (1983). Inhalated adenosine and guanosine on airway resistance in normal and asthmatic subjects. *Br. J. Clin. Pharmacol.* 15, 161–165.

Cushley, M. J., Tattersfield, A. E., and Holgate, S. T. (1984). Adenosine-induced bronchoconstriction in asthma: Antagonism by inhalated theophylline. *Am. Rev. Respir. Dis.* 129, 38–44.

Daly, W. J. (1982). Adenosine receptors: Target and future drugs. *J. Med. Chem.* 25, 197–207.

Daval, J.-L., Nicolas, F., and Doriat, J.-F. (1996). Adenosine physiology and pharmacology: How about A2 receptors? *Pharmacol. Ther.* 71, 325–335.

De Sánchez, V. C., Brunner, A., and Piña, E. (1972). *In vivo* modification of the energy change in the liver cell. *Biochem. Biophys. Res. Commun.* 46, 1441–1445.

Di Minno, G., Villa, S., Berele, V., and Gaetano, G. (1980). Dipyridamole as antithrombotic agent: An intricate mechanism of action. *In* "Diet and Drugs in Atherosclerosis" (G. Noseda, B. Lewis, and R. Paoletti, Eds.), pp. 121–124. Raven Press, New York.

Dinarello, C. A., Gelfand, J. A., and Wolff, S. M. (1993). Anticytokine strategies in the treatment of the systemic inflammatory response syndrome. *J. Am. Med. Assoc.* 269, 1829–1835.

Dobbins, J. W., Laurenson, J. P., and Forrest, J. N., Jr. (1984). Adenosine and adenosine analogues stimulate adenosine cyclic $3',5'$-monophosphate-dependent chloride secretion in the mammalian ileum. *J. Clin. Invest.* 74, 929–935.

Dorfinger, L. J., and Schonbrunn, A. (1985). Adenosine inhibits prolactin and growth hormone secretion in a clonal pituitary cell line. *Endocrinology* 117, 2330–2338.

Driver, A. G., Kukoly, C. A., Metzger, W. J., and Mustafa, S. J. (1991). Bronchial challenge with adenosine causes the release of serum neutrophil chemotactic factor in asthma. *Am. Rev. Respir. Dis.* 143, 1002–1007.

Driver, A. G., Kukoly, C. A., Ali, S., and Mustafa, S. J. (1993). Adenosine in bronchoalveolar lavage fluid in asthma. *Am. Rev. Respir. Dis.* 148, 91–97.

Dubey, R. K., Gillespie, D. G., Mi, A., and Jackson, E. K. (1997). Exogenous and endogenous adenosine inhibits fetal calf serum-induced growth of rat cardiac fibroblasts: Role of A_{2B} receptors. *Circulation* 96, 2656–2666.

Eigler, A., Greten, T. F., Sinha, B., Haslberger, C., Sullivan, G. W., and Endres, S. (1997). Endogenous adenosine curtails lipopolysaccharide-stimulated tumour necrosis factor synthesis. *Scand. J. Immunol.* 45, 132–139.

Ekas, R. D., Jr., Steenberg, M. L., Eikenburg, D. C., and Lockhandwala, M. F. (1981). Presynaptic inhibition of sympathetic neurotransmission by adenosine in the rat kidney. *Eur. J. Pharmacol.* 76, 301–307.

Epsinal, J., Challiss, R. A., and Newsholme, E. A. (1983). Effect of adenosine deaminase and an adenosine analogue on insulin sensitivity in soleus muscle of the rat. *FEBS Lett.* 158, 103–106.

Feoktistov, I., and Biaggioni, I. (1995). Adenosine A_{2B} receptors evoke IL-8 secretion in human mast cells. *J. Clin. Invest.* 96, 1979–1986.

Firestein, G. S., Boyle, D., Bullough, D. A., Gruber, H. E., Sajjadi, F. G., Montag, A., Sambol, G., and Mullane, K. M. (1994). Protective effect of an adenosine kinase inhibitor in septic shock. *J. Immunol.* 12, 5853–5858.

Firestein, G. S., Bullough, D. A., Erion, M. D., Jimenez, R., Ramirez-Weinhouse, M., Barankiewicz, J., Smith, C. W., Gruber, H. E., and Mullane, K. M. (1995). Inhibition of neutrophil adhesion by adenosine and an adenosine kinase inhibitor. The role of selectins. *J. Immunol.* 154, 326–334.

Fisher, J. W., and Nakajima, J. (1992). The role of hypoxia in renal production of erythropoietin. *Cancer* 70, 928–939.

Fredholm, B. B., and Sollevi, A. (1986). Cardiovascular effects of adenosine. *Clin. Physiol.* 6, 1–21.

Fredholm, B. B., Abbracchio, M. P., Burnstock, G., Daly, J. W., Harden, T. K., Jacobson, K. A., Leff, P., and Williams, M. (1994). Nomenclature and classification of purinoceptors. *Pharm. Rev.* 46, 143–156.

Funaya, H., Kitakaze, M., Node, K., Minamino, T., Komamura, K., and Hori, M. (1997). Plasma adenosine levels increase in patients with chronic heart failure. *Circulation* 95, 1363–1365.

Gerber, J. G., Nies, A. S., and Payne, N. A. (1985). Adenosine receptors on canine parietal cells modulate gastric acid secretion to histamine. *J. Pharmacol. Exp. Ther.* 233, 623–627.

Gerber, J. G., and Payne, N. A. (1988). Endogenous adenosine modulates gastric acid secretion to histamine in canine parietal cells. *J. Pharmacol. Exp. Ther.* 244, 190–194.

Girbert, E. R., Anderson, J. E., Cohen, F., Polara, B., and Meuwissen, H. J. (1972). Adenosine-deaminase deficiency in two patients with severely impaired cellular immunity. *Lancet* 2, 1067–1069.

Granger, C. B. (1997). Adenosine for myocardial protection in acute myocardial infarction. *Am. J. Pharmacol.* 79, 44–48.

Grisham, M. B., Hernandez, L. A., and Granger, D. N. (1989). Adenosine inhibits ischemia–reperfusion-induced leukocyte adherence and extravasation. *Am. J. Physiol.* 257, H1334–H1339.

Gruber, H. E., Hoffer, M. E., McAllister, D. R., Laikind, P. K., Lane, T. A., Schmid-Schoenbein, G. W., and Engler, R. L. (1989). Increased adenosine concentration in blood from ischemic myocardium by AICA riboside. Effects on flow, granulocytes, and injury. *Circulation* 80, 1400–1411.

Gustafsson, L. E. (1984). Adenosine antagonism and related effects of theophylline derivatives in guinea pig ileum longitudinal muscle. *Acta Physiol. Scand.* 122, 191–198.

Haas, J. A., and Osswald, H. (1981). Adenosine induced fall in glomerular capillary pressure. Effect of ureteral obstruction and aortic constriction in the Munich–Wistar rat kidney. *Naunyn-Schmiedeberg's Arch. Pharmacol.* 317, 86–89.

Headrick, J. P. (1996). Ischemic preconditioning: Bioenergetic and metabolic changes and the role of endogenous adenosine. *J. Mol. Cell. Cardiol.* 28, 1227–1240.

Hedqvist, P., and Fredholm, B. B. (1976). Effects of adenosine on adrenergic neurotransmission: Prejunctional inhibition and postjunctional enhancement. *Naunyn-Schmiedebrg's Arch. Pharmacol.* 293, 217–223.

Heseltine, L., Webster, J. M., and Taylor, R. (1995). Adenosine effects upon insulin action on lipolysis and glucose transport in human adipocytes. *Mol. Cell. Biochem.* 144, 147–151.

Hillaire-Buys, D., Bertrand, G., Gross, B. G., and Loubatieres-Mariani, M. M. (1987). Evidence for an inhibitory A_1 type adenosine receptor on pancreatic insulin-secreting cells. *Eur. J. Pharmacol.* 136, 109–112.

Hillaire-Buys, D., Chapal, J., Bertrand, G., Pettit, P., and Loubatieres-Mariani, M. M. (1994). Purinergic receptors on insulin-secreting cells. *Fundam. Clin. Pharmacol.* 8, 117–127.

Hirschhorn, R. (1995). Adenosine deaminase deficiency: Molecular basis and recent developments. *Clin. Immunol. Immunopathol.* 76, S219–S227.

Hom, G. J., and Lokhandwala, M. F. (1981a). Presynaptic inhibition of vascular sympathetic neurotransmission by adenosine. *Eur. J. Pharmacol.* 69, 101–106.

Hom, G. J., and Lokhandwala, M. F. (1981b). Effect of dipyridamole on sympathetic nerve function: Role of adenosine and presynaptic purinergic receptors. *J. Cardiovasc. Pharmacol.* 3, 391–401.

Hopper, A. H., Tindall, H., and Davies, J. A. (1989). Administration of aspirin–dipyridamole reduces proteinuria in diabetic nephropathy. *Nephrol. Dial. Transplant.* 4, 140–143.

Hori, M., Tamai, J., Kitakaze, M., Iwakura, K., Gotoh, K., Iwaki, K., Koretsune, Y., Kagiya, T., Kitabatake, A., and Kamada, T. (1989). Adenosine-induced heperemia attenuates myocardial ischemia in coronary microembolization in dogs. *Am. J. Physiol.* **257**, H244–H251.

Huang, S., Apasov, S., Koshiba, M., and Sitkovsky, M. (1997). Role of A_{2A} extracellular adenosine receptor-mediated signaling in adenosine-mediated inhibition of T-cell activation and expansion. *Blood* **90**, 1600–1610.

Hughes, P. J., Holgate, S. T., and Church, M. K. (1984). Adenosine inhibits and potentiates IgE-dependent histamine release from human lung mast cells by an A_2-purinoceptor mediated mechanism. *Biochem. Pharmacol.* **33**, 3847–3852.

Joost, H. G., and Steinfelder, H. J. (1982). Modulation of insulin sensitivity by adenosine. Effects on glucose transport, lipid synthesis, and insulin receptors of the adipocytes. *Mol. Pharmacol.* **22**, 614–616.

Jordan, J. E., Zhao, Z.-Q., Sato, H., Taft, S., and Vinten-Johansen, J. (1997). Adenosine A_2 receptor activation attenuates reperfusion injury by inhibiting neutrophil accumulation, superoxide generation and coronary endothelial adherence. *J. Pharmacol. Exp. Ther.* **280**, 301–309.

Kamikawa, Y., and Shimo, Y. (1989). Adenosine selectively inhibits noncholinergic transmission in guinea pig bronchi. *J. Appl. Physiol.* **66**, 2084–2091.

Karasawa, A., Rochester, J. A., and Lefer, A. M. (1992). Effects of adenosine, an adenosine-A_1 antagonist and their combination in splanchnic occlusion shock in rats. *Circ. Shock* **36**, 154–161.

Kitakaze, M., Funaya, H., Minamino, T., Node, K., Sato, H., Ueda, Y., Okuyama, Y., Kuzuya, T., Hori, M. and Yoshida, K. (1997). Role of protein kinase C-alpha in activation of ecto-5′ nucleotidase in the preconditioned canine myocardium. *Biochem. Biophys. Res. Commun.* **239**, 171–175.

Kloor, D., Stumvoll, W., Faust, B., Delabar, U., Mühlbauer, B., and Osswald, H. (1996). Does *S*-adenosylhomocysteine (SHA) accumulate in the ischemic rat kidney? *Naunyn-Schmiedeberg's Arch. Pharmacol.* **353**, R11.

Knight, D., Zheng, X., Rocchini, C., Jacobson, M., Bai, T., and Walker, B. (1997). Adenosine A_3 receptor inhibits migration of human eosinophils. *J. Leuk. Biol.* **62**, 465–468.

Knowles, M. R., Clarke, L. L., and Boucher, R. C. (1991). Activation by extracellular nucleotides of chloride secretion in the airway epithelia of patients with cystic fibrosis. *N. Engl. J. Med.* **325**, 533–538.

Koper, W. J., Yeaman, S. J., and Honnor, R. C. (1988). Adenosine effects on hormone-stimulated steroidogenesis in isolated bovine adrenal zona fasciculata cells. *J. Steroid Biochem.* **29**, 179–183.

Koshiba, M., Kojima, H., Huang, S., Apasov, S., and Sitkovsky, M. V. (1997). Memory of extracellular adenosine A_{2A} purinergic receptor-mediated signaling in murine T cells. *J. Biol. Chem.* **41**, 25881–25889.

Law, W. R., and Raymond, R. M. (1988). Adenosine potentiates insulin-stimulated myocardial glucose uptake *in vivo*. *Am. J. Physiol.* **254**, H970–H975.

LeBlanc, J., and Soucy, J. (1994). Hormonal dose-response to an adenosine receptor agonist. *Can. J. Physiol. Pharmacol.* **72**, 113–116.

LeBlanc, J., Richard, D., and Racotta, I. S. (1995). Metabolic and hormone-related responses to caffeine in rats. *Pharmacol. Res.* **32**, 129–133.

Ledent, C., Vaueosis, J.-M., Schiffmann, S. N., Pedrazzini, T., Yacoubi, M. E., Vanderhaeghen, J.-J., Costentin, J., Heath, J. K., Vassart, G., and Parmentier, M. (1997). Aggressiveness, hypoalgesia and high blood pressure in mice lacking the adenosine A_{2A} receptor. *Nature* **388**, 674–678.

Le Moine, O., Stordeur, P., Schandene, L., Marchant, A., de Goote, D., Goldman, M., and Deviere, J. (1996). Adenosine enhances IL-10 secretion by human monocytes. *J. Immunol.* **156**, 4408–4414.

Levens, N., Beil, M., and Schulz, R. (1991). Intrarenal actions of the new adenosine agonist CGS 21680A, selective for the A_2 receptor. *J. Pharmacol. Exp. Ther.* 257, 1013–1019.

Li, Y.-O., and Fredholm, B. B. (1985). Adenosine analogues stimulate cyclic AMP formation in rabbit cerebral microvessels via adenosine A_2-receptors. *Acta Physiol. Scand.* 124, 253–259.

Macallum, C. E., Walker, R. M., Barsoum, N. J., and Smith, G. S. (1991). Preclinical toxicity studies of an adenosine agonist, N-(2,2-diphenylethyl)adenosine. *Toxicology* 67, 21–35.

Manzini, S., and Ballati, L. (1990). 2-Chloroadenosine induction of vagally-mediated and atropine-resistant bronchomotor responses in anesthetized guinea pigs. *Br. J. Pharmacol.* 100, 251–256.

Marquardt, D. L., Parker, C. W., and Sullivan, T. J. (1978). Potentiation of mast cell mediator release by adenosine. *J. Immunol.* 120, 871–878.

Martin, B. J., McClanahan, T. B., Van Wylen, D. G., and Gallagher, K. P. (1997). Effects of ischemia, preconditioning, and adenosine deaminase inhibition on interstitial adenosine levels and infarct size. *Basic Res. Cardiol.* 92, 240–251.

Masuda, M., Demeulemeester, A., Chang-Chun, C., Hendrikx, M., VanBelle, H., and Flameng, W. (1991). Cardioprotective effects of nucleoside transport inhibition in rabbit hearts. *Ann. Thoracic Surg.* 52, 1300–1305.

Mathie, R. T., Alexander, B., Ralevic, V., and Burnstock, G. (1991). Adenosine-induced dilatation of the rabbit hepatic arterial bed is mediated by A_2-purinoceptors. *Br. J. Pharmacol.* 103, 1103–1107.

McQueen, D. S., and Ribeno, T. A. (1981). Effect of adenosine on carotid chemoreceptor activity in the rat. *Br. J. Pharmacol.* 74, 129–136.

Meade, C. J., Mierau, J., Leon, I., and Ensinger, H. A. (1996). *In vivo* role of the adenosine A_3 receptor: N^6-2-(4-Aminophenyl)ethyladenosine induces bronchospasm in BDE rats by a neurally mediated mechanism involving cells resembling mast cells. *J. Pharmacol. Exp. Ther.* 279, 1148–1156.

Merkel, L. A., Lappe, R. W., River, L. M., Cox, B. F., and Perrone, M. H. (1992). Demonstration of vasorelaxant activity with an A_1-selective adenosine agonist in porcine coronary artery: Involvement of potassium channels. *J. Pharmacol. Exp. Ther.* 260, 437–443.

Minamino, T., Kitakaze, M., Asanuma, H., Tomiyama, Y., Shiraga, M., Sato, H., Ueda, Y., Funaya, H., Kuzuya, T., Matsuzawa, Y., and Hori, M. (1998). Endogenous adenosine inhibits P-selectin-dependent formation of coronary thromboemboli during hypoperfusion in dogs. *J. Clin. Invest.* 101, 1643–1653.

Mizumoto, H., and Karasawa, A. (1993). Renal tubular site of action of KW-3902, a novel adenosine A_1-receptor antagonist, in anesthetized rats. *Jpn. J. Pharmacol.* 31, 251–253.

Mizumoto, H., Karasawa, A., and Kubo, K. (1993). Diuretic and renal protective effects of 8-(noradamantan-3-yl)-1,3-dipropylxanthine (KW-3902), a novel adenosine A_1-receptor antagonist, via pertussis toxin insensitive mechanism. *J. Pharmacol. Exp. Ther.* 266, 200–206.

Moroz, C., and Twig, S. (1985). The regulatory role of adenosine activated T-lymphocyte subset on the immune response in humans. II. Adenosine induced expression of T8 antigen. *Biomed. Pharmacother.* 39, 145–150.

Muller, M. J., and Paton, D. M. (1979). Presynaptic inhibitory action of 2-substituted adenosine derivatives on neurotransmission in rat vas deferens: Effects of inhibitors of adenosine uptake and deamination. *Naunyn-Schmiedeberg's Arch. Pharmacol.* 306, 23–28.

Murray, J. L., Mehta, K., and Lopez-Berestein, G. (1988). Induction of adenosine deaminase and 5'-nucleotidase activity in cultured human blood monocytes and monocytic leukemia (THP-1) cells by differentiating agents. *J. Leukoc. Biol.* 44, 205–211.

Nagashima, K., Kusaka, H., and Karasawa, A. (1995). Protective effects of KW-3902, an adenosine A_1-receptor antagonist, against cisplatin-induced acute renal failure in rats. *Jpn. J. Pharmacol.* 67, 349–357.

Nagashima, K., and Karasawa, A. (1996). Modulation of erythropoietin production by selective adenosine agonists and antagonists in normal and anemic rats. *Life Sci.* **59**, 761–771.

Nosaka, K., Takahashi, T., Nishi, T., Imaki, H., Suzuki, T., Suzuki, K., Kurokawa, K., and Endou, H. (1997). An adenosine deaminase inhibitor prevents puromycin aminonucleoside nephrotoxicity. *Free Radic. Biol. Med.* **22**, 597–605.

Nyce, J. W., and Metzger, W. J. (1997). DNA antisense therapy for asthma in an animal model. *Nature* **385**, 721–725.

Okada, S., Kurata, N., Ota, Z., and Ofuji, T. (1981). Effect of dipyridamole on proteinuria of nephrotic syndrome. *Lancet* **1**, 719–720.

Oliver, A., Lamas, S., Rodriguez-Puyol, D., and López-Novao, J. M. (1989). Adenosine induces mesangial cell contraction by an A_1-type receptor. *Kidney Int.* **35**, 1300–1305.

Olsson, R. A., and Pearson, J. D. (1990). Cardiovascular purinoceptors. *Physiol. Rev.* **70**, 761–845.

Ondo, J. G., Walker, M. W., and Wheeler, D. D. (1989). Central actions of adenosine on pituitary secretion of prolactin, leuteinizing hormone and thyrotropin. *Neuroendocrinology* **49**, 654–658.

Osswald, H., Schmitz, H. J., and Kemper, R. (1977). Tissue content of adenosine, inosine and hypoxanthine in the rat kidney after ischemia and postischemic recirculation. *Pflügers. Arch.* **371**, 45–49.

Osswald, H., M.hlbauer, B., and Vallon, V. (1997). Adenosine and tubuloglomerular feedback. *Blood Purif.* **15**, 243–252.

Palmer, T. M., and Stiles, G. L. (1995). Neurotransmitter receptors. VII. Adenosine receptors. *Neuropharmacology* **34**, 683–694.

Pares-Herbute, N., Hillaire-Buys, D., Etienne, P., Gross, R., Loubatieres-Mariani, M. M., and Monnier, L. (1996). Adenosine inhibitory effect on enhanced growth of aortic smooth muscle cells from streptozotocin-induced diabetic rats. *Br. J. Pharmacol.* **118**, 783–789.

Peachell, P. T., Columbo, M., Kagey-Sobotka, A., Lichtenstein, L. M., and Marone, G. (1988). Adenosine potentiates mediator release from human lung mast cells. *Am. Rev. Respir. Dis.* **138**, 1143–1151.

Pitarys, C. J., II, Virmani, R., Vildibill, H. D., Jr., Jackson, E. K., and Forman, M. B. (1991). Reduction of myocardial reperfusion injury by intravenous adenosine administered during the early reperfusion period. *Circulation* **83**, 237–247.

Plotsky, P. M., Otto, S., and Sapolsy, R. M. (1986). Inhibition of immunoreactive CRF secretion into hypophysial-portal circulation by delayed glucocorticoid feedback. *Endocrinology* **119**, 1126–1130.

Polosa, R., Phillips, G. D., Rajakulasingam, K., and Holgate, S. T. (1991). The effect of inhaled ipratropium bromide alone and in combination with oral terfenadine on bronchoconstriction provoked by adenosine 5′-monophosphate and histamine in asthma. *J. Allergy Clin. Immunol.* **87**, 939–947.

Polosa, R., and Holgate, S. T. (1997). Adenosine bronchoprovocation: A promising marker of allergic inflammation in asthma? *Thorax* **52**, 919–923.

Richardson, P. J. (1997). Antisense therapy for asthma. *Expert Opin. Invest. Drugs* **6**, 1143–1147.

Richardt, G., Waas, W., Kranzhofer, R., Mayer, E., and Schomig, A. (1987). Adenosine inhibits exocytotic release of endogenous noradrenaline in rat heart: A protective mechanism in early myocardial ischemia. *Circ. Res.* **61**, 117–123.

Riches, D. W. H., Watkins, J. L., Henson, P. M., and Stanworth, D. R. (1985). Regulation of macrophage lysosomal secretion by adenosine, adenosine phosphate esters, and related structural analogues of adenosine. *J. Leukoc. Biol.* **37**, 545–557.

Rodríguez-Nodal, F., San Román, J. I., López-Novoa, J. M., and Calvo, J. J. (1995). Effect of adenosine and adenosine agonists on amylase release from rat pancreatic lobules. *Life Sci.* **57**, 253–258.

Rongen, G. A., Floras, J. S., Lenders, W. M., Thien, T., and Smith, P. (1997). Cardiovascular pharmacology of purines. *Clin. Sci.* **92**, 13–24.

Rose, F. R., Hirschhorn, R., Weissmann, G., and Cronstein, B. C. (1988). Adenosine protects neutrophil chemotaxis. *J. Exp. Med.* **167**, 1186–1194.

Rubino, A., Mantelli, L., Amerini, S., and Ledda, F. (1990). Adenosine modulation of nonadrenergic non-cholinergic neurotransmission in isolated guinea-pig atria. *Naunyn-Schmiedeberg's Arch. Pharmacol.* **342**, 520–522.

Rubino, A., Reevic, V., and Burnstock, G. (1993). The P_1-purinoceptors that mediate the prejunctional inhibitory effect of adenosine on capsaicin-sensitive nonadrenergic noncholinergic neurotransmission in the rat mesenteric arterial bed are of the A_1 type. *J. Pharmacol. Exp. Ther.* **267**, 1100–1104.

Rudnick, M. R., Berns, J. S., Cohen, R. M., and Goldfarb, S. (1996). Contrast media-associated nephrotoxicity. *Curr. Opin. Nephrol. Hypertens.* **5**, 127–133.

Sajjadi, F. G., Takabayashi, K., Foster, A. C., Domingo, R. C., and Firestein, G. S. (1996). Inhibition of TNF- expression by adenosine: Role of A3 adenosine receptors. *J. Immunol.* **156**, 3435–3442.

Savic, V., Stefanovic, V., Ardaillou, N., and Ardaillou, R. (1990). Induction of ecto-5'-nucleotidase of rat cultured mesangial cells by interleukin-1β and tumor necrosis factor. *Immunology* **70**, 324–326.

Schnermann, J., Weihprecht, H., and Briggs, J. P. (1990). Inhibition of tubuloglomerular feedback during adenosine $_1$ receptor blockade. *Am. J. Physiol.* **258**, F553–F561.

Schrier, D. J., Lesch, M. E., Wright, C. D., and Gilbertsen, R. B. (1990). The antiinflammatory effects of adenosine receptor agonists on the carrageenan-induced pleural inflammatory response in rats. *J. Immunol.* **145**, 1874–1879.

Shinozuka, K., Maeda, T., and Hayashi, E. (1985). Effects of adenosine on ^{45}Ca uptake and [^3H]acetylcholine release in synaptosomal preparation from guinea-pig myenteric plexus. *Eur. J. Pharmacol.* **113**, 417–424.

Siragy, H. M., and Linden, J. (1996). Sodium intake markedly alters renal interstitial fluid adenosine. *Hypertension* **27**, 404–407.

Spielman, W. S., and Arend, L. J. (1991). Adenosine receptors and signaling in the kidney. *Hypertension* **17**, 117–130.

Stehle, J. H., Rivkees, S. A., Lee, J. J., Weaver, D. R., Deeds, J. D., and Reppert. S. M. (1992). Molecular cloning and expression of the cDNA for a novel A_2-adenosine receptor subtype. *Mol. Endocrinol.* **6**, 384–393.

Stone, T. W., Collis, M. G., Williams, M., Miller, L. P., Karasawa, A., and Hillaire-Buys, D. (1995). Adenosine: Some therapeutic applications and prospects. *In* "Pharmacological Sciences: Perspectives for Research and Therapy in the Late 1990s" (A. C. Cuello and B. Collier, Eds.). Birkhäuser Verlag, Basel, pp. 303–309.

Takeda, M., Yoshitomi, K., and Imai, M. (1993). Regulation of $NaCO_3$ transport in rabbit proximal convoluted tubule via adenosine A1 receptor. *Am. J. Physiol.* **265**, F511–F519.

Tally, K. J., Hrnjez, B. J., Smith, J. A., Mun, E. C., and Matthews, J. B. (1996). Adenosine scavenging: A novel mechanism of chloride secretory control in intestinal epithelial cells. *Surgery* **120**, 248–254.

Tamaoki, J., Tagaya, E., Chiyotani, A., Takemura, H., Nagai, A., Konno, K., Onuki, T., and Nitta, S. (1997). Effect of adenosine on adrenergic neurotransmission and modulation by endothelium in canine pulmonary artery. *Am. J. Physiol.* **272**, H1100–H1105.

Thorn, J. A., and Jarvis, S. M. (1996). Adenosine transporters. *Gen. Pharmacol.* **27**, 613–620.

Thornton, J. D., Liu, G. S., Olsson, R. A., and Downey, J. M. (1992). Intravenous pretreatment with A_1-selective adenosine analogues protects the heart against infarction. *Circulation* **85**, 659–665.

Tomaru, A., Ishii, A., Kishibayashi, N., and Karasawa, A. (1993). Colonic giant migrating contractions induced by glycerol enema in anesthetized rats. *Jpn. J. Pharmacol.* **63**, 525–528.

Tomaru, A., Ishii, A., Kishibayashi, N., Shimada, J., Suzuki, H., and Karasawa, A. (1994). Possible physiological role of endogenous adenosine in defecation in rats. *Eur. J. Pharmacol.* **264**, 91–94.

Tomaru, A., Ina, Y., Kishibayashi, N., and Karasawa, A. (1995). Excitation and inhibition via adenosine receptors of the twitch response to electrical stimulation in isolated guinea pig ileum. *Jpn. J. Pharmacol.* **69**, 429–433.

Tritsche, G. L., and Niswander, P. W. (1983). Modulation of macrophage superoxide release by purine metabolism. *Life Sci.* **32**, 1359–1362.

Tulin-Silver, J., Schteingart, D. E., and Mathews, K. P. (1981). Effect of theophylline on cortisol secretion. *J. Allegy Clin. Immunol.* **67**, 45–50.

Utterback, D. B., Staples, E. D., White, S. E., Hill, J. A., and Belardinelli, L. (1994). Basis for the selective reduction of pulmonary vascular resistance in humans during infusion of adenosine. *J. Appl. Physiol.* **76**, 724–730.

Vallon, V., and Osswald, H. (1994). Dipyridamole prevents diabetes-induced alterations of kidney function in rats. *Naunyn-Schmiedeberg's Arch. Pharmacol.* **349**, 217–222.

Van Galen, P. J., Stiles, G. A., Michaels, G., and Jacobson, K. A. (1992). Adenosine A_1 and A_2 receptors: Structure–function relationships. *Med. Res. Rev.* **12**, 423–471.

Wang, J., Su, S. F., Dresser, M. J., Schaner, M. E., Washington, C. B., and Giacomini, K. M. (1997). Na(+)-dependent purine nucleoside transport from human kidney: Cloning and functional characterization. *Am. J. Physiol.* **273**, F1058–1065.

Ward, P. A., Cunningham, T. W., McCulloch, K. K., and Johnson, K. J. (1988). Regulatory effects of adenosine and adenine nucleotide on oxygen radical responses of neutrophils. *Lab. Invest.* **58**, 438–447.

Westerberg, V. S., and Geiger, J. D. (1989). Adenosine analogs inhibit gastric acid secretion. *Eur. J. Pharmacol.* **160**, 275–281.

Weyrich, A. S., Ma, X.-1., Lefer, D. J., Albertine, K. H., and Lefer, A. M. (1993). *In vivo* neutralization of P-selectin protects feline heart and endothelium in myocardial ischemia and reperfusion injury. *J. Clin. Invest.* **91**, 2620–2629.

Wiklund, N. P., Cederqvist, B., Matsuda, H., and Gustafsson, L. E. (1987). Adenosine can excite pulmonary artery. *Acta. Physiol. Scand.* **131**, 477–478.

Wilbur, S. L., and Marchlinski, F. E. (1997). Adenosine as an antiarrythmic agent. *Am. J. Cardiol.* **79**, 30–37.

Williams, M. (1987). Purine receptors in mammalian tissues: Pharmacology and functional significance. *Annu. Rev. Pharmacol. Toxicol.* **27**, 315–345.

Wollner, A., Wollner, S., and Smith, J. B. (1993). Acting via A_2 receptors, adenosine inhibits the upregulation of Mac-1 (CD11b/CD18) expression on FMLP-stimulated neutrophils. *Am. J. Resp. Cell. Mol. Biol.* **9**, 179–185.

Woo, K. T. (1996). Recent concepts in the pathogenesis and therapy of IgA nephritis. *Ann. Acad. Med. (Singapore)* **22**, 265–269.

Yamagishi, F., Hommma, N., Haruta, K., Iwatsuki, K., and Chiba, S. (1985). Adenosine potentiates secretin-stimulated pancreatic exocrine secretion in the dog. *Eur. J. Pharmacol.* **118**, 203–209.

Yao, K., Kusaka, H., Sano, J., Sato, K., and Karasawa, A. (1994a). Diuretic effects of KW-3902, a novel adenosine A_1-receptor antagonist, in various models of acute renal failure in rats. *Jpn. J. Pharmacol.* **64**, 281–288.

Yao, K., Kusaka, H., Sato, K., and Karasawa, A. (1994b). Protective effects of KW-3902, a novel adenosine A_1-receptor antagonist, against gentamycin-induced acute renal failure in rats. *Jpn. J. Pharmacol.* **65**, 167–170.

Yao, S. Y., Ng, A. M., Muzyka, W. R., Grigiths, M., Cass, C. E., Baldwin, S. A., and Young, D. J. (1997). Molecular cloning and functional characterization of nitrobenzylthioinosine (NBMPR)-sensitive (es) and NBMPR-insensitive (ei) equilibrative nucleoside transporter proteins (rENT1 and rENT2) from rat tissues. *J. Biol. Chem.* **272**, 28423–28430.

Zhang, Y., and Lautt, W. (1992). Arterial and venous plasma concentrations during haemorrhage. *Br. J. Pharmacol.* **105**, 765–767.

Zhao, A.-Q., Nakanishi, K., MacGee, D. S., Tan, P., and Vinten-Johansen, J. (1994). A_1-receptor mediated myocardial infarct size reduction by endogenous adenosine is exerted during ischemia. *Cardiovasc. Res.* **28**, 270–279.

Zhou, Q. Y., Li, C., Olah, M. E., Johnson, R. A., Stiles, G., and Civelli, O. (1992). Molecular cloning and characterization of an adenosine receptor: The A_3 adenosine receptor. *Proc. Natl. Acad. Sci. U.S.A.* **89**, 7432–7436.

CHAPTER 5

Biochemical Characterization of Adenosine Agonists and Antagonists

HIROMI NONAKA AND MICHIO ICHIMURA

Biochemistry, Pharmaceutical Research Institute, Kyowa Hakko Kogyo Co., Ltd., Sunto-gun, Shizuoka, Japan

I. INTRODUCTION

Adenosine modulates a variety of physiological functions by stimulating specific cell surface receptors both in the central nervous system (CNS) and in peripheral tissues. Adenosine receptors were initially divided into A_1 and A_2 subtypes based on their ability to inhibit and stimulate cyclic adenosine monophosphate (cAMP) accumulation, respectively. (van Calker *et al.,* 1979). Currently, four different adenosine receptor subtypes are recognized, designated A_1, A_{2A}, A_{2B}, and A_3. The classification is based on both cDNA cloning and their affinity for agonists and antagonists (Linden *et al.,* 1991; Palmer and Stiles, 1995; Zhou *et al.,* 1992). In addition, the receptors can be classified according to the mechanism of signal transduction. A_1 and A_3 adenosine receptors interact with pertussis toxin-sensitive G-proteins of the G_i and G_o family, whereas A_{2A} and A_{2B} adenosine receptors stimulate adenylyl cyclase via G_s protein (Palmer and Stiles, 1995). It has become clear that adenosine receptors are also coupled to effectors other than adenylyl cyclase.

The identification of adenosine receptor subtypes has been made according to the order of affinity and/or functional activity of the receptor ligands. This method can be useful in combination with molecular biology because most cells and tissues express at least two subtypes of adenosine receptors. Functional studies of the subtypes both *in vitro* and *in vivo* have progressed by the use of selective agonists and antagonists. The adenosine A_1 receptor is perhaps the most extensively characterized because selective agonists (e.g., N^6-cyclohexyladenosine [CHA], R-N^6-phenylisopropyladenosine [PIA], N^6-cyclopentyladenosine [CPA] have been used since the mid-1980s (Olssen, 1984; Trivedi *et al.*, 1989) and the selective antagonist, 8-cyclopentyl-1, 3-dipropylxanthine (DPCPX) has been available since the late 1980s (Lohse *et al.*, 1987). Until more recently, the lack of selective ligands, especially selective receptor antagonists, hampered the pharmacological characterization of adenosine A_{2A} receptors. However, the selective A_{2A} agonist $[^3H]$ 2-[p-(2-carboxyethyl)phenethyl-amino]-5′-N-ethylcarboxamido-adenosine (CGS21680) enabled the investigation of A_{2A} receptor sites (Jarvis *et al.*, 1989a), and important progress has been made with the development of selective A_{2A} receptor antagonists. The use of both selective agonists and antagonists has provided a lot of information on the function of A_{2A} receptors. In contrast, there are no agents that exhibit high selectivity and affinity for A_{2B} receptors as of yet. As a consequence, adenosine A_{2B} receptors are typically identified using negative evidence, that is, by a low sensitivity to A_1- and A_{2A}-selective ligands such as CPA and CGS21680, respectively. Some selective agonists and antagonists have been found for A_3 receptors, although our understanding of these receptors has been limited by the marked species differences in receptor sensitivity to various ligands (Linden, 1994).

The development of selective agonists and antagonists for the A_1 and A_{2A} adenosine receptor subtypes has opened the possibility that these receptors could be promising molecular targets for therapeutics in disorders such as cardiovascular disease, Parkinson's disease, inflammatory disease, and so on.

This chapter describes the binding characterization of adenosine receptor ligands and the signal transduction for each subtype. Emphasis is placed on adenosine A_{2A} receptor antagonists and the biochemical basis of their application to the therapy of Parkinson's disease.

II. LIGANDS FOR ADENOSINE RECEPTOR SUBTYPES

Several research groups have found various adenosine receptor agonists and antagonists. The adenosine receptor subtypes and their ligands are summarized in Table I. In 1986, Pharmaceutical Research Institute of Kyowa Hakko Kogyo started a program for exploring adenosine antagonists that could be applicable to some human diseases. As a consequence, a selective A_1 receptor antagonist, KW-3902 (a xanthine derivative, Fig. 1A) was found (Mizumoto

TABLE I   Adenosine Receptor Subtypes and Ligands

Sub-type	Distribution in CNS	Peripheral tissue	Transmembrane signaling	Agonist	Antagonist
High affinity for adenosine ($<10^{-6}$ M)					
A_1	Widely distributed	Myocyte Kidney	Adenylyl cyclase $\downarrow$ PLC $\uparrow$ K^+ channel $\uparrow$ Ca^{2+} channel $\downarrow$	CHA CPA R-PIA	DPCPX KW-3902
A_{2A}	Striatum Nucleus accumbens Olfactory tubercle	Platelet Coronary artery	Adenylyl cyclase $\uparrow$	CGS21680 APEC	KF17837 SCH58261 CSC ZM241385 KW-6002
Low affinity for adenosine ($>10^{-6}$ M)					
A_{2B}	Widely distributed (low density)	Colon Ceacum Urinary bladder	Adenylyl cyclase $\uparrow$	NECA	CGS15943
A_3	Widely distributed (low density)	Lung Eosinophil Testis	Adenylyl cyclase $\downarrow$ PLC $\uparrow$	2-CI-IB-MECA	MRS-1191 BW-A522

A

KW-3902

B

KW-6002; R = CH$_3$CH$_2$
KF17837; R = CH$_3$CH$_2$CH$_2$

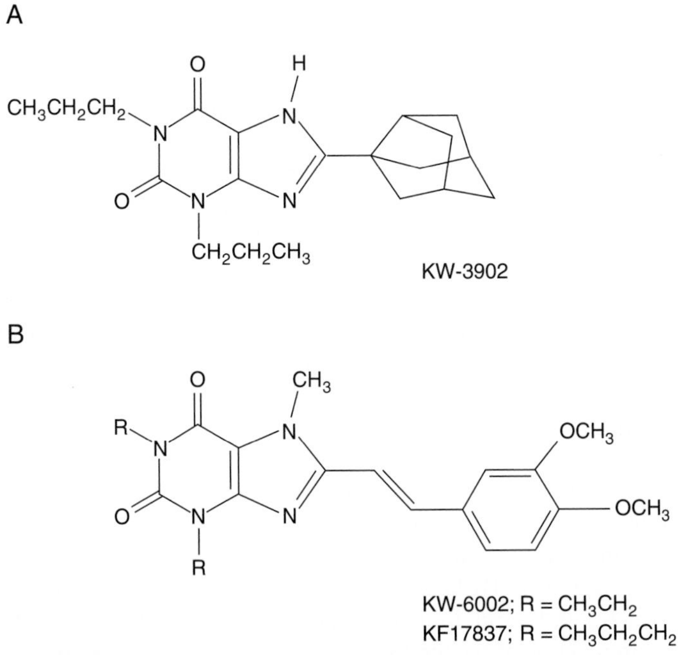

FIGURE 1   Structures of (A) KW-3902 and (B) KW-6002 and KF17837.

et al., 1993; Nonaka et al., 1996; Shimada et al., 1992a; see Chapter 3). KW-3902 is currently under clinical trials for a cardiovascular disorder. Moreover, in the course of the derivatization of A_1 receptor antagonists, several compounds that possessed selectivity for the A_{2A} receptors were discovered. One of them, KF17837 (a xanthine derivative, Fig. 1B) is a representative compound with a high affinity and selectivity for A_{2A} receptors (Nonaka et al., 1994a; Shimada et al., 1992b; see Chapter 3). The biochemical and pharmacological effects of KF17837 were thoroughly investigated, which resulted in the demonstration that KF17837 possesses a unique pharmacological activity (i.e., anti-Parkinson's disease activity in an in vivo animal model) (Kanda et al., 1994; Richardson et al., 1997). The details of this activity are described in Chapter 11. KW-6002 (Shimada et al., 1997; see Fig. 1B), a derivative of KF17837, is currently under clinical trial for Parkinson's disease.

A. BINDING CHARACTERIZATION OF ADENOSINE RECEPTOR LIGANDS

1. A_1 receptor

Because A_1 receptor selective agonists were discovered earlier than other receptor ligands, many binding studies have been performed on a variety of mammalian tissues and cells. The potency profile of adenosine agonists at the A_1 receptor is as follows; R-PIA = CHA = CPA > 5'-N-ethylcarboxamido-adenosine or ethyl-carboxamidoadenosine (NECA) > S-PIA. [^{3}H]CPA bound to rat brain membranes with high affinity to a single site (K_d value; 0.48 ± 0.08 nM and B_{max} value; 416 ± 46 fmol/mg protein). The kinetics were slow, showing that the specific binding reached saturation in approximately 90 min and the $t_{1/2}$ was about 60 min (Williams et al., 1986). DPCPX, which exhibits a high selectivity and affinity for the A_1 receptors, has been a widely used antagonist in the characterization of A_1 receptors (Lohse et al., 1987).

The A_1 receptor selective antagonist KW-3902 has potent diuretic and renal protective activities in rats at very low doses (Mizumoto et al., 1993; Nonaka et al., 1996; Shimada et al. 1992; see Chapter 3). This compound possesses a higher affinity ($K_i = 0.19 \pm 0.04$ nM in rat brain) and selectivity for the A_1 receptor than DPCPX (see Tables II and III). The tritiated compound [^{3}H]KW-3902 was used for the analysis of the binding properties to rat forebrain membranes. Association and dissociation kinetic rate constants were as follows: $k_{obs} = 0.41 \pm 0.022$ min^{-1}, $k_1 = 0.019 \pm 0.00099$ min^{-1}, $t_{1/2} = 37 \pm 2.0$ min. $K_{+1} = 0.68 \pm 0.088$ min^{-1} nM^{-1}, and $K_d = 0.030$ nM. Saturation studies with [^{3}H]KW-3902 revealed that it bound with a high affinity ($K_d = 77 \pm 5.5$ pM) and limited capacity ($B_{max} = 470 \pm 23$ fmol/mg protein) to a single class of recognition sites (Fig. 2). A high positive correlation

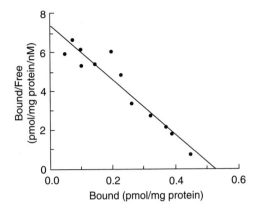

FIGURE 2 Representative Scatchard plot for [^{3}H]KW-3902 binding to rat forebrain membranes. A K_d value of 0.077 ± 0.0055 nM and a B_{max} value of 470 ± 23 fmol/mg protein were determined. These K_d and B_{max} values indicate means ± standard errors from four experiments. From Nonaka et al. (1996).

was observed between the pharmacological profile of adenosine ligands to inhibit the binding of [^{3}H]KW-3902 and that of [^{3}H]CHA (Nonaka et al., 1996).

With G-protein coupled receptors, agonists generally label both low- and high-affinity states of the receptors, depending on the receptor–G-protein coupling, whereas antagonists equally label both states of the receptors. The competition curves for agonists versus binding of [^{3}H]KW-3902 were biphasic in the absence of guanosine triphosphate (GTP) (i.e., K_{iH}, of 2.7 nM, and K_{iL}, of 64 nM for R-PIA) (Fig. 3). The K_{iH} was similar to the K_i for [^{3}H]CHA binding (1.1 nM) suggesting that the high-affinity site corresponded to the A_1 receptor recognized by [^{3}H]CHA. The addition of GTP resulted in a rightward shift of the inhibition curve for R-PIA with a Hill coefficient of 0.86 (see Fig. 3). The inhibition curve of the antagonist KW-3902 was not affected by GTP (see Fig. 3). The rightward shift of the agonist competition curve by GTP, but no shift of the antagonist curve, indicated that the [^{3}H]KW-3902 binding sites were coupled to G-proteins. The K_i value of R-PIA in the presence of GTP corresponded to the K_{iL}. This suggests that R-PIA recognizes both the low- and high-affinity states modulated by GTP.

KW-3902 exhibited species difference in diuretic activity (i.e., the threshold dosages having significant diuretic activity were 0.001 mg/kg po in rat and 1 mg/kg po in dog) (Kobayashi et al., 1993). Several other xanthine antagonists have been reported to show higher binding affinities for rat A_1 receptors than for guinea pig A_1 receptors (Ferkany et al., 1986; Ukena et al., 1986). We further demonstrated that the affinity of xanthine antagonists for

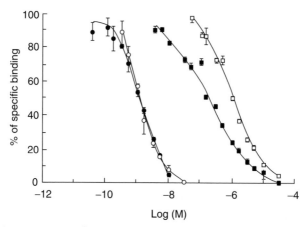

FIGURE 3 Competition of [³H]KW-3902 binding to rat forebrain membranes by *R*-PIA (square) and KW-3902 (circle). Specific binding of [³H]KW-3902 in the presence (open symbols) and in the absence (closed symbols) of 100 μM GTP was determined at various concentrations of *R*-PIA or KW-3902. Data points represent means ± standard errors from at least three separate experiments conducted in duplicate. From Nonaka *et al.* (1996).

A_1 receptors labeled with [³H]CHA was lower in dog than in guinea pig (Table II). Thus, KW-3902 showed K_i values of 0.19, 1.3, and 10 nM for rat, guinea pig, and dog A_1 receptors, respectively. The difference in the A_1 affinity of KW-3902 apparently contributed to the difference in the diuretic activities. Moreover, Jockers *et al.* (1994) showed that not only the affinity of the A_1 receptor ligands, but also the specificity of the interaction between the A_1 receptors and G-proteins, varied among species. In [¹²⁵I]HPIA binding to bovine

TABLE II Equlibrium Binding Constants of [³H]CHA Binding to Mammalian Forebrain and Inhibition Constants of KW-3902 and Other Adenosine Antagonists[a]

	K_d (nM)	K_i (nM)			
Species	[³H]CHA	KW-3902	DPCPX	CGS15943	XAC
Rat	1.2 ± 0.19	0.19 ± 0.042	0.49 ± 0.06	2.1 ± 0.49	1.1 ± 0.043
Guinea pig	7.5 ± 0.28	1.3 ± 0.12	6.4 ± 0.35	9.6 ± 0.44	11 ± 0.28
Dog	28 ± 5.2	10 ± 2.6	17 ± 6.5	8.2 ± 1.1	16 ± 1.8

[a]Values are means ± standard errors of three to five separate experiments performed in duplicate. From Nonaka *et al.* (1996).

brain membranes, $G_{i\alpha\text{-}3}$ was the most potent among $G_{2\alpha\text{-}1}$, $G_{i\alpha\text{-}2}$ $G_{i\alpha\text{-}3}$, and $G_{o\alpha}$, whereas in human membranes, $G_{i\alpha\text{-}1}$, $G_{i\alpha\text{-}2}$, and $G_{i\alpha\text{-}3}$ were equipotent and $G_{o\alpha}$ was less potent. Subtle differences in the primary sequence of A_1 receptors have been shown to affect the ligand binding profile of species homologues (Olah et al., 1992; Tucker et al., 1994). Similar small differences in amino acid sequence could affect the specificity of G-protein binding.

2. A_{2A} Receptor

In early studies, brain A_{2A} receptors were characterized using the nonselective agonist [^{3}H]NECA and the nonselective antagonist [^{3}H]PD115,199, in combination with an appropriate concentration of either A_1-selective agonist CPA or the A_1-selective antagonist DPCPX to block A_1 sites (Bruns et al., 1986, 1987). These binding experiments showed similar pharmacological profiles and regional distributions and were consistent with the specific labelling of the high-affinity brain A_{2A} receptor (Bruns et al., 1986, 1987; Jarvis et al., 1989b). However, [^{3}H]NECA binds to different states and/or subtypes of the adenosine receptors (Bruns et al., 1986; Stone et al., 1988), as well as to other proteins, such as adenotin (Bruns et al., 1986; Hutchison and Fox, 1989;. Lohse et al., 1988a). In 1989, the agonist CGS21680, an analogue of NECA, was reported by Jarvis and colleagues (1989a) to have a high affinity and selectivity for rat striatal adenosine A_{2A} receptors. [^{3}H]CGS21680 has the ability to label the A_{2A} receptor without the need for A_1-selective ligands to block A_1 receptors. The binding of [^{3}H]CGS21680 in rat striatal membranes reached equilibrium after approximately 90 min and the $t_{1/2}$ for dissociation at 23°C was 21.3 min (Jarvis et al., 1989a). In saturation experiments, [^{3}H]CGS21680 bound to a single class of receptors with a K_d value of 15.5 $\pm$ 2 nM and a B_{max} value of 375 $\pm$ 14 fmol/mg of protein (Jarvis et al., 1989a). Further investigation has made clear that CGS21680 binds not only A_{2A} sites but also other low-affinity non-A_{2A} sites (James et al., 1992: Wan et al., 1990).

In binding studies, the use of an antagonist radioligand is usually preferred to an agonist because the affinity of an antagonist is independent of the receptor –G-protein coupling state. The xanthine derivative [^{3}H]KF17837S has been reported as the first A_{2A} receptor selective antagonist radioligand (Nonaka et al., 1994b). Although KF17837 in solid state is stable to light, the compound in dilute solution was rapidly isomerized by exposure to visible light to form the stable equilibrium mixture, KF17837S (i.e., the E-isomer 18% and the Z-isomer 82%, see Chapter 3). Both KF17837 and KF17837S were found to have high affinity and selectivity for rat striatal adenosine A_{2A} receptors labeled by [^{3}H]CGS21680 with K_i values of 1.0 $\pm$ 0.057 nM and 7.9 $\pm$ 0.055 nM, respectively, whereas the Z-isomer was virtually inactive (Nonaka et al., 1994a). Figure 4 shows competitive inhibition of

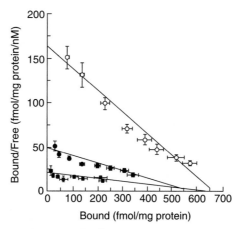

FIGURE 4 Competition of KF17837 for [³H]CGS21680 binding to adenosine A_{2A} receptors on rat striatal membranes. Scatchard analysis of [³H]CGS21680 binding in the presence or absence of KF17837. Open circle, control; closed circle, in the presence of 3 nM KF17837; closed triangle, in the presence of 10 nM KF17837. Values are means ± standard errors of three or four separate experiments performed in duplicate. From Nonaka *et al.* (1996).

[³H]CGS21680 binding by KF17837. Well-known xanthine compounds (e.g., theophylline and caffeine), which are A_{2A} receptor antagonists, have many pharmacological effects. However, KF17837S appears not to interact with other adenosine transporters or neurotransmitter receptors, including α_1-, α_2, and β-adrenoceptors, dopamine D_1 and D_2 receptors, histamine H_1 and H_2 receptors, muscarinic M_1 receptors, nicotinic receptors, and 5-HT$_{1A}$ and 5-HT$_2$ receptors. Moreover, unlike other xanthines, such as caffeine and theophylline, no effect is seen on phosphodiesterases at a concentration of 10 μM (Nonaka *et al.*, 1994a). [³H]KF17837S-specific binding reached equilibrium after approximately 10 min at a radioligand concentration of 1.0 nM. With the addition of 1 μM KF17837S, [³H]KF17837S binding rapidly reversed. Association and dissociation kinetic rate constants were as follows: $k_{obs} = 0.45 \pm 0.073$ min^{-1}, $k_{-1} = 0.39 \pm 0.091$ min^{-1}, $t_{1/2} = 2.5 \pm 1.0$ min, and $k_{+1} = 0.041$ min^{-1}nM^{-1}. These values gave a kinetic dissociation constant, K_d, of 9.6 nM (Nonaka *et al.*, 1994b). Saturation studies showed that the binding of [³H]KF17837S occurred at a single site with a high affinity (K_d: 7.1 ± 0.91 nM) and limited capacity (B_{max}: 1.3 ± 0.23 pmol/mg protein). Adenosine antagonists competed for the binding of [³H]KF17837S with the following order of activity: CGS15943 > KF17837S > PD115,199 xanthine amine congener (XAC) > DPCPX > KW-3902 > caffeine (Table III). Adenosine agonists inhibited [^{3}H]KF17837S binding in the following order: NECA CGS21680 > CV-1808 R-PIA > CPA > S-PIA (see Table III). The K_i values of the antagonists for [^{3}H]KF17837S binding and the rank order of potency were similar to those of [^{3}H]CGS21680 binding. The affinities of the agonists were lower in [^{3}H]KF17837S binding than in [^{3}H]CGS21680 binding. However, a strong positive correlation ($r = 0.98$) was observed between the pharmacological profile of these two radioligand experiments, and the results are similar to those observed using a new nonxanthine A_{2A} receptor antagonist [^{3}H]SCH58261 (Zocchi *et al.*, 1996). The antagonists produced steep inhibition curves (i.e., Hill coefficients not significantly different from unity) (see Table III). In contrast, the Hill coefficients of the agonists were between 0.43 and 0.83 in [^{3}H]KF17837S displacement (see Table III). Addition of 100 μM GTP, which would be expected to cause dissociation of the receptor–G-protein complex, slightly shifted the inhibition curve of CGS21680 in

TABLE III   Comparison of Inhibition by Various Adenosine Agonists and Antagonists for Binding of [^{3}H]KF17837S and [^{3}H]CGS21680 to Rat Striatal Membranes[a]

	[^{3}H]KF17837S		[^{3}H]CGS21680
	K_i(nM)	nH[b]	K_i(nM)
Agonists			
NECA	59 ± 9.4	0.69 ± 0.15	3.1 ± 0.40
CGS21680	130 ± 38	0.43 ± 0.011	4.5 ± 1.1
CV1808	340 ± 71	0.79 ± 0.058	44 ± 2.4
R-PIA	510 ± 75	0.71 ± 0.10	54 ± 2.9
CPA	1500 ± 240	0.67 ± 0.057	230 ± 31
S-PIA	6400 ± 1100	0.84 ± 0.058	660 ± 54
Antagonists			
CGS15943	0.39 ± 0.013	1.00 ± 0.19	0.39 ± 0.13
KF17837S	9.7 ± 1.7	0.97 ± 0.17	7.9 ± 0.055
PD115,199	9.8 ± 2.9	1.02 ± 0.087	5.7 ± 0.88
XAC	21 ± 4.0	0.95 ± 0.13	14 ± 4.0
DPCPX	160 ± 35	1.03 ± 0.18	120 ± 9.1
KW-3902	230 ± 12	0.96 ± 0.080	170 ± 16
Caffeine	11000 ± 2100	1.28 ± 0.26	19000 ± 910

[a]Values are means ± standard errors of three to five separate experiments performed in duplicate.
[b]nH, Hill coefficient.
From Nonaka *et al.* (1996).

[³H]KF17837 binding to the right (Fig. 5), resulting in an apparent K_i value for CGS21680 approximately three times larger than that seen in the absence of GTP. These results suggest the [³H]KF17837S labels two agonist coupling states without distinction. The differing susceptibility of [³H]CGS21680 and [³H]KF17837S to displacement by agonists supports the concept that A$_{2A}$ receptors exist in two agonist coupling states, with [³H]KF17837S labeling both states and [³H]CGS21680 mainly labeling the high-affinity state for the agonists. Despite the rightward shift of the inhibition curve, the addition of GTP hardly affected the slope factor (see Fig. 5). Although the exact reason is unknown, this may be related to a tight coupling of the A$_{2A}$ receptor and G-proteins, which is modulated by Mg^{2+} (Nanoff and Stiles, 1993; Parkinson and Fredholm, 1992). Luthin et al. (1995) have shown the shift from two affinity states in the absence of GTPγS to a single lower-affinity state in the presence of GTPγS using [¹²⁵I] 2-[2-(4-aminophenyl)ethylamino]adenosine (APE) in rat striatal membranes. They suggested that the magnitude of the shift in binding produced by the addition of GTPγS depends on the concentration of the radioligand (i.e, the high-affinity state would be selectively labeled by low concentrations of radiologand and, thus, the apparent shift in affinity would

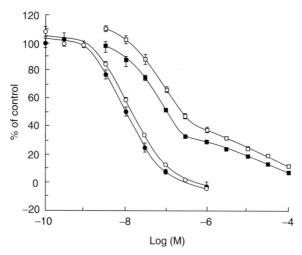

FIGURE 5 Competition by CGS21680 (squares) and KF17837S (circles) with [³H]KF17837S binding to rat striatal membranes. Specific binding of [³H]KF17837S in the presence (open symbols) and in the absence (closed symbols) of 100 μM GTP was determined at various concentrations of CGS21680 or KF17837S. Data points represent means ± standard errors from at least four separate experiments conducted in duplicate.
From Nonaka et al. (1994b).

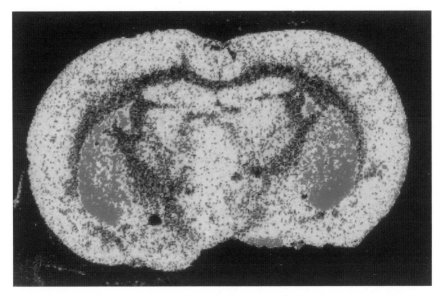

FIGURE 6 Linearized autoradiographic image of 10nM[³H]KF17837S binding to a rat brain section.

be greater) (Luthin *et al.*, 1995). Therefore, unsuitable concentrations of [^{3}H]CGS21680 may mask the appearance of two affinity states, whereas they can be detected with [^{125}I]APE.

In rat brain coronal sections, [^{3}H]KF17837S binding was highly localized in the striatum. Lower levels of the binding were observed in the globus pallidus, whereas the superficial layers of the cortex were also weakly labeled (Fig. 6). This localization is similar to that of A_{2A} receptors reported in the autoradiograms using [^{3}H]CGS21680 and *in situ* hybridization using a probe for the mRNA coding for a cloned A_{2A} receptor (Jarvis and Williams, 1989; Parkinson and Fredholm, 1990; Schiffmann *et al.*, 1991; see Chapter 2), although the binding of [^{3}H]KF17837S in nucleus accumbens and olfactory tubercle, where A_{2A} receptors are also highly localized, remains to be investigated. James *et al.* (1992) and Johansson *et al.* (1993) have characterized the low level of specific binding of [^{3}H]CGS21680 in rat and human cerebral cortex, the binding properties of which appeared to be A_{2A}-like but different from the striatal A_{2A} receptors. Other pharmacological agents tested that cause less than 50% inhibition of [^{3}H]KF17837S binding site in rat striatal membranes (at 10 μM) include dopamine, the dopamine D_1 receptor antagonist SCH23390   [(R-(+)-8-chloro-2,3,4,5-tetrahydro-3-methyl-5-phenyl-1H-3-benzazepine-7-ol], the dopamine D_1 receptor agonist SKF38393 [2,3,4,5-tetrahydro-7,8-dihydroxy-1-phenyl-1H-3-benzazepine HCl], the dopamine D_1/D_2 receptor antagonist haloperidol, the muscarinic acetylcholine receptor antagonist atropine, the α_1-adrenergic receptor antagonist prazosin, the α_2-adrenergic receptor agonist clonidine, and the Ca^{2+} channel antagonists nifedipine and nitrendipine.

KW-6002, under clinical trial for Parkinson's disease, has similar biochemical properties to those of KF17837. The K_i values of KW-6002 are 2.2 $\pm$ 0.34 nM to rat striatal A_{2A} receptors and 150 $\pm$ 22 nM to rat forebrain A_1 receptors, respectively (Shimada *et al.*, 1997).

The nonxanthine antagonists, [^{3}H]SCH58261 and [^{125}I]ZM241385, have also been shown to label brain and recombinant A_{2A} receptors (Palmer and Stiles, 1995; Zocchi *et al.*, 1996). In addition, [^{3}H]SCH58261 was reported to recognize the A_{2A} receptors in peripheral tissues, including human platelets (Dionisotti *et al.*, 1996), lymphocytes (Varani *et al.*, 1997), neutrophil (Varani *et al.*, 1998), and porcine coronary arteries (Belardinelli *et al.*, 1996).

3. A_{2B} Receptor

A_{2B} receptor binding can be detected using the nonselective agonist [^{3}H]NECA in bovine chromaffin cells (Casadó *et al.*, 1992). However, [^{3}H]NECA does not have a high affinity for the A_{2B} receptor (IC$_{50}$ = 1.0 μM) and shows a higher affinity for the A_1 and A_{2A} receptors than the A_{2B} receptor.

A cAMP response stimulated by NECA, but a lesser extent response by CGS21680, is considered to be a more reliable indicator of the A_{2B} receptor than that observed with [^{3}H]NECA binding. Linden *et al.* (1998) reported the A_{2B} receptor binding assay using [^{3}H]1,3-diethyl-8-phenylxanthine to human recombinant A_{2B} receptors overexpressed in HEK-293 cells. The K_d value of [^{3}H]1,3-diethyl-8-phenylxanthine was 30 nM. Owing to the absence of selective A_{2B} receptor agonists, the precise pharmacological properties of the A_{2B} receptor are still largely unknown.

4. A_3 Receptor

The A_3 receptor was identified only after molecular cloning (Zhou *et al.*, 1992). Some A_3 receptor selective agonists and antagonists have been discovered by binding studies using CHO cells transfected with the cloned A_3 receptor. Special attention must be paid to the species being studied because xanthine binding to A_3 receptors exhibits marked species differences. Ji *et al.* (1994) reported that the affinities of 8-arylxanthines at the rat, rabbit, and gerbil brain A_3 receptors, labelled by [^{125}I]AB-MECA in the presence of 1.0 μM XAC, an A_1 and A_{2A} receptor antagonist, were much less than that at the cloned sheep and human A_3 receptors (Linden *et al.*, 1993 Salvatore *et al.*, 1993). [^{125}I]AB-MECA, [^{125}I]ABA, and [^{125}I]APNEA have been used to label the A_3 receptors (Linden, 1994; Olah *et al.*, 1994), however, these compounds also bind to A_1 receptors. [^{125}I]AB-MECA showed high affinity to membranes prepared from CHO cells stably expressing the rat A_3 receptors with K_d and B_{max} values of 1.48 $\pm$ 0.33 nM and 3.06 $\pm$ 0.21 pmol/mg of protein, respectively (Olah *et al.*, 1994). In 1994, 2-Cl-IB-MECA was introduced as the first highly selective A_3 receptor agonist (Kim *et al.*, 1994). This compound has been shown to have high affinity (K_i = 0.33 nM) and selectivity (2500- and 1400-fold for A_3 vs A_1 and A_{2A} receptors, respectively) for the rat A_3 receptor and has enabled study of the pharmacological effects of A_3 receptors.

The first report of the tissue distribution of mRNA for rat A_3 receptors showed that the most abundant message was found in testis and moderate amounts in lung, kidney, and heart (Zhou *et al.*, 1992). Because the apparent tissue distribution in the rat was different from that observed in humans and sheep, it was suggested that the distribution pattern of the A_3 receptor was species specific. In contrast, Dixon *et al.* (1996) detected widespread expression of the A_3 receptor in the rat, showing moderate amounts in testis, which was similar to that observed for this receptor in humans and sheep. These differing results may be due to quantitative rather than qualitative differences in the abundance of the transcript (see Chapter 2).

III. SIGNAL TRANSDUCTION

A. A_1 RECEPTOR

A_1 receptors are negatively linked to adenylyl cyclase via a pertussis toxin-sensitive G-protein. The A_1 receptor modulation of phospholipase C (PLC) activity has exhibited confusing results; that is, A_1 receptor agonists stimulated (Gerwins and Fredholm, 1992a), inhibited (Long and Stone, 1987), or had no effect (Nanoff et al., 1990) on inositol phosphate formation or mobilization of $[Ca^{2+}]_i$. Studies in DDT_1MF-2 smooth muscle cells suggested a stimulation of PLC via A_1 receptors in addition to a stimulation of the effects induced by adenosine triphosphate (ATP) (Gerwins and Fredholm, 1992a) or bradykinin (Gerwins and Fredholm, 1992b). It had remained unclear whether the stimulation of PLC via A_1 receptors was a direct effect or whether adenosine enhanced only the effects elicited via other receptors. Some reports have provided the answer that A_1 receptors transfected into CHO cells couple to PLC followed by mobilization of $[Ca^{2+}]_i$ via a pertussis toxin-sensitive G-protein (Freund et al., 1994; Iredale et al., 1994). The ability of purified G-protein $\beta\gamma$ subunits to stimulate PLC in DDT_1MF-2 cell membrane preparation has shown an effect markedly dependent on Ca^{2+} concentrations (Dickenson et al., 1995). This finding might indicate the amplification of the PLC signal via A_1 receptors.

In addition, it is known that A_1 receptors are functionally coupled to K^+_{ATP} channels, which can depress Ca^{2+} entry when activated (Kirsch et al., 1990). K^+_{ATP} channel openers have been shown to be cardioprotective (Grover, 1994), and the effects of adenosine can be attenuated by K^+_{ATP} channel blockers (Toombs et al., 1993). The function of the A_1 receptor could contribute to the cardioprotective effect of adenosine because transgenic mice bearing rat A_1 receptor cDNA under control of the cardiac-specific α-myosin heavy chain promoter significantly improved contractile recovery from ischemic injury (Matherne et al., 1997). Moreover, A_1 receptor activation caused a glibenclamide sensitive inhibition of the basal ^{45}Ca influx and basal myocyte contractile amplitude, consistent with the coupling of the A_1 receptor to K_{ATP} channels in the myocytes (Liang, 1996). These data indicate that myocyte K_{ATP} channel is a downstream effector of the A_1 receptor.

Increasing evidence shows that adenosine may be an important mediator of bronchial asthma (Ali et al., 1994; Church and Holgate, 1986). In a rabbit allergic model, the administration of the A_1 receptor antisense DNA improved dynamic compliance and bronchial hyperresponsiveness in response to histamine challenge (Nyce and Metzger, 1997). This result indicates the A_1 receptor block might be capable of ameliorating asthma.

B. A$_{2A}$ RECEPTOR

The A$_{2A}$ receptor was identified from the canine thyroid library as an orphan receptor RDC8 having the character of elevating adenylyl cyclase activity (Maenhaut *et al.*, 1990). The stimulation of A$_{2A}$ receptors results in the activation of G$_s$, which has a stimulatory effect on adenylyl cyclase. Olah (1997) reported, using chimeric A$_1$/A$_{2A}$ receptors, that the coupling of A$_{2A}$ receptor–G-protein is predominantly dictated by the segment of NH$_2$-terminal of the third intracellular loop of the A$_{2A}$ receptor. The rat adrenal cell line PC12 has been often used to evaluate the function of the A$_{2A}$ receptor, although it has been shown that this cell line coexpresses the A$_{2B}$ receptor by polymerase chain reaction-based analysis (Chern *et al.*, 1993; Ploeg *et al.*, 1996). CGS21680 showed a concentration-dependent stimulation of the intracellular level of cAMP in PC12 cells (Fig. 7A), with an EC$_{50}$ value of 97 ± 37 nM, consistent with a previous report (Hide *et al.*, 1992). The effect of 1 μM CGS21680 was dose-dependently antagonized by KF17837S with an IC$_{50}$ value of 53 ± 10 nM (Fig. 7B). KF17837S alone had no effect on the basal levels. These results indicate that KF17837S is a functional A$_{2A}$ antagonist with no partial agonistic activity. In addition, the cAMP response of KF17837S was assessed using rat striatal slices because the A$_{2A}$ receptor is enriched in striatum where it may have an important functional role (see Chapter 2). In rat striatal slices, KF17837S concentration-dependently inhibited cAMP accumulation induced by CGS21680 (Fig. 8), as well as that observed in PC12 cells.

Related signal transduction pathways of the A$_{2A}$ receptor have been reported. Kleppisch and Nelson (1995) showed, using the whole-cell patch-clamp technique, the adenosine can activate K$_{ATP}$ currents in arterial smooth muscle cells through the A$_{2A}$-stimulated adenylyl cyclase and protein kinase A activation. Adenosine and CGS21680, but not the A$_1$ receptor agonist CCPA, induced the currents that were inhibited by glibenclamide, a selective inhibitor of K$_{ATP}$ channels, and that currents were reduced by the protein kinase A inhibitor H-89. A$_{2A}$ receptor activation in vascular beds elicits vasodilation with accumulation of cAMP (Cushing *et al.*, 1991). It is suggested that this phenomenon explains the mechanism of K$_{ATP}$ channel activation via the A$_{2A}$ receptor.

Adenosine acts as a mitogen on several cell types (Ethier *et al.*, 1993; Meininger and Granger, 1990; Van Daele *et al.*, 1992). In primary endothelial cells, the stimulation of the A$_{2A}$ receptor activates mitogen-activated protein kinase (MAP kinase), that is, an increase in tyrosine phosphorylation of the p42 isoform and to a lesser extent of p44 isoform (Sexl *et al.*, 1997). This is not mediated by G$_s$ protein because no alteration was caused by pretreatment of the cells with cholera toxin, whereas PD098059, an inhibitor of MAP

A

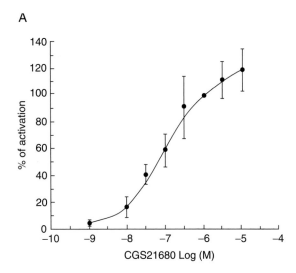

B

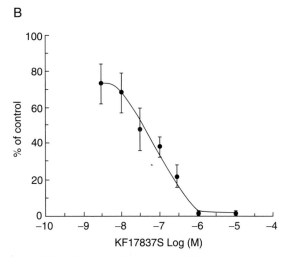

FIGURE 7   Effects of CGS21680 and KF17837S on cAMP content in intact PC12 cells. (A) Concentration–response curve of CGS21680 for the elevation of cAMP levels. The results are expressed as percentage of the 1 μM CGS21680-elevated cAMP levels (13 $\pm$ 3.6 pmol/10^6 cells). The basal cAMP levels are 0.98 $\pm$ 0.19 pmol/10^6 cells. The EC_{50} value is 97 $\pm$ 37 nM. (B) Concentration–response curve of KF17837S for the attenuation of 1 μM CGS21680-elevated cAMP levels. The results are expressed as percentage of the 1 μM CGS21680-elevated cAMP levels. The IC_{50} value is 53 $\pm$ 10 nM. The values shown are means $\pm$ standard errors of three or four separate experiments performed in duplicate. From Nonaka et al. (1994a).

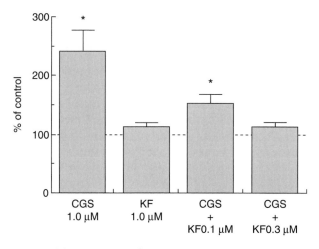

FIGURE 8 cAMP accumulation in rat striatal slices induced by adenosine A_{2A} receptors. CGS21680-induced cAMP accumulation was dose-dependently blocked by KF17837S. Data represent percentage of control and mean ± standard errors of three separate experiments. cAMP level in 12 striatal slices for control was 15 ± 1.1 pmol/mg protein. *$p < 0.05$ versus control.

kinase kinase 1 (MEK1), blocked this pathway. NECA also increased the level of GTP bound type $p21^{ras}$. Thus, the mitogenic activation via the A_{2A} receptor is not due to G_s protein-related pathway but $p21^{ras}$–MAP kinase pathway.

The desensitization mechanism of the A_{2A} receptor has been reported. cAMP accumulation is reduced by long-term agonist treatment; however, the binding capacity, the affinity of the agonist, and the level of the transcription of A_{2A} receptors do not change during desensitization (Chern *et al.*, 1993; Ramkumar *et al.*, 1991). Lai *et al.* (1997) reported that a calcium-independent, novel PKC phosphorylates adenylyl cyclase type VI in PC12 cells and, as a result, a reduction of the activity of the enzyme is induced during the A_{2A} receptor desensitization. In addition, it has been suggested that the A_{2A} receptor desensitization is mediated by G-protein coupled receptor kinase 2 (GRK2) in NG108-15 cells overexpressing the dominant negative mutant GRK2 (Mundell *et al.*, 1997). Multiple phosphorylation reactions involving at least two enzymes are implicated in A_{2A} receptor desensitization.

C. A_{2B} RECEPTOR

The presence of low-affinity A_2 (termed A_{2B}) receptors was originally suggested by the atypical properties of some adenosine analogues in the control of cAMP accumulation in whole cells (Bruns et al., 1986; Stiles, 1992). Adenosine A_{2B} receptor cDNAs have been cloned, which has confirmed that the A_{2B} receptors and abundant in ceacum, large intestine, and urinary bladder (Stehle et al., 1992). The A_{2B} receptors couple with G_S protein and the stimulation of this receptor results in activation of adenylyl cyclase in a similar manner to the A_{2A} receptors. The mouse fibroblast cell line NIH-3T3, human T-cell line Jurkat, and human embryonic kidney (HEK293) cell have all been shown to exhibit A_{2B} receptor-mediated stimulation of cAMP levels (Brackett and Daly, 1994; Cooper et al., 1997; Nonaka et al., 1994a; Ploeg et al., 1996). NECA, the nonselective adenosine receptor agonist, dose-dependently induced an accumulation of cAMP in Jurkat cells with an EC_{50} value of 960 ± 140 nM whereas CGS21680 exhibited only a slight effect on cAMP accumulation (Fig. 9A). The results are consistent with those of Kvanta et al. (1991), and confirm that Jurkat cells predominantly express A_{2B} receptors. KF17837S inhibited cAMP elevation stimulated by 10 μM NECA with an IC_{50} value of 1500 ± 290 nM (Fig. 9B), whereas the antagonist had no effect on the basal cAMP levels in Jurkat cells (Nonaka et al., 1994a). It is strongly suggested by the results of the cAMP response and of the autoradiography of [^{3}H]KF17837S in rat brain (Nonaka et al., 1994b) that KF17837S exerts its striatal effects by blocking the A_{2A} receptor even though the striatum expresses all adenosine receptor subtypes (Dixon et al., 1996).

The A_{2B} receptor had been shown to be coupled to PLC in Xenopus oocytes injected with the cRNA (Yakel et al., 1993). Furthermore, it was shown that IP_3 accumulation, one indicator of intracellular calcium mobilization, was elicited by NECA in HEK-293 cells stably transfected with human A_{2B} receptors (Linden et al., 1998). PLC activation via the A_{2B} receptor has also been reported in the human mast cell line HMC-1 where the activation led to IL-8 release (Feoktistov and Biaggioni, 1995). In addition to the mobilization of intracellular calcium via PLC, it has been reported that A_{2B} receptors are coupled to Ca^{2+} channel via G_S proteins without an accompanying increase in cAMP (Mirabet et al., 1997). In canine BR mastocytoma cells, A_{2B} receptors have been found to mainly regulate degranulation (Auchampach et al., 1997), suggesting that A_{2B} receptors may also be involved in the effects of adenosine in asthma (see Chapter 4).

Adenosine also has effects as a secretagogue in ileum and colon (Dobbins et al., 1984; Grasl and Turnheim, 1984). Neutrophils release 5'-AMP, which is converted by ecto-5'-nucleotidase on the apical membrane of the intestinal

A

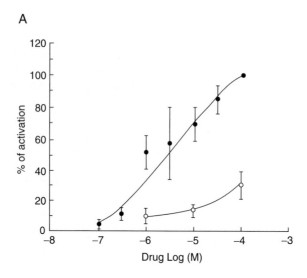

B

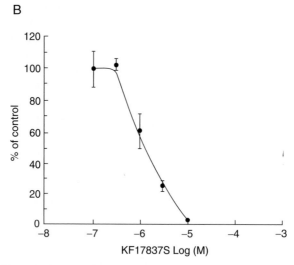

FIGURE 9   Effects of NECA and KF17837S on cAMP content in intact Jurkat cells. (**A**) Concentration–response curves of NECA (closed circle) and CGS21680 (open circle) for the elevation of cAMP levels. The results are expressed as percentage of the 100 μM NECA-elevated cAMP levels (21 $\pm$ 9.2 pmol/10^6 cells). The basal cAMP levels are 1.7 $\pm$ 0.76 pmol/10^6 cells. The EC_{50} value of NECA is 960 $\pm$ 140 nM. (**B**) Concentration–response curve of KF17837S for the attenuation of 10 μM NECA-elevated cAMP level. The results are expressed as percentage of the 10 μM NECA-elevated cAMP levels (14 $\pm$ 5.0 pmol/10^6 cells). The IC_{50} value is 1500 $\pm$ 290 nM. The values shown are means $\pm$ standard errors of four or five separate experiments performed in duplicate. From Nonaka *et al.* (1994a).

epithelial cell to adenosine (Madara *et al.*, 1993). In the case of intestinal inflammation, activated neutrophils accumulate in the colonic crypt, the site of electrogenic chloride secretion (Kumar *et al.*, 1982). In the polarized human intestinal epithelial cell line T84, adenosine and its analogues elicited Cl^- secretion via an increase in cAMP, and this pathway was inhibited by a protein kinase A inhibitor H-89 (Strohmeier *et al.*, 1995). The effect of adenosine and its analogues might be mediated via the A_{2B} receptors. The distribution of the A_{2B} receptor, abundantly expressed in colon, and the Cl^- secretion pathway might indicate that the A_{2B} receptor has an important function in secretary diarrhea associated with inflammation.

D. A_3 RECEPTOR

The A_3 receptor sequence was first cloned from a rat testis cDNA library, and functional expression showed A_3 receptor-mediated inhibition of adenylyl cyclase (Meyerhof *et al.*, 1991). A_3 receptors expressed in CHO cells inhibited this enzyme with a maximal inhibition of about 50% (Linden *et al.*, 1993; Salvatore *et al.*, 1993; Zhou *et al.*, 1992).

In the rat mast cell line RBL-2H3, A_3 receptors have been found to cause inhibition of adenylyl cyclase and activation of PLC leading to formation of inositol-1,4,5-triphosphate, with an accompanying increase in intracellular calcium levels (Ramkumar *et al.*, 1993). Adenosine and its analogues alone do not induce secretion in mast cells, but they do potentiate secretion induced by other stimulants (Gilfillan *et al.*, 1990; Lohse *et al.*, 1988b; Marquardt *et al.*, 1978). The enhancement activity of adenosine analogues for the antigen-stimulated degranulation showed a similar rank order to the binding affinity for the A_3 receptors (Ramkumar *et al.*, 1993). The expression of the A_3 receptor on RBL-2H3 was also shown by the radioligand binding and reverse transcription polymerase chain reaction (RT-PCR) (Ramkumar *et al.*, 1993). However, the A_{2A} and A_{2B} receptors were also detected in these cells (Marquardt *et al.*, 1994), indicating adenosine-induced mast cell degranulation might not be necessarily mediated solely by A_3 receptors. The distribution of A_3 receptors in lung is of interest from a therapeutic point of view because they could be potential targets for antiasthmatic or antiinflammatory drugs. For example, the mean amount of A_3 receptor transcripts is more abundant in lung tissue from patients with airway inflammation than in normal lung (Walker *et al.*, 1997). Walker *et al.* (1997) identified the A_3 receptor in mesenchymal cells and eosinophils within the lamina propia of the airways and the adventitia of blood vessels but not human mast cells. A_3 receptor transcripts were highly expressed in peripheral blood eosinophils purified from atopic donors in comparison with neutrophils or mononuclear cells. Moreover, an A_3 receptor agonist inhibited platelet-activating factor-induced eosinophil chemotaxis, and the effect was eliminated by addition of an A_3 receptor selective antagonist (Walker et al., 1997). Further investigations using RBL-2H3 cells and other mast cells are necessary to clarify the function of the A_3 receptor in this cell type.

McWhinney et al. (1996) proposed that activation of A_3 receptors inhibits induction of the cytokine tumor necrosis factor-α (TNF-α) gene and TNF-α protein expression, induced by endotoxin in the macrophage cell line J774.1. This result might imply a novel cross-talk between the A_3 receptor and the endotoxin CD14 receptor.

There are several complicated reports of the effect of the A_3 receptor in the CNS. An A_3 agonist administered just prior to forebrain ischemia caused cell death and reduced survival rates in gerbils (von Lubitz et al., 1994). In contrast, chronic administration of an A_3 agonist produced decreasing neuronal cell death and improving survival rates (von Lubitz et al., 1994). PLC activation occurs as a very early response to brain ischemia (Lin et al., 1991; Rudolphi, 1991), and Abbracchio et al. (1995) reported that the A_3 receptor agonists induced PLC activation in rat brain. Further investigation of the PLC pathway regulated by the A_3 receptor in the CNS may explain these complicated phenomena. Another study demonstrated that, in the CA1 region of rat hippocampus, adenosine (30 μM) normally acts on the A_1 receptors to inhibit synaptically evoked excitatory responses. In this system, activation of A_3 receptors with Cl-IB-MECA (100 nM) antagonized the A_1 receptor-mediated inhibition of excitatory neurotransmission. The effects of Cl-IB-MECA were blocked by a selective A_3 antagonist, MRS 1191 (Dunwiddie et al., 1997). Due to the low affinity of A_3 receptors for adenosine, they are unlikely to be activated under normal conditions when both A_1 and A_{2A} receptors show some tonic activity. However, in ischemia, brain adenosine concentrations increase and A_3 receptors are expected to be activated. This activation of A_3 receptors might counteract the A_1 receptor-mediated inhibition of excitatory neurotransmission and lead to a deleterious effect on survival rates of neuronal cells.

IV. BIOCHEMICAL BASIS OF THE USE OF A_{2A} ANTAGONISTS IN PARKINSON'S DISEASE

A selective adenosine A_{2A} receptor antagonist showed an anti-Parkinson's disease activity in vivo animal model (Kanda et al., 1994; Richardson et al., 1997). From the point of view of drug resistance, antagonists have advantages compared with agonists (e.g., A_{2A} antagonists are not expected to induce drug resistance after chronic administration). The details of the pharmacology *in vivo* is described in Chapters 10 to 12, In this section, the biochemical aspects of the anti-Parkinson's disease activity of A_{2A} receptor antagonists are described.

It is clear that Parkinson's disease is caused by the specific degeneration of dopaminergic nigrostriatal neurons in the basal ganglia. As described in the previous section of this chapter, the A_{2A} receptor is highly concentrated in the striatum, nucleus accumbens, and olfactory tubercle. It appears that in the striatum, which is a major component of basal ganglia, the A_{2A} receptor mRNA exists mainly in the medium spiny neurons (MSNs) as detected by *in situ* hybridization (Schiffmann *et al.*, 1991). Because the striatum is involved in regulating movement, this distribution suggests a specific function of the A_{2A} receptor in the neuronal networks controlling movement. There exist two major output pathways from the basal ganglia. One is the *direct* (from striatum to internal segments of globus pallidus/substantia nigra) and the other is *indirect* (from striatum to internal segments of globus pallidus/substantia nigra via the external segments of globus pallidus and subthalamic nucleus), which are responsible for smooth and coordinated movement (see Figure 1 of Chapter 1). The MSNs, which constitute 90–95% of striatal neurons, are the major output neurons of this brain region and form the direct pathway and the first part of the indirect pathway. These MSNs, which release γ-aminobutyric acid (GABA), are controlled by inhibitory feedback from recurrent collateral axons within the striatal region. They receive glutamatergic excitatory inputs from the cerebral cortex and also possess modulatory inputs from dopaminergic neurons (nigrostriatal neurons), which die in Parkinson's disease. In this neuronal network, the level of output activity between the direct and the indirect pathway is well balanced, and this balance is believed to control well-coordinated movement. Dopamine controls both pathways via D_1 (direct pathway) and D_2 (indirect pathway) receptors. In Parkinson's disease, the effect of dopamine denervation gives rise to an imbalance in the activity of the output pathways, and this imbalance (hyperactive in the indirect pathway) is supposed to be involved in induction of the dysfunction in Parkinson's disease (Gerfen, 1992).

Electrophysiological studies of a rat striatal slices revealed that the A_{2A} selective agonist CGS21680 suppressed GABAergic neurotransmission onto these MSNs and that the A_{2A} selective antagonist KF17837S blocked the inhibitory effect of CGS21680 (Mori *et al.*, 1996; see Chapter 6). This effect of the A_{2A} receptor antagonist on GABA neurotransmission was also confirmed by neurochemical experiments. In nerve terminals derived from the striatum, the A_{2A} agonist, CGS21680, inhibited [^{3}H]GABA release evoked by 15 mM KCl (Kirk and Richardson, 1994). KF17837S blocked the CGS21680-induced inhibition of GABA release (Kurokawa *et al.*, 1994; Chapter 7).

Considering the relationship between hyperactivity of the indirect pathway in Parkinson's disease and the suppression of GABAergic neurotransmission by the A_{2A} receptor, it is likely that the A_{2A} antagonists decrease the activity of the output neurons (MSNs) in the indirect pathway by increasing the GABAergic transmission from the recurrent collaterals. This effect of A_{2A} antagonists is due to disinhibition of the inhibitory collateral inputs and, thus, compensates for the imbalance of the two pathways induced by dopamine denervation. Adenosine may also tonically modulate the GABAergic synaptic transmission among MSNs.

With respect to the signal transduction of the A_{2A} receptor for GABAergic neurotransmission within striatum MSNs, in rat striatal slices, CGS21680 (1 μM) increased cAMP accumulation from the control level of 15.1 ± 1.1 pmol/mg protein to 32.2 ± 4.8 pmol/mg protein. KF17837S ($0.1-0.3$ μM) dose-dependently suppressed this increase. This result suggests that cAMP is the second messenger for the synaptic regulation of GABAergic transmission by the A_{2A} receptors (Fig. 8). In addition, the suppression of GABAergic transmission via the A_{2A} receptor was mimicked by membrane-permeable cAMP analogues, such as dibutyryl cAMP or 8-Br cAMP, and this result strongly suggests the involvement of cAMP in adenosine modulation of the synaptic transmission (Mori *et al.*, 1996).

Similar regulation of neurotransmitter release by cAMP has been reported in the hippocampal slices. The calcium channels in presynaptic sites are phosphorylated by cAMP-dependent protein kinase (PKA) in response to endogenous electrical stimulation, and this regulation by PKA may be involved in the control of neurotransmitter release (Hell *et al.*, 1995). Other reports on isolated pyramidal neurons from the CA3 region of the guinea pig hippocampus indicated another effect of adenosine receptor activation on Ca^{2+} currents induced by depolarization. Activation of A_1 receptors inhibited the N-type Ca^{2+} current, whereas activation of A_{2B} receptors resulted in potentiation of ω-agatoxin-sensitive P-type Ca^{2+} current. In the case of activation of A_{2B} receptors, internal application of the specific inhibitor peptide, WIPTIED, prevented the potentiation of Ca^{2+} current (Mogul *et al.*, 1993). This result suggests that potentiation of Ca^{2+} current by A_{2B} receptor activation is due to augmentation of cAMP level. However, the reports on molecular mechanism of the A_{2A} receptor regulation for GABA neurotransmission are controversial in terms of cAMP involvement (Kirk and Richardson 1995; Mori *et al.*, 1996). Kirk and Richardson (1995) reported that the A_{2A} receptor inhibition of potassium (15 mM)-evoked GABA release from striatal nerve terminals was not mediated by cAMP elevation because activation of adenylyl cyclase by forskolin antagonized the receptor action and a selective PKA inhibitor HA-

1004 was not able to block the effect. They also implied the involvement of N-type Ca^{2+} channels and protein kinase C for this mechanism. More precise investigations might be necessary to determine whether cAMP is the second messenger for the regulation of GABA synaptic transmission in striatum by A_{2A} receptors.

V. CONCLUSION

The molelcular cloning of adenosine receptors (A_1, A_{2A}, A_{2B}, A_3 subtypes) and discovery of their selective ligands have revealed the biochemical characteristics and the physiological roles of adenosine and its receptors in mammals. Moreover, pharmacological investigations using the ligands have led to the recognition of adenosine receptors as one of the more promising molecular targets for therapeutics. Our adenosine receptor antagonists may have a possibility as novel drugs for the treatment of cardiovascular or CNS disease (especially, Parkinson's disease).

REFERENCES

Abbracchio, M.P., Brambilla, R., Ceruti, S., Kim, H.O., Von Lubitz, J.E., Jacobson, K.A., and Cattabeni, F. (1995). G protein-dependent activation of phospholipase C by adenosine A_3 receptors in rat brain. Mol Pharmacol 48, 1038–1045.

Ali, S., Mustafa, S.J., and Metzger, W.J. (1994). Adenosine receptor-mediated bronchoconstriction and bronchial hyperresponsiveness in allergic rabbit model. Am J Physiol 266, L271–L277.

Auchampach, J.A., Jin, X., Wan, T.C., Caughey, G.H., and Linden, J. (1997). Canine mast cell adenosine receptors: cloning and expression of the A_3 receptor and evidence that degranulation is mediated by the A_{2B} receptor. Mol Pharmacol 52, 846–860.

Belardinelli, L., Shryock, J.C., Ruble, J., Monopoli, A., Dionisotti, S., Ongini, E., Dennis, D.M., and Baker, S.P. (1996) Binding of the novel non-xanthine A_{2A} adenosine receptor antagonist (^{3}H)-SCH 58261 to coronary artery membranes. Circ Res 79, 1153–1160.

Brackett, L.E., and Daly, J.W. (1994) Functional characterization fo the A_{2B} adenosine receptor in NIH 3T3 fibroblasts. Biochem Pharmacol 47, 801–814.

Bruns, R.F., Lu, G.H., and Pugsley, T.A. (1986). Characterization of the A_2 adenosine receptor labeled by [^{3}H]NECA in rat striatal membranes. Mol Pharmacol 29, 331–346.

Bruns, R.F., Fergus, J.H., Badger, E.W., Bristol, J.A., Santay, L.A., and Hays, S.J. (1987). PD115,199: an antagonist ligand for adenosine A_2 receptors. Naunyn-Schmiedeberg's Arch Pharmacol 335, 64–69.

Casadó, V., Casillas, T., Mallol, J., Canela, E.I., Lluis, C., and Franco, R. (1992). The adenosine receptors present on the plasma membrane of chromaffin cells are of the A_{2B} subtype. J Neurochem 59, 425–431.

Chern, Y., Lai, H.-L., Fong, J.C., and Liang, Y. (1993). Multiple mechanism for desensitization of A_{2A} adenosine receptor-mediated cAMP elevation in rat pheochromocytoma PC12 cells. Mol Pharmacol 44, 950–958.

Church, M.K., and Holgate, S.T. (1986). Adenosine and asthma. *Trends Pharmacol Sci* 7, 49–50.

Cooper, J., Hill, S.J., and Alexander, S.P.H. (1997). An endogenous A_{2B} adenosine receptor coupled to cyclic AMP generation in human embryonic kidney (HEK) cells. *Br J Pharmacol* 122, 546–550.

Cushing, D.J., Brown, G.L., Sabouni, M.H., and Mustafa, S.J. (1991). Adenosine receptor-mediated coronary artery relaxation and cyclic nucleotide production. *Am J Physiol* 261, H343–H348.

Dickenson, J.M., Camps, M., Gierschik, P., and Hill, S.J. (1995). Activation of phospholipase C by G-protein beta gamma subunits in DDT1 MF-2 cells. *Eur J Pharmacol* 288, 393–398.

Dionisotti, S., Ferrara, S., Molta, C., Zocchi, C., and Ongini, E. (1996). Labeling of A_{2A} adenosine receptors in human platelets using the new non-xanthine antagonist radioligand [^{3}H]-SCH 58261. *J Pharmacol Exp Ther* 298, 726–732.

Dixon, A.K., Gubitz, A.K., Sirinathsinghji, D.J.S. Richardson, P.J., and Freeman, T.C. (1996). Tissue distribution of adenosine receptor mRNAs in the rat. *Br J Pharmacol* 118, 1461–1468.

Dobbins, J.W., Laurenson, J.P., and Forrest, J.N., Jr. (1984). Adenosine and adenosine analogues stimulate adenosine cyclic 3′,5′-monophosphate-dependent chloride secretion in the mammalian ileum. *J Clin Invest* 74, 929–935.

Dunwiddie, T.V., Diao, L., Kim, H.O., Jiang, J.-L., and Jacobson, K.A. (1997). Activation of hippocampal adenosine A_3 receptors produces a desensitization of A_1 receptor-mediated response in rat hippocampus. *J Neurosci* 17, 607–614.

Ethier, M.F., Chander, V., and Dobson, J.G. (1993). Adenosine stimulates proliferation of human endothelial cells in culture. *Am J Physiol* 265, H131–H138.

Feoktistov, I., and Biaggioni, I. (1995). Adenosine A_{2B} receptors evoke interleukin-8 secretion in human mast cells. *J Clin Invest* 96, 1979–1986.

Ferkany, J.W., Valentine, H.L., Stone, G.A., and Williams, M. (1986). Adenosine A_1 receptors in mammalian brain: species differences in their interactions with agonists and antagonists. *Drug Dev Res* 9, 85–93.

Freund, S., Ungerer, M., and Lohse, M.J. (1994). A_1 adenosine receptors expressed in CHO-cells couple to adenylyl cyclase and to phospholipase C. *Naunyn-Schmiedeberg's Arch Pharmacol* 350, 49–56.

Gerfen, C.R. (1992). The neostriatal mosaic: multiple levels of compartmental organization in the basal ganglia. *Annu Rev Neurosci* 15, 285–320.

Gerwins, P., and Fredholm, B.B. (1992a). ATP and its metabolite adensine act synergistically to mobilize intracellular calcium via the formation of inositol 1,4,5-trisphosphate in a smooth muscle cell line. *J Biol Chem* 267, 16081–16087.

Gerwins, P., and Fredholm, B.B. (1992b). Stimulation of adenosine A_1 receptors and bradykinin receptors, which act via different G proteins, synergistically raises inositol 1,4,5-trisphosphate and intracellular free calcium in DDT_1 MF-2 smooth muscle cells. *Proc Natl Acad Sci USA* 89, 7330–7334.

Gilfillan, A.M., Wiggan, G.A., and Welton, A.F. (1990). Pertussis toxin pretreatment reveals differential effects of adenosine analogs on IgE-dependent histamine and peptidoleukotriene release from RBL-2H3 cells. *Biochim Biophys Acta* 1052, 467–474.

Grasl, M., and Turnheim, K. (1984). Stimulation of electrolyte secretion in rabbit colon by adenosine. *J Physiol* 346, 93–110.

Grover, G.J. (1994). Protective effects of ATP sensitive potassium channel openers in models of myocardial ischemia. *Cardiovasc Res* 28, 778–782.

Hell, J.M., Yokoyama, C.T., Breeze, L.J., Chavkin, C., and Catterall, W.A. (1995). Phosphorylation of presynaptic and postsynaptic calcium channels by cAMP-dependent protein kinase in hippocampal neurons. *EMBO J* 14, 3036–3044.

Hide, I., Padgett, W.L., Jacobson, K.A., and Daly, J.W. (1992). A_{2A} adenosine receptors from rat striatum and rat pheochromocytoma PC12 cells: characterization with radioligand binding and by activation of adenylate cyclase. *Mol Pharmacol* **41**, 352–359.

Hutchison, K.A., and Fox, I.H. (1989). Purification and characterization of the adenosine A_2-like binding site from human placental membranes. *J Biol Chem* **264**, 19898–19903.

Iredale, P.A., Alexander, S.P.H. and Hill, S.J. (1994). Coupling of a transfected human brain A_1 adenosine receptor in CHO-K1 cells to calcium mobilization via a pertussis toxin-sensitive mechanism. *Br J Pharmacol* **111**, 1252–1256.

James, S., Xuereb, J.H., Askalan, R., and Richardson, P.J. (1992). Adenosine receptors in post-mortem human brain. *Br J Pharmacol* **105**, 238–244.

Jarvis, M.F., Schulz, R., Hutchison, A.J., Do, U.H., Sills, M.A., and Williams, M. (1989a). [^{3}H]CGS21680, a selective A_2 adenosine receptor agonist directly labels A_2 receptors in rat brain. *J Pharmacol Exp Ther* **251**, 888–893.

Jarvis, M.F., Jackson, R.H., and Williams, M. (1989b). Autoradiographic characterization of high-affinity adenosine A_2 receptors in the rat brain. *Brain Res* **484**, 111–118.

Jarvis M.F., and Williams, M. (1989). Direct autoradiographic localization of adenosine A_2 receptors in the rat brain using the A_2-selective agonist, [^{3}H]CGS21680. *Eur J Pharmacol* **168**, 243–246.

Ji, X.D., von Lubitz, D., Olah, M.E., Stiles, G.L., and Jacobson, K.A. (1994). Species differences in ligand affinity at central A_3-adenosine receptors. *Drug Dev Res* **33**, 51–59.

Jockers, R., Linder, M.E., Hohenegger, M., Nanoff, C., Bertin, B., Strosberg, A. D., Marullo, S., and Freissmuth, M. (1994). Species differences in the G protein selectivity of the human and bovine A_1-adenosine receptor. *J Biol Chem* **269**, 32077–32084.

Johansson, B., Georgiev, V., Parkinson, F.E., and Fredholm, B.B. (1993). The binding of the adenosine A_2 receptor selective agonist [^{3}H]CGS21680 to rat cortex differs from its binding to rat striatum. *Eur J Pharmacol* **247**, 103–110.

Kanda, K., Shiozaki, S., Shimada, J., Suzuki, F., and Nakamura, J. (1994). KF17837: a novel selective adenosine A_{2A} receptor antagonist with anticataleptic activity. *Eur J Pharmacol* **256**, 263–268.

Kim, O.H., Ji, X.D., Siddiqi, S.M., Olah, M.E., Stiles, G.L., and Jacobson, K.A. (1994). 2-Substitution of N^6-benzyladenosine-5′-uronamides enhances selectivity for A_3 adenosine receptors. *J Med Chem* **37**, 3614–3621.

Kirk, I.P., and Richardson, P.J. (1994). Adenosine A_{2A} receptor mediated modulation of striatal [^{3}H]-GABA and [^{3}H]ACh release. *J Neurochem* **62**, 960–966.

Kirk, I.P., and Richardson, P.J. (1995). Inhibition of striatal GABA release by the adenosine A_{2A} receptor is not mediated by increase in cyclic AMP. *J Neurochem* **64**, 2801–2809.

Kirsch, G.E., Codina, J., Birnbaumer, L., and Brown, A.M. (1990). Coupling of ATP-sensitive K^+ channels to A_1 receptors by G proteins in rat ventricular myocytes. *Am J Physiol* **259**, H820–H826.

Kleppisch, T., and Nelson, M.T. (1995). Adenosine activates ATP-sensitive potassium channels in arterial myocytes via A_2 receptors and cAMP-dependent protein kinase. *Proc Natl Acad Sci USA* **92**, 12441–12445.

Kobayashi, T., Mizumoto, H., and Karasawa, A. (1993). Diuretic effects of KW-3902 (8-(no-radamantan-3-yl)-1,3-dipropylxanthine), a novel adenosine A_1 receptor antagonist, in conscious dogs. *Biol Pharm Bull* **16**, 1231–1235.

Kumar, N.B., Nostrant, T.T., and Appleman, H.D. (1982). The histologic spectrum of acute self limited colitis (acute infectious-type colitis). *Am J Surg Pathol* **6**, 523–529.

Kurokawa, M., Kirk, I.P., Kirkpatrick, K.A., Kase, H., and Richardson, P.J. (1994). Inhibition by KF17837 of adenosine A_{2A} receptor-mediated modulation of striatal GABA and ACh release. *Br J Pharmacol* **113**, 43–48.

Kvanta, A., Jondal, M., and Fredholm, B.B. (1991). CD3-dependent increase in cyclic AMP in human T-cells following stimulation of the CD2 receptor. *Biochim Biophys Acta* **1093**, 178–183.

Lai, H.-L., Yang, T.-H., Messing, R.O., Ching, Y.-H., Lin, S.-C., and Chern, Y. (1997). Protein kinase C inhibits adenylyl cyclase type VI activity during desensitization of the A_{2A}-adenosine receptor-mediated cAMP response. *J Biol Chem* **272**, 4970–4977.

Liang, B.T. (1996). Direct preconditioning of cardiac ventricular myocytes via adenosine A_1 receptor and K_{ATP} channel. *Am J Physiol* **271**, H1769-H1777.

Lin, T.N., Liu T.H., Xu, J., Hsu, C.Y., and Sun, G.Y. (1991). Brain polyphosphoinositide metabolism during focal ischemia in rat cortex. *Stroke* **22**, 495–498.

Linden, J., Taylor, H.E., Robeva, A.S., Tucker, A.L., Stehle, J.H., Rivkees, S.A., Fink, J.S., and Reppert, S.M. (1993). Molecular cloning and functional expression of a sheep A_3 adenosine receptor with widespread tissue distribution. *Mol Pharmacol* **44**, 524–532.

Linden, J., Tucker, A.L., and Lynch, K.R. (1991). Molecular cloning of adenosine A_1 and A_2 receptors. *Trends Pharmacol Sci* **12**, 326–328.

Linden, J. (1994). Cloned adenosine A_3 receptors: pharmacological properties, species differences and receptor functions. *Trends Pharmacol Sci* **15**, 298–306.

Linden, J., Auchampach, J.A., Jin, X., and Figler, R.A. (1998). The structure and function of A_1 and A_{2B} adenosine receptors. *Life Sci* **62**, 1519–1524.

Lohse, M.J., Klotz, K.-N. Lindenborn-Fotinos, J., Reddington, M., Schwabe, U., and Olsson, R.A. (1987). 8-Cyclopentyl-1,3-dipropylxanthine (DPCPX)—a selective high affinity antagonist radioligand for A_1 adenosine receptors. *Naunyn-Schmiedeberg's Arch Pharmacol* **336**, 204–210.

Lohse, M.J., Elger, B., Lindenborn-Fotinos, J., Klotz, K.-N. and Schwabe, U. (1988a). Separation of solubilized A_2 adenosine receptors of human platelets from non-receptor [^{3}H]NECA binding sites by gel filtration. *Naunyn-Schmiedeberg's Arch Pharmacol* **337**, 64–68.

Lohse, M., Klotz, K.-N., Salzer, M.J., and Schwabe, U. (1988b). Adenosine regulates the Ca^{2+} sensitivity of mast cell mediator release. *Proc Natl Acad Sci USA* **85**, 8875–8879.

Long, C.J., and Stone, T.W. (1987). Adenosine reduces agonist-induced production of inositol phosphates in rat aorta. *J Pharm Pharmacol* **39**, 1010–1014.

Luthin, D.R., Olsson, R.A., Thompson, R.D., Sawmiller, D.R., and Linden, J. (1995). Characterization of two affinity states of adenosine A_{2A} receptors with a new radioligand, 2-[2-(4-amino-3-[^{125}I]iodophenyl)ethylamino]adenosine. *Mol Pharmacol* **47**, 307–313.

Madara, J.L., Patapoff, T.W., Gillece-Castro, B., Colgan, S.P., Parkos, C.A., Delp, C., and Mrsny, R.J. (1993). 5'-Adenosine monophosphate is the neutrophil-derived paracrine factor that elicits chloride secretion from T84 intestinal epithelial cell monolayers. *J Clin Invest* **91**, 2320–2325.

Maenhaut, C., Van Sande, J., Libert, F., Abramowicz, M., Parmentier, M., Vanderhaegen, J.-J., Dumont, J.E., Vassart, G., and Schiffmann, S. (1990). RDC8 codes for an adenosine A_2 receptor with physiological constitutive activity. *Biochem Biophys Res Commun* **173**, 1169–1178.

Marquardt, D.L., Parker, C.W., and Sullivan, T.J. (1978). Potentiation of mast cell histamine release by adenosine. *J Immunol* **120**, 871–878.

Marquardt, D.L., Walker, L.L., and Heinemann, S. (1994). Clonning of two adenosine receptor subtypes from mouse bone marrow-derived mast cells. *J Immunol* **152**, 4508–4515.

Matherne, G.P., Linden, J., Byford, A.M., Gauthier, N.S., and Headrick, J.P. (1997). Transgenic A_1 adenosine receptor overexpression increases myocardial resistance to ischemia. *Proc Natl Acad Sci USA* **94**, 6541–6546.

McWhinney, C.D., Dudley, M.W., Bowlin, T.L., Peet, N.P., Schook, L., Bradshaw, M., De, M., Borcherding, D.R., and Edwards, C.K. III, (1996). Activation of adenosine A_3 receptors on macrophages inhibits tumor necrosis factor-α. *Eur J Pharmacol* **310**, 209–216.

Meininger, C.J., and Graner, H.J. (1990). Mechanisms leading to adenosine-stimulated proliferation of microvascular endothelial cells. *Am J Physiol* **258**, H198–H206.

Meyerhof, W., Muller-Brechlin, R., and Richter, D. (1991). Molecular cloning of a novel putative G-protein coupled receptor expressed during rat spermiogenesis. *FEBS Lett* **284**, 155–160.

Mirabet, M., Mallol, J., and Franco, R. (1997). Calcium mobilization in Jurkat cells via A_{2B} adenosine receptors. *Br J Pharmacol* **122**, 1075–1082.

Mizumoto, H., Karasawa, A., and Kubo, K. (1993). Diuretic and renal protective effects of 8-(noradamantan-3-yl)-1,3-dipropylxanthine (KW-3902), a novel adenosine A_1-receptor antagonist, via pertussis toxin insensitive mechanism. *J Pharmacol Exp Ther* **266**, 200–206.

Mogul, D.J., Adams, M.E., and Fox, A.P. (1993). Differential activation of adenosine receptors decrease N-type but potentiates P-type Ca^{2+} current in hippocampal CA3 neurons. *Neuron* **10**, 327–334.

Mori, A., Shindou, T., Ichimura, M., Nonaka, H., and Kase, H. (1996). The role of adenosine A_{2A} receptors in regulating GABAergic synaptic transmission in striatal medium spiny neurons. *J Neurosci* **16**, 605–611.

Mundell, S.J., Benovic, J.L., and Kelly, E. (1997). A dominant negative mutant of the G protein-coupled receptor kinase 2 selectively attenuates adenosine A_2 receptor desensitization. *Mol Pharmacol* **51**, 991–998.

Nanoff, C., Freissmuth, M., Tuisl, E., and Schütz, W. (1990). P_2-, but not P_1- purinoceptors mediate formation of 1,4,5-inositol triphosphate and its metabolites via a pertussis toxin-insensitive pathway in the rat renal cortex. *Br J Pharmacol* **100**, 63–68.

Nanoff, C., and Stiles, G.L. (1993). Solubilization and characterization of the A_2- adenosine receptor. *J Recep Res* **13**, 961–973.

Nonaka, H., Ichimura, M., Takeda, M., Nonaka, Y., Schimada, J., Suzuki, F., Yamaguchi, K., and Kase, H. (1994a). KF17837 ((E)-8-(3,4-dimethoxystyryl)-1,3-dipropyl-7-methylxanthine), a potent and selective adenosine A_2 receptor antagonist. *Eur J Pharmacol* **267**, 335–341.

Nonaka, H., Mori, A., Ichimura, M., Shindou, T., Yanagawa, K., Shimada, J., and Kase, H. (1994b). Binding of [^{3}H]KF17837S, a selective adenosine A_2 receptor antagonist, to rat brain membranes. *Mol Pharmacol* **46**, 817–822.

Nonaka, H., Ichimura, M., Takeda, M., Kanda, T., Shimada, J., Suzuki, F., and Kase, H. (1996). KW-3902, a selective high affinity antagonist for adenosine A_1 receptors. *Br J Pharmacol* **117**, 1645–1652.

Nyce, J.W., and Metzger, W.J. (1997). DNA antisense therapy for asthma in an animal model. *Nature* **385**, 721–725.

Olah, M.E., Ren, H., Ostrowski, J., Jacobson K.A., and Stiles, G.L. (1992). Cloning, expression, and characterization of the unique bovine A_1 adenosine receptor. *J Biol Chem* **267**, 10764–10770.

Olah, M.E., Gallo-Rodriguez, C., Jacobson, K.A., and Stiles, G.L. (1994). [^{125}I]AB-MECA, a high affinity radioligand for the rat A_3 adenosine receptor. *Mol Pharmacol* **45**, 978–982.

Olah, M.E. (1997). Identification of A_{2A} adenosine receptor domain involved in selective coupling to G_s. Analysis of chimeric A_1/A_{2A} adenosine receptors. *J Biol Chem* **272**, 337–344.

Olssen, R.A. (1984). Structure of the coronary artery adenosine receptor. *Trends Pharmacol Sci* **5**, 113–116.

Palmer, T.M., and Stiles, G.L. (1995). Adenosine receptors. *Neuropharmacol* **34**, 683–694.

Parkinson, F.E., and Fredholm, B.B. (1990). Autoradiographic evidence for G-protein coupled A_2-receptors in rat neostriatum using [^{3}H]CGS21680 as a ligand. *Naunyn-Schmiedeberg's Arch Pharmacol* **342**, 85–89.

Parkinson, F.E., and Fredholm, B.B. (1992). Differential effect of magnesium on receptor–G-protein coupling of adenosine A_1 and A_2 receptors: a quantitative autoradiographical study. *Mol Neuropharmacol* **1**, 179–186.

Ramkumar, V., Olah, M.E., Kenneth, O., Jacobson, K.A., and Stiles, G.L. (1991). Distinct pathways of desensitization of A_1- and A_2-adenosine receptors in DDT1MF-2 cells. *Mol Pharmacol* **40**, 639–647.

Ramkumar V., Stiles, G.L., Beaven, M., and Ali, H. (1993). The adenosine A_3 receptor is the unique adenosine receptor which facilitates release of allergic mediators in mast cells. *J Biol Chem* **268**, 16667–16670.

Richardson, P.J., Kase, H., and Jenner, P.J. (1997). Adenosine A_{2A} receptor antagonists as new agents for the treatment of Parkinson's disease. *Trends Pharmacol Sci* **18**, 338–344.

Rudolphi, K.A. (1991). Manipulation of purinergic tone as a mechanism for controlling ischemic brain damage. *In* "Adenosine and Adenine Nucleotides as Regulators of Cellular Function" (J.W. Phillis, ed.), pp. 423–436. CRC Press, Boca Raton.

Salvatore C.A., Jacobson, M.A., Taylor, H.E., Linden, J., and Johnson, R.G. (1993). Molecular cloning and characterization of the human A_3 adenosine receptor. *Proc Natl Acad Sci USA* **90**, 10365–10369.

Schiffmann, S.N., Libert, F., Vassart, G., and Vanderhaeghen, J.-J. (1991). Distribution of adenosine A_2 receptor mRNA in the human brain. *Neurosci Lett* **130**, 177–181.

Sexl, V., Mancusi, G., Höller, C., Gloria-Maercker, E., Schütz, W., and Freissmuth, M. (1997). Stimulation of the mitogen-activated protein kinase via the A_{2A} adenosine receptor in primary human endothelial cells. *J Biol Chem* **272**, 5792–5799.

Shimada, J., Koike, N., Nonaka, H., Shiozaki, S., Yanagawa, K., Kanda, T., Kobayasi, H., Ichimura, M., Nakamura, J., Kase, H., and Suzuki, F. (1997). Adenosine A_{2A} antagonists with potent anti-cataleptic activity. *Bioorg Medicinal Chem Lett* **7**, 2349–2352.

Shimada, J., Suzuki, F., Nonaka, H., and Ishii, A. (1992a). 8-Polycycloalkyl-1,3-dipropylxanthines as potent and selective antagonists for A_1-adenosine receptors. *J Med Chem* **35**, 924–930.

Shimada, J., Suzuki, F., Nonaka, H., Ishii, A., and Ichikawa, S. (1992b). (E)-1,3-Dialkyl-7-methyl-8-(3,4,5-trimethoxystyryl) xanthines: potent and selective adenosine A_2 antagonists. *J Med Chem* **35**, 2342–2345.

Stehle, J.H., Rivkees, S.A., Lee, J.J., Weaver, D.R., Deeds, J.D., and Reppert, S.M. (1992). Molecular cloning and expression of the cDNA for a novel A_2-adenosine receptor subtype. *Mol Endocrinol* **6**, 384–393.

Stiles, G.L. (1992). Adenosine receptors. *J Biol Chem* **267**, 6451–6454.

Stone, G.A., Jarvis, M.F., Sills, M.A., Weeks B., Snowhill, E.W., and Williams, M. (1988). Species differences in high-affinity adenosine A_2 binding sites in striatal membranes from mammalian brain. *Drug Dev Res* **15**, 31–46.

Strohmeier, G.R., Reppert, S.M., Lencer, W.I., and Madara, J.L. (1995). The A_{2B} adenosine receptor mediates cAMP responses to adenosine receptor agonists in human intestinal epithelia. *J Biol Chem* **270**, 2387–2394.

Toombs, C.F., McGee, D.S., Johnston, W.E., and Vinten-Johansen, J. (1993). Protection from ischaemic-reperfusion injury with adenosine pretreatment is reversed by inhibition of ATP sensitive potassium channels. *Cardiovasc Res* **27**, 623–629.

Trivedi, B.K., Bridges, A.J., Patt, W.C., Priebe, S.R., and Bruns, R.F. (1989). N^6-Bicycloalkyladenosines with unusually high potency and selectivity for the adenosine A_1 receptor. *J Med Chem* **32**, 8–11

Tucker, A.L., Robeva, A.S., Taylor, H.E., Holeton, D., Bockner, M., Lynch, K.R., and Linden, J. (1994). A_1 adenosine receptors. *J Biol Chem* **269**, 27900–27906.

Ukena, D., Jacobson, K.A., Padgett, W.L., Ayala, C., Shamim, M.T., Kirk, K.L., Olsson, R.O., and Daly, J.W. (1986). Species differences in structure–activity relationships of adenosine agonists and xanthine antagonists at brain A_1 adenosine receptors. *FEBS Lett* **209**, 122–128.

van Calker, D., Müller, M., and Hamprecht, B. (1979). Adenosine regulates via two different types of receptors, the accumulation of cyclic AMP in cultured brain cells. *J. Neurochem* **33**, 999–1005.

Van Daele, P., Van Coevorden, P.P.R., and Boeynaems, J.M. (1992). Effects of adenine nucleotides on the proliferation of aortic endothelial cells. *Circ Res* **70**, 82–90.

Van der Ploeg, I., Ahlberg, S., Parkinson, F.E., Olsson, R.A., and Fredholm, B.B. (1996). Functional characterization of adenosine A_2 receptors in Jurkat cells and PC12 cells using adenosine receptor agonists. *Naunyn-Schmiedeberg's Arch Pharmacol* **353**, 250–260.

Varani, K., Gessi, S., Dalpiaz, A., Ongini, E., and Borea, P.A. (1997). Characterization of A_{2A} adenosine receptors in human lymphocyte membranes by [^{3}H]-SCH 58261 binding. *Br J Pharmacol* **122**, 386–392.

Varani, K., Gessi, S., Dionisotti, S., Ongini, E., and Borea, P.A. (1998). [^{3}H] SCH58261 lebelling of functional A_{2A} adenosine receptors in human neutrophil membranes. *Br J Pharmacol* **123**, 1723–1731.

von Lubitz, D.K.J.E., Lin, R.C.S., Popik, P., Carter, M.F., and Jacobson, K.A. (1994). Adenosine A_3 receptor stimulation and cerebral ischemia. *Eur J Pharmacol* **263**, 59–67.

Walker, B.A.M., Jacobson, M.A., Knight, D.A., Salvatore, C.A., Weir, T., Zhou, D., and Bai, T.R. (1997). Adenosine A_3 receptor expression and function in eosinophils. *Am J Respir Cell Mol Biol* **16**, 531–537.

Wan, W., Sutherland, G.R., and Gieger, J.D. (1990). Binding of the adenosine A_2 receptor ligand [^{3}H]CGS21680 to human and rat brain: evidence for multiple affinity sites. *J Neurochem* **55**, 1763–1771.

Williams, M., Braunwalder, A., and Erickson, T.J. (1986). Evaluation of the binding of the A-1 selective adenosine radioligand, cyclopentyladenosine (CPA), to rat brain tissue. *Naunyn-Schmiedeberg's Arch Pharmacol* **332**, 179–183.

Yakel, J.L., Warren, R.A., Reppert, S.M., and North, R.A. (1993). Functional expression of adenosine A_{2B} receptor in Xenopus oocytes. *Mol Pharmacol* **43**, 277–280.

Zocchi, C., Ongini, E., Ferrara, S., Baraldi, P.G., and Dionisotti, S. (1996). Binding of the radioligand [^{3}H]-SCH 58261, a new non-xanthine A_{2A} adenosine receptor antagonist, to rat striatal membranes. *Br J Pharmacol* **117**, 1381–1386.

Zhou, Q.-Y., Li, C., Olah, M.E., Johnson, R.A., Stiles, G.L., and Civelli, O. (1992). Molecular cloning and characterization of an adenosine receptor: the A_3 adenosine receptor. *Proc Natl Acad Sci USA* **89**, 7432–7436.

CHAPTER **6**

Physiology of Adenosine Receptors in the Striatum

Regulation of Striatal Projection Neurons

AKIHISA MORI

Pharmaceutical Research & Development Center, Kyowa Hakko Kogyo Co., Ltd., Chiyodaku, Tokyo, Japan

TOMOMI SHINDOU

Pharmaceutical Research Institute, Kyowa Hakko Kogyo Co., Ltd., Shuntogun, Shizuoka, Japan

I. INTRODUCTION

The basal ganglia, as well as other brain regions, are governed by an intricate balance between excitation and inhibition, modulation of which has substantial effects on both the physiology and pathology of these brain areas. The striatum is a major component of the basal ganglia, which is a conspicuous complex of nuclei believed to work in strict synergy with the cerebral cortex regulating motor as well as motivational functions. Advances in our understanding of the anatomy and physiology of the basal ganglia are starting to reveal the nature of the neuronal organization of the striatum. In the striatum, the activity of the major output neurons (i.e., medium spiny neurons) is regulated both by excitatory inputs from the cortex and thalamus and by inhibitory inputs from the striatal interneurons and medium spiny neurons. However, lack of fundamental knowledge about the medium spiny neurons has hampered the understanding of striatal function and of motor diseases caused by abnormalities in basal ganglia function.

Considerable attention has been focused on the role of striatal adenosine and the effects caused by A_{2A} receptor stimulation. This is not only because the

A_{2A} receptor is highly expressed in the striatum (see Chapter 2) but also because of findings that adenosine (via the A_{2A} receptor) suppresses intrastriatal inhibitory synaptic transmission (Mori *et al.*, 1996). This differs from the previous belief that, in the mammalian central nervous system (CNS), adenosine suppresses excitatory synaptic transmission through A_1 receptors. In addition to this action of striatal adenosine on medium spiny neurons, A_{2A} receptors have also been shown to regulate cholinergic interneurons (see Chapter 7).

This chapter concentrates on A_{2A} receptor modulation of inhibitory synaptic transmission and relates this to the more general role of adenosine in basal ganglia physiology. Finally, a hypothetical mechanism of action of A_{2A} receptor antagonists in the treatment of Parkinson's disease is proposed.

II. STRIATAL CELL SUBTYPES

Striatal neurons are divided into subgroups according to the transmitter used and their firing patterns. There are 31 million spiny GABAergic projection neurons in the caudate nucleus and putamen of primates, which represent 90–95% of striatal neuronal population (Francois *et al.*, 1996). The somatodendritic and axonal morphology of these neurons has been extensively studied by Golgi and intracellular labeling techniques. These neurons have a medium-size soma $(10-20\ \mu)$ with a large, centrally located smooth nucleus and a thin rim of cytoplasm, and their dendrites are studded with approximately 5000 spines (Wilson, 1990). They are thus referred to as medium spiny neurons. In addition to γ-aminobutyric acid (GABA), they synthesize neuropeptides, including substance P (SP), dynorphin, and enkephaline (Enk). *In vivo*, the spiny cells do not fire tonically, but rather transiently for up to several seconds, and respond directly to stimulation from the cortex and thalamus.

In addition to spiny projection cells containing SP, dynorphin, or Enk, there are three main classes of aspiny interneurons: cholinergic large aspiny cells, parvalbumin-containing GABAergic aspiny cells, and somatostatin/nitric oxide synthase (NOS)-containing aspiny cells. Cholinergic cells represent only 1–5% of the total population of striatal neurons (Aosaki *et al.*, 1995; Kawaguchi *et al.*, 1995). They have large polygonal or fusiform cell bodies with two to five primary dendrites that branch extensively. *In vivo*, they fire tonically but irregularly in response to excitatory synaptic inputs. Parvalbumin cells are GABAergic interneurons and have axons with very dense collateral arborizations within or near their dendritic fields. *In vivo*, they fire more phasically at higher frequencies in response to cortical stimulation than do other striatal cells. Dendrites of somatostatin/NOS cells are not ramified as are the cholinergic or parvalbumin cells, but their axon collaterals extend further than those of other classes of striatal cells. They also contain neuropeptide Y. In addition to these subtypes, there are smaller numbers of striatal cells that have not been physiologically detailed (Kawaguchi, 1997). Also, the existence of intrinsic glutamatergic neurons has been postulated (Mori *et al.*, 1994a, 1994b). Figure 1 in Chapter 1 shows the basic neural connections among the cerebral cortex, basal ganglia, and thalamus.

III. THE STRIATAL MEDIUM SPINY NEURONS

The striatal medium spiny neurons, which are of major physiological importance in regulating voluntary movement, can be subdivided into two main populations. The striatopallidal neurons contain GABA and Enk and project to the external segment of the globus pallidus (GPe) in primates. The other population are the striatonigral and striatoentopeduncular neurons, which contain GABA, SP, and dynorphin and project to the substantial nigra pars reticulata (SNr) and the internal segment of the globus pallidus (GPi) in primates. These two projections can be considered as the origins of the two major output pathways of the basal ganglia-thalamo-cortical circuitry.

Striatal spiny projection neurons receive massive glutamatergic inputs from the cerebral cortex and thalamus. These neurons also receive various intrastriatal GABAergic, cholinergic, and dopaminergic inputs, the latter from the mesencephalic nigra (see review by Alexandar and Crucher, 1990; Gerfen, 1992; Graybiel, 1990). Another synaptic input from glutamatergic interneurons has been suggested (Mori *et al.*, 1994a, 1994b), although this remains to be confirmed anatomically. Characterization of glutamatergic and GABAergic response of spiny projection cells to intrastriatal and cortical stimulation indicates that the main synaptic driving forces of these cells include AMPA/kainate (non-NMDA), N-methyl-D-aspartate (NMDA), and $GABA_A$ responses (Kita, 1996).

Glutamatergic afferent fibers from the cortex and thalamus run straight in the striatum and form en passant synaptic contacts with spine heads of the medium spiny neurons (Fox *et al.*, 1971; Kemp and Powell, 1971), forming a cruciform axodendritic pattern. Thousands of cortical neurons may synapse on a single striatal neuron (Wilson, 1990). The heads of the dendritic spines have both glutamatergic non-NMDA and NMDA receptors (Albin *et al.*, 1992; Kita, 1996).

The GABAergic input onto medium spiny neurons is intrinsic and originates from both their own extensive axon collaterals and GABAergic interneurons, forming intrastriatal inhibitory circuits. The boutons that arise from the local collaterals of spiny neurons form symmetrical inhibitory synapses onto the stalks of dendritic spines, dendritic shafts, somata, and the initial segments of axons of medium spiny neurons (reviewed by Wilson, 1990). GABA released from the axon collaterals would produce strong local mutual inhibition and thereby, provide a mechanism for concentrating the diffuse pattern of the various inputs onto the relevant striatal target system.

Against the common view that the intrastriatal inhibitory feedback circuit is a central organizing principle of striatum function, Jaegar *et al.* (1994) reported that the mutual inhibition among medium spiny neurons is weak or nonexistent in striatal slice preparation *in vitro*. Data (Stern *et al.*, 1998) using intracellular recording from pairs of spiny neurons *in vivo* is compatible with this. Based on the result, it has been proposed that dominant GABAergic response on spiny cells is not feedback but feedforward circuit from GABAergic interneurons onto spiny cells (Kita, 1996; Smith *et al.*, 1998). The axons of the GABAergic interneurons form synapses with the soma and proximal dendrites of spiny neurons (Kita *et al.*, 1990) and GABA released at these synapses may thus serve as part of a striatal feedforward circuit, providing another intrastriatal inhibition mechanism (Kita, 1993, 1996).

In both feedback and feedforward circuits, the release of GABA appears to be tightly regulated by an unidentified neuroactive substance(s) (see review by Kita, 1993). However, the precise roles of these collaterals and interneurons have not been determined or have the mechanisms regulating GABA release from their nerve terminals been described. We have demonstrated that adenosine is one such neuroactive substance regulating the release of GABA in the striatum.

IV. A_{2A} RECEPTOR-MEDIATED SUPPRESSION OF GABAERGIC TRANSMISSION ONTO MEDIUM SPINY NEURONS

A_{2A} receptor immunoreactivity in the rat striatum was shown to be associated primarily with dendritic shafts and spines but was also detected in glia and axon terminals (Rosin *et al.*, 1997, 1998). Immunoreactive terminals often formed symmetric inhibitory synapses and are likely to be those of medium spiny neuron axon collaterals.

It has been revealed, by both neurochemistry (see Chapter 7) and electrophysiology, that the A_{2A} receptor directly serves to suppress intrastriatal GABAergic transmission. In particular, electrophysiological findings demonstrated that A_{2A} receptor modulation is attributable to presynaptic site. This disinhibitory modulation is likely to occur in surround inhibitory inputs among medium spiny neurons through A_{2A} receptors on terminals of recurrent axon collaterals.

A. A_{2A} RECEPTOR SUPPRESSION OF IPSPS AND IPSCS IN MEDIUM SPINY NEURONS

Intracellular recordings of evoked inhibitory postsynaptic potentials (IPSPs) elicited by focal stimulation were made from neurons in slices of adult rat striatum (Mori et al., 1996). The A_{2A} receptor selective agonist CGS 21680 (see Chapter 5) at 1 μM significantly reduced the peak IPSP amplitude to approximately 80% of control without changing the resting membrane potential or the time course of the IPSP. The amplitude was minimally affected by the A_1 receptor selective agonist (S)ENBA (Trivedi et al., 1989) at 0.3 μM. These results suggest that adenosine A_{2A} receptors serve to suppress GABA receptor-mediated inhibitory inputs onto striatal neurons.

To verify this finding, we measured evoked inhibitory postsynaptic currents (IPSCs) with whole-cell patch clamp recording from medium spiny neurons. CGS 21680 significantly reduced the averaged amplitude of evoked IPSCs (Fig. 1A), without affecting the time course of the IPSCs. After drug removal, the IPSC amplitude slowly recovered. The suppression of IPSCs by CGS 21680 was concentration dependent and saturated at 1 μM: 76 ± 8% ($n = 11$, $p < 0.05$), 66 ± 10% ($n = 7$, $p < 0.01$), and 68 ± 10% ($n = 3$) of control at 0.3 μM, 1.0 μM, and 10 μM CGS 21680, respectively (Fig. 1C). The A_{2A} receptor selective antagonist KF17837 (see Chapter 5), when applied together with 1 μM CGS 21680, blocked the inhibitory effect of CGS 21680 in a concentration-dependent fashion: the IPSC amplitudes were 86 ± 7% (N = 6) and 103 ± 4% (N = 8) of control at 0.1 μM and 1 μM of KF17837, respectively. Two different A_1 receptor selective antagonists, DPCPX and KF15372 (both at 0.1 μM), had no effect on the CGS 21680 (1 μM)-induced suppression of the IPSCs at 0.1 μM (Fig. 1B and 1C). For both antagonists, this concentration is sufficient to block A_1 receptors (Lohse et al., 1987; Suzuki et al., 1992). These results demonstrate the existence of A_{2A} receptor-mediated modulation of striatal GABA transmission in the medium spiny neurons. Furthermore, KF17837 alone dose-dependently enhanced the IPSC amplitude: 107 ± 16% ($n = 3$), 122 ± 14% ($n = 4$), and 140 ± 19% ($n = 4$) of control at 1, 3, and 10 μM, respectively. This indicated that endogenous adenosine, present within the striatal slice, suppressed GABA receptor-mediated inhibitory input onto striatal neurons (Mori et al., 1996).

B. PRESYNAPTIC A_{2A} RECEPTOR MODULATION

The A_{2A} receptor-mediated suppression of GABAergic transmission onto medium spiny neurons was shown to be presynaptic by the analysis of spontaneous miniature synaptic events (Mori et al., 1996). In the presence of

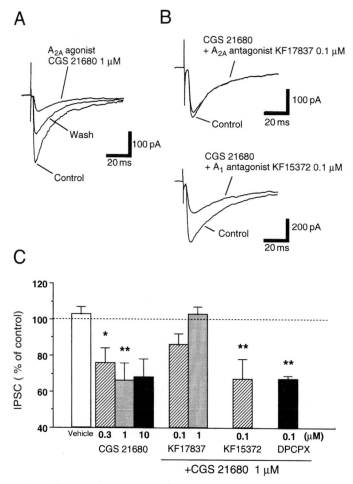

FIGURE 1 The adenosine A_{2A} receptor selectively suppresses GABAergic IPSCs in striatal medium spiny neurons. Effects of CGS 21680 alone and coapplication of CGS 21680 with the A_1 receptor antagonist KF15372 or DPCPX or with the A_{2A} receptor antagonist KF17837 on striatal GABAergic IPSCs, recorded by using the whole-cell patch clamp method from the medium spiny neurons in striatal slices. (A) Superimposed traces of an average of consecutive IPSCs (15 traces) before (control), during, and after (wash) the application of CGS 21680 (1 μM). (B) Typical superimposed traces of average of consecutive IPSCs (12 traces) before (control) and during coapplication of CGS 21680 (1 μM) with KF17837 (0.1 μM) (upper) or with KF15372 (0.1 μM) (lower). (C) Pooled data showing that the suppression by CGS 21680 of IPSCs were dose dependent (0.3–1 μM) and selectively blocked by KF17837. Data represent percentage of control and mean ± SEM (bars) values. Vehicle application had no effect on amplitude of IPSCs (103 ± 4% of control; $n = 15$). $*p < 0.05$, $**p < 0.01$ versus vehicle by Scheffe test. All pooled data were obtained by making a comparison between averaged IPSCs (12–15 traces) before and during drug applications. (From Mori et al., 1996.)

tetrodotoxin to block the propagation of action potentials to the terminals, spontaneous GABA release from presynaptic terminals can be detected as spontaneous miniature inhibitory synaptic currents (mIPSCs). The frequency of these synaptic currents indicates the number of GABA release events from presynaptic terminals, whereas the amplitude indicates the activity of postsynaptic GABA receptor ion channels.

CGS 21680 (1 μM) decreased the mean frequency to approximately 60% of control, whereas the mean amplitude was not changed (Fig. 2A [inset] and 2B). The decrease in the mean frequency slowly recovered after drug removal. In four cells, we were able to collect sufficient numbers of currents for a distribution analysis. There was no significant change in these mIPSC amplitude distributions by assessment of the Kolmogorov–Smirnov test. The typical data are shown in Figure 2A. In striking contrast to the effects of CGS 21680 on mIPSCs, 10 μM KF17837 increased the mean frequency of mIPSCs to approximately 140% of control. In these cells, KF17837 gave no significant

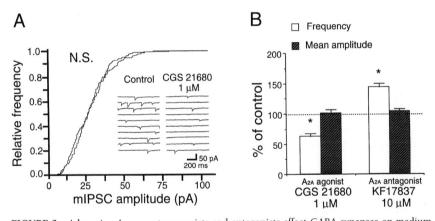

FIGURE 2   Adenosine A_{2A} receptor agonists and antagonists affect GABA synapses on medium spiny neurons at pre- but not postsynaptic sites. (A) (Inset) Typical traces of spontaneous mIPSCs recorded from a medium spiny neuron shown with 10 sweeps in left (control) and right (during CGS 21680 1 μM application). Cumulative probability distributions of mIPSC amplitude in control (175 events) and in 1 μM CGS 21680 (142 events), constructed from the same data, are shown at the inset. There was no statistically significant difference among these distributions as assessed by the Kolmogorov–Smirnov test ($p > 0.4$). The frequencies (Hz) and amplitudes (mean $\pm$ SD, pA) of mIPSCs were 1.05 and 27.5 $\pm$ 11.8 in control, and 0.66 and 27.7 $\pm$ 13.2 in CGS 21680 application, respectively. (B) Pooled data showing that CGS 21680 (1 μM) decreased and KF17837 (10 μM) increased the mean frequency, without affecting the mean amplitude of mIPSCs. Data represent percentage of control and mean $\pm$ SEM (bars) values. Control values of the frequency (Hz) and mean amplitude (pA) of mIPSCs were 0.79 $\pm$ 0.13 and 23.4 $\pm$ 2.5 with CGS 21680 experiment (six cells) and 0.71 $\pm$ 0.13 and 19.7 $\pm$ 1.00 with KF17837 experiment (four cells), respectively. *$p < 0.01$, $n = 4$–6. (From Mori et al., 1996.)

change in either the mean amplitude (Fig. 2B) or the amplitude distribution. These results indicated that CGS 21680 reduced and KF17837 increased the quantal release of transmitter from the presynaptic terminals.

We also examined the effect of CGS 21680 on GABA-induced hyperpolarization (Mori et al., 1996). Using intracellular recording from striatal slices, this was shown to be bicuculline sensitive and thus mediated by GABA$_A$ receptors. Repetitive bath application of 10 mM GABA-induced reproducible responses of a similar amplitude to the evoked IPSPs. CGS 21680 had no effect on the peak amplitude of GABA-induced depolarizing action at both 1 μM and 10 μM. These results demonstrated that the suppression of GABAergic synaptic transmission in the medium spiny neurons was due to presynaptic, but not postsynaptic, A$_{2A}$ receptors.

Presynaptic modulation of GABA release by the A$_{2A}$ appeared to be mediated by the cyclic AMP signaling pathway because CGS 21680 at 1 μM induced both IPSC suppression (Mori et al., 1996) and cyclic AMP accumulation in the striatal slice (see Chapter 5) and cyclic AMP analogues 8-bromo-cyclic AMP and dibutyryl cyclic AMP suppressed IPSCs (Mori et al., 1996).

C. PHYSIOLOGICAL SIGNIFICANCE OF A$_{2A}$ RECEPTOR MODULATION OF GABAERGIC SYNAPTIC TRANSMISSION IN MEDIUM SPINY NEURONS

Both the intrastriatal GABAergic feedback circuit and the feedforward circuit play important roles in the temporal and spatial filtering of inputs from the cortex, other parts of the brain, and striatal interneurons, thus regulating striatal output activity (Groves, 1983; Kita, 1993).

How does A$_{2A}$ receptor-mediated modulation of collateral GABA inputs influence the projection neurons? Kita (1996) proposed a physiological role for the GABAergic input onto the medium spiny neurons. In a simplified schematic representation of the relationship between synaptic input and the membrane potential, the current–voltage relationship of a spiny projection neuron (which possesses strong inward and outward membrane rectifiers) shows the large sigmoid-shaped curve (Fig. 3). The response mediated via GABA$_A$ receptors has a reversal potential near the spike threshold potentials and acts mainly to shunt the glutamatergic inputs. Thus, the GABA input plays a significant role in determining the degree of depolarization of spiny projection neurons. A$_{2A}$ receptor activation could weaken the shunting effect caused by GABA receptor activation, thereby causing the membrane to shift to a depolarizing state. A$_{2A}$ receptor-mediated suppression of IPSPs and IPSCs in the medium spiny neurons was approximately 20–30% (see Fig. 1C). Us-

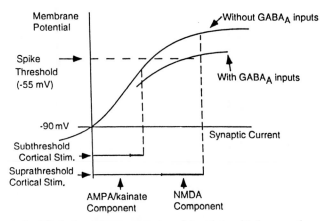

FIGURE 3 A simplified schematic representation of the relationship between the synaptic input and the membrane potential change of medium spiny neurons. The ordinate and abscissa are the membrane potential and total synaptic current, respectively. The large sigmoid-shaped curve represents the current–voltage relationship of a spiny projection neuron, which exhibits strong inward and outward membrane rectification. When weak (subthreshold) cortical stimulation was applied, the main synaptic deriving force was an AMPA/kainate response. In contrast, when strong repetitive (suprathreshold) cortical stimulation was applied, the NMDA response became a significant factor due to relief of the NMDA receptors from Mg-block. The GABA$_A$ receptor response has a reversal potential near the spike threshold potentials and acts mainly to shunt the glutamatergic inputs. For simplification, some details, such as the decrease of the input resistance due to activation of glutamatergic inputs, are ignored in this scheme. (From Kita, 1996.)

ing Kita's model, this degree of modulation would be enough to cause a spiny cell to depolarize to the spike threshold. Interestingly, spiny cells do not fire frequently, but are very active in maintaining subthreshold excitatory potentials. Thus, these cells are not quiet, but busy in determining whether or not to fire at depolarizing episodes (Kawaguchi, 1997). This model therefore suggests a means by which A$_{2A}$ receptor-mediated control of inhibitory inputs onto striatal output cells could exert profound physiological effects on these cells.

There is also the possibility that the A$_{2A}$ receptor controls the feedforward regulation mechanism mediated by the GABA interneurons, but as yet there has been no evidence for these neurons expressing the A$_{2A}$ receptor (Schiffmann *et al.*, 1991a, 1991b).

What does the disinhibition by A$_{2A}$ receptors on recurrent inputs among spiny cells mean physiologically? Because the A$_{2A}$ receptor mRNA is expressed predominantly in the striatopallidal spiny neurons (Schiffmann *et al.*, 1991a), A$_{2A}$ receptor modulation presumably occurs at the synapses formed by collateral axon terminals of striatopallidal medium spiny neurons.

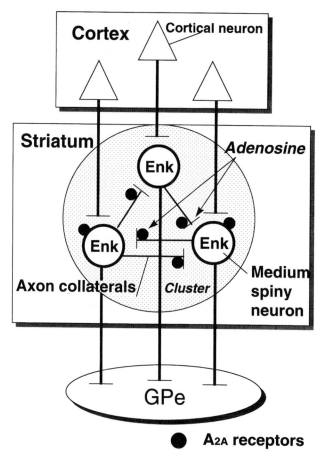

FIGURE 4 Intrastriatal disinhibitory modulation by adenosine via A_{2A} receptors expressed in terminals of recurrent axons of striatopallidal spiny projection neurons. Within a small cluster, Enk-containing neurons projecting to GPe form inhibitory feedback circuits. Endogenous adenosine via A_{2A} receptors in recurrent collaterals tonically suppress GABAergic inhibition, resulting in disinhibition of neurons within the clusters. Thus, adenosine increases the activity of the indirect pathway. This figure also shows that the A_{2A} receptor is expressed in postsynaptic membrane, including soma and dendrites of spiny cells.

Interestingly, SP- and Enk-containing cells are distributed uniformly within the striatum, but spiny cells with the same projection sites may be aggregated into small clusters of cells (Kawaguchi et al., 1990; Loopuijt and van der Kooy, 1985; Paskevich et al., 1991). Therefore, this intrastriatal modulation via A_{2A} receptors may selectively increase the neuronal activity of the striatopallidal indirect pathway by relief of intrastriatal disinhibition within such clusters of GPe-projection neurons (Fig. 4).

Finally, as mentioned previously, no direct synaptic inhibition or electrical interaction among striatal spiny cells has been detected *in vitro* or *in vivo*, using intracellular recordings (Jaeger *et al.*, 1994; Stern *et al.*, 1998). It is possible that endogenous adenosine (via A_{2A} receptors) prevented the detection of mutual inhibition, selectively attenuating recurrent inhibition within striatal projection cell clusters. The activity of adenosine within brain slices is variable but often high (e.g., the A_{2A} receptor antagonist KF17837 enhanced on IPSCs and mIPSCs in striatal slices) (see Fig. 2B). Further analysis of surround inhibition in such clusters should therefore be performed in the presence of A_{2A} receptor antagonists and/or adenosine deaminase.

V. ADENOSINE RECEPTOR MODULATION OF GLUTAMATERGIC SYNAPTIC TRANSMISSION IN THE STRIATUM

The A_1 receptor is widely distributed in the CNS, at both postsynaptic and presynaptic sites, where its stimulation inhibits neurotransmitter release (Fredholm, 1995). In the striatum, as well as in the nucleus accumbens (Uchimura and North, 1991), adenosine has been suggested to presynaptically inhibit synaptic transmission in cortical afferents (Melenka and Kocsis, 1988). Furthermore, A_1, but not A_{2A}, receptor activation has been shown to mimic the depressant effects of adenosine on excitatory synaptic transmission in striatal slices during both whole-cell and field potential recording (Lovinger and Choi, 1995). Flagmeyer *et al.* (1997) reported that adenosine and the A_1 agonist N^6-cyclopentyl adenosine reduced EPSPs of both cortical and thalamic origin by more than 50%. An A_1 antagonist blocked these effects, and the site of action was suggested to be presynaptic. The A_{2A} agonist 5'-(N-cyclopropyl)-carboxamidoadenosine had no effect on excitatory synaptic transmission (Flagmeyer *et al.*, 1997). We have also demonstrated that adenosine receptor activation suppressed glutamatergic EPSCs in striatal medium spiny neurons, an effect blocked by an A_1 receptor antagonist but not by an A_{2A} receptor antagonist (unpublished data). It was therefore concluded that adenosine (via the A_1 receptor on the presynapse) suppressed glutamatergic synaptic transmission onto spiny projection cells. Because the glutamatergic input is the main extrinsic driving force of striatal projection neurons (Kita, 1996), this role of A_1 receptor will be important in the regulation of striatal output activity.

As mentioned, although A_2 receptor activation is likely to have no effect on glutamatergic input to striatal neurons, it remains to be investigated whether postsynaptic A_{2A} receptors on the dendrites and spines of the striatopallidal neurons (Rosin *et al.*, 1997, 1998) regulate the response to the excitatory input. It has been reported that A_{2A} receptor activation by the agonist CGS 21680 inhibits NMDA-induced inward current in medium spiny neurons of rat striatal slices. The mechanism has been suggested to be due to a direct effect on medium spiny neurons rather than to an indirect effect via neighboring presynaptic structures (e.g., corticostriatal afferents) (Norenberg *et al.*, 1997). Furthermore, Norenberg *et al.* (1997) suggested that A_{2A} receptors appear to negatively modulate NMDA receptor channel conductance via the phospholipase C/inositoltriphosphate/Ca^{2+} pathway rather than the adenylate cyclase/ PKA pathway (Norenberg *et al.*, 1998). Chase *et al.* (1998) suggested that the subunit composition and/or phosphorylation state of the NMDA receptors, expressed on the dendritic spines of striatal medium spiny neurons, changes in ways that affect motor performance. It has been proposed that blockade of A_{2A} receptors can therefore affect the internal signaling of striatopallidal neurons and thus elicit antiparkinsonian and/or antidyskinetic activity (Chase, 1998). It is clear that when considering the role of the A_{2A} receptor in the control of motor function, effects on glutamatergic and cholinergic (see Chapter 7) systems, as well as the GABA system outlined in this chapter, should be borne in mind.

VI. INFLUENCE OF ADENOSINE RECEPTOR ACTIVATION ON MEMBRANE PROPERTIES OF MEDIUM SPINY NEURONS

Adenosine, when applied to brain slices, has been reported to have no effects on the membrane properties of striatal neurons (Flagmeyer *et al.*, 1997), including spiny projection neurons (Calabresi *et al.*, 1997). The A_{2A} receptor agonist CGS 21680 (100 nM), the A_1 agonist 2-chloro-N^6-cyclopentyladenosine (CCPA: 10 μM) and the nonselective P1 purinoceptor antagonist 8-(*p*-sulphophenyl)-theophylline (8-SPT: 100 μM) did not alter the resting membrane potential, the threshold current necessary to elicit an action potential, the amplitude of spikes, their rise time, amplitude of the afterhyperpolarization (AHP), or the time to peak of AHP (Norenberg *et al.*, 1997). The lack of adenosine effects on the membrane properties of striatal neurons is incompatible with a previous study showing that adenosine hyperpolarizes striatal neurons cultured from embryonic mice, probably via the activation of an A_1 receptor (Trussel and Jackson, 1985). The effects of adenosine on membrane properties and ion channels of spiny cells are incompletely characterized and still need to be investigated.

VII. ANTIPARKINSONIAN EFFECTS OF A_{2A} RECEPTOR ANTAGONISTS

Parkinson's disease is a common disorder arising from the degeneration of dopaminergic nigrostriatal neurons, and its symptoms are related to abnormal functioning of the basal ganglia (Albin et al., 1989; Chesselet and Delfs, 1996). Two major output pathways from the basal ganglia, the direct striatonigral and indirect striatopallidal pathway, are responsible for smooth and well-coordinated movement (Gerfen, 1992). Dopamine exerts regulatory control on both pathways, mainly via dopamine D_1 receptors on the striatonigral spiny cells and D_2 receptors on the striatopallidal spiny cells (Gerfen et al., 1990), although the specific expression of dopamine receptors by these neurons is probably not absolute (Surmeier et al., 1992). Parkinsonian symptoms can be reproduced in primates treated with the dopaminergic neurotoxin MPTP (1-methyl-4-phenyl-1,2,3,6-tetrahydropyridine; see Chapters 11 and 12). The biochemical, anatomical, and clinical changes produced by systemic treatment of primates by MPTP resemble those found in humans with Parkinson's disease. The introduction of this reliable animal model has considerably advanced the experimental study of parkinsonism (DeLong, 1990). MPTP-induced destruction of the substantia nigra pars compacta (SNc) in monkeys causes increased neuronal firing in GPi and the substantia nigra pars reticulata (SNr) and decreased firing in GPe. This was due to reduced D_1-dopaminergic excitation of the inhibitory striatonigral pathway and to reduced D_2-dopaminergic inhibition of excitatory striatopallidal pathway (Filion et al., 1991). This imbalance has been believed to be the neural correlate of the motor dysfunction in Parkinson's disease.

Current models of the pathophysiology of parkinsonism emphasize changes of the overall activity in the indirect pathway (Albin et al., 1989; DeLong, 1990; Obeso et al., 1997). These models are based on electrophysiological and metabolic studies in macaques (Filion and Tremblay, 1991; Filion et al., 1988; Miller and DeLong, 1988; Mitchell et al., 1989), which provide evidence that a reduction of tonic neuronal activity in GPe by the loss of striatal dopamine leads to disinhibition of the subthalamic nucleus (STN) and, subsequently, to excessive subthalamopallidal drive (Fig. 5). This results in decreased facilitation of cortical motor areas and subsequent development of akinesia and bradykinesia (Obeso et al., 1997; Wichmann and DeLong, 1993).

A_{2A} receptor antagonists may be a promising new therapy for Parkinson's disease (Chapters 9–12). A possible mechanism for the antiparkinsonian efficacy of A_{2A} receptor antagonists, focusing on the regulation of striatopallidal neuronal activity, is outlined in Figure 6. Physiologically, striatal adenosine tonically suppresses GABAergic feedback inhibition via A_{2A} receptors on the

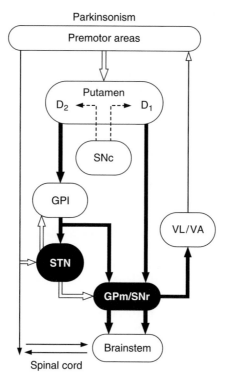

FIGURE 5 Functional modifications associated with lesion of the SNc after MPTP intoxication in monkeys and in Parkinson's disease in humans. Aurgumented excitatory output from STN leads to exaggerated activation of the GPm (the medial globus pallidum: GPi) and SNr, which translates as increased inhibition of the thalamus and brainstem. GPl (the lateral globus pallidus: GPe) excitability is reduced by inhibition from the striatopallidal (D_2 receptor-mediated) projection. (From Obeso *et al.*, 1997.)

collateral axon terminal of striatopallidal medium spiny neurons within small clusters. In the normal state, the inputs onto medium spiny neurons, including both the dopaminergic input via D_2 receptors and the glutamatergic input, are in balance, resulting in appropriate control of the striatopallidal pathway (Fig. 6A). In the parkinsonian state, following loss of the nigrostriatal dopaminergic input, an increase in the rate of firing of the striatopallidal neurons could occur (Fig. 6B), resulting in an imbalance in the activities of the striatopallidal and striatonigral pathways. A_{2A} receptor antagonists block the striatal A_{2A} receptor-induced disinhibition among striatopallidal spiny cells, resulting in increased inhibition, thus suppressing excessive activation of indirect pathway (Fig. 6C) and shifting the striatopallidal/striatonigral neuronal balance toward the normal state. This mechanism of action is

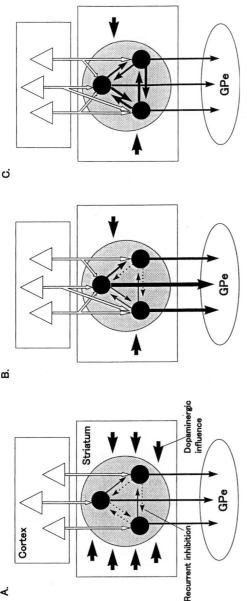

FIGURE 6 Schematic diagram to explain the proposed mechanism of antiparkinsonian efficacy of A$_{2A}$ receptor antagonists in the regulation of striatopallidal neuronal activity. (A) Normal condition, (B) Parkinson's disease, and (C) treatment with A$_{2A}$ antagonists in Parkinson's disease are shown. This figure is based on Figure 4. Open triangles in cortex and closed circles represent cortical neurons and Enk-containing striatopallidal spiny neurons, respectively. The shadow areas in the striatum represent a cluster of cells. Excitatory inputs are depicted as white arrows, and both inhibitory inputs and inhibitory influences are represented by black arrows. In both (B) and (C), the number of arrows representing the dopaminergic influence is reduced, compared with (A), indicating degeneration of the dopaminergic input. Each state leads to different changes in activities of both recurrent inhibition among Enk-containing spiny cells and their projections to the GPe, which is indicated by the thickness of the black arrows. A$_{2A}$ antagonists relieve the intrastriatal disinhibition among projection cells of a cluster, resulting in a more normal output activity (C). Branching of white arrows in (B) and (C) represses the synchronization of spiny cells by changes in glutamatergic input. The synchronization in parkinsonian state might be helpful for the action of A$_{2A}$ antagonist to simultaneously influence on neurons in the cluster.

intrinsically different from that of the dopamine-related modulators used in most parkinsonian therapies.

Synchronization of a neural network can be the result of an external common drive and/or functional connections inside the network. Interestingly, Bergman et al. (1994) reported that, although the firing of neurons in the globus pallidus of normal monkeys is almost always uncorrelated, after dopamine depletion and induction of parkinsonism by treatment with MPTP, oscillatory activity and the firing of many neurons became correlated. As a result, strong rhythmic burst discharges occur in the STN and GPi. Furthermore, in MPTP-treated monkeys, the spiking activity of the tonically active neurons (TANs, identified as striatal cholinergic interneurons; Aosaki et al., 1995; Kawaguchi et al., 1995; Wilson et al., 1990) are also synchronized (Raz et al., 1996). In the pallidum, dopaminergic depletion results in increased coupling of neuronal activity (Nini et al., 1995; Tremblay et al., 1989). From these results, it has been proposed that dopamine acts as a source of desynchronization of spiking activity of the basal ganglia and that a pathophysiological consequence of dopamine depletion in Parkinson's disease is increased synchronization of basal ganglia activity. After the development of parkinsonian symptoms, the networks of basal ganglia lose their ability to maintain previously inhibitory cross-connections between parallel subcircuits. Most dopaminergic synapses in the striatum target the head or neck of a dendritic spine, always with a second, probably cortical, synapse located on the same spine head. Dopamine can therefore modulate the cross-connection among different corticostriatal glutamatergic modules, facilitating independent action of striatopallidal modules in the normal state. Treatment with MPTP results in both increased synchronization and the appearance of oscillatory activity in the pallidum. This suggests that the normal dopaminergic system supports segregation of the functional subcircuits of the basal ganglia and that a breakdown of this independent processing is a hallmark of Parkinson's disease (see Fig. 7 and the review by Bergman et al., 1998). It has been suggested that oscillatory bursting in STN and GPi found in these experiments might be secondary to tonic disinhibition of both structures. Tonic inhibition from the GPe may be reduced after loss of dopamine in the striatum (Raz et al., 1996).

From this consideration of information processing in the basal ganglia of normal and parkinsonian primates, it appears that in the parkinsonian state the corticostriatal glutamatergic input drives neuronal activity of certain spiny projection cells to be synchronized. Recurrent collateral inhibition would be strengthened by such synchronization. Then, A_{2A} receptor antagonists would be more influential on striatopallidal neuronal activity when these cells were synchronized (and firing action potential along recurrent collateral axons), than in the normal state when few of the (unsynchronized cells) would be ac-

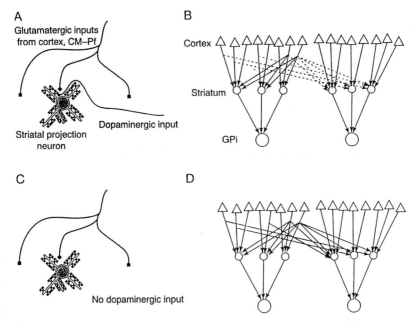

FIGURE 7 Dopamine modulation of functional connectivity in the basal ganglia—a working hypothesis: the main action of dopamine is to regulate the coupling level between the subcircuits of the basal ganglia. In normal state (**A**), dopamine endings on striatal spines can veto divergent glutamatergic inputs to the striatum, thereby reducing the efficacy of cross-connections between channels. (**B**) Diagrammatic model of the resulting segregated channels in the normal state. Broken arrows represent cross-channel connections with reduced efficacy. Following dopamine depletion (**C**) this segregation of afferent channels is lost, resulting in synchronized activation of pallidal cells (**D**). CM-Pf, centromedian-parafascicular nuclei. (From Bergman *et al.*, 1998.)

tive (see Fig. 6). Furthermore, it is possible that adenosine via A_{2A} receptors directly contributes to the appearance of synchronized activity in the parkinsonian state, although little has been known about pathophysiological relationship between adenosine A_{2A} receptors and Parkinson's disease.

VIII. CONCLUSION

This chapter focused on the physiological significance of striatal adenosine acting via A_{2A} receptors. Based on the hypothesis for the functional role of adenosine in the striatopallidal pathway, we propose a mechanism of action of A_{2A} receptor antagonists in their control of motor behavior. The extensive work on striatal adenosine and basal ganglia physiology have introduced new insights into our understanding of the relationship between adenosine and motor control and suggested a new therapeutic approach for Parkinson's disease. However, a number of aspects require further investigation: 1) the precise loci of adenosine receptor subtypes on medium spiny neurons; 2) long-term regulation of synaptic input, in particular, the glutamatergic system via adenosine receptors; 3) the function of A_{2A} receptors expressed in the soma and postsynaptic membrane of medium spiny neurons; and 4) pathophysiological evidence for the mechanism of antiparkinsonian efficacy of A_{2A} receptor antagonists proposed in this chapter.

REFERENCES

Albin, R.L., Makowiec, R.L., Hollingsworth, Z.R., Dure, L.S., IV, Penny, J.B., and Young, A.B. (1992). Excitatory amino acid binding sites in the basal ganglia of the rat. *Neurosci* **46**, 35–48.

Albin, R.L., Young, A.B., and Penny, J.B. (1989). The functional anatomy of basal ganglia disorders. *Trends Neurosci* **12**, 366–375.

Alexander, G.E., and Crutcher, M.D. (1990). Functional architecture of basal ganglia circuits: neuronal substrates of processing. *Trends Neurosci* **13**, 266–271.

Aosaki, T., Kimura, M., and Graybiel, A.M. (1995). Temporal and spatial characteristics of tonically active neurons of the primate's striatum. *J Neurophysiol* **73**, 1234–1252.

Bergman, H., Wichmann, T., Karmon, B., and DeLong, M.R. (1994). The primate subthalamic nucleus. II: neuronal activity in the MPTP model of parkinsonism. *J Neurophysiol* **72**, 507–520.

Bergman, H., Feingold, A., Nini, A., Raz, A., Slovin, H., Abeles, M., and Vaadia, E. (1998). Physiological aspects of information processing in the basal ganglia of normal and parkinsonian primates. *Trends Neurosci* **21**, 32–38.

Calabresi, P., Centonze, D., Pisani, A., and Bernardi, G. (1997). Endogenous adenosine mediates the presynaptic inhibition induced by aglycemia at corticostriatal synapses. *J Neurosci* **17**, 4509–4516.

Chase, T.N. (1998). Novel approaches to the palliation of Parkinson's disease. *Movement Disorder* **13**, M39.

Chase, T.N., Oh, J.D., and Blanchet, P.J. (1998). Neostriatal mechanism in Parkinson's disease. *Neurology* **51**, S30–S35.

Chesselet, M.F., and Delfs, J.M. (1996). Basal ganglia and movement disorder: an update. *Trends Neurosci* **19**, 417–422.

DeLong, M.R. (1990). Primate model of movement disorders of basal ganglia origin. *Trends Neurosci* **13**, 281–285.

Filion, M., and Tremblay, L. (1991). Abnormal spontaneous activity of globus pallidus neurons in monkeys with MPTP-induced parkinsonism. *Brain Res* **547**, 142–151.

Filion, M., Tremblay, L., and Bedard, P.J. (1988). Abnormal influences of passive limb movement on the activity of globus pallidus neurons in parkinsonian monkeys. *Brain Res* **444**, 165–176.

Filion, M., Tremblay, L., and Bedard, P.J. (1991). Effects of dopamine agonists on the spontaneous activity of globus pallidus neurons in monkeys with MPTP-induced parkinsonism. *Brain Res* **547**, 152–161.

Flagmeyer, I., Haas, H.L., and Stevens, D.R. (1997). Adenosine A_1 receptor-mediated depression of corticostriatal and thalamostriatal glutamatergic synaptic potentials in vitro. Brain Res. 778, 178–185.

Fox, C.A., Andrade, A.N., Hillman, D.E., and Schwyn, R.C. (1971). The spiny neurons in the primate striatum: a Golgi and electron microscopes study. J fur Hirnforshung 13, 181–201.

Francois, C., Yelink, J., Arecchi-Bouchhioua, P., and Percheron, G. (1996). Branching pattern and geometrical properties of dendritic and axonal arborizations in the striato-pallido-thalamic system in macaques. In "The Basal Ganglia V" (C. Ohye, Mi. Kumura, and J.S. McKenzie, eds.), pp. 43–58, Prenum Press, New York.

Fredholm, B.B. (1995). Purinoceptors in the nervous system. Pharmacol Toxicol 76, 228–239.

Gerfen, C.R. (1992). The neostriatal mosaic: multiple levels of compartmental organization in the basal ganglia. Ann Rev Neurosci 15, 285–320.

Gerfen, C.R., Engber, T.M., Mahan, L.C., Susel, Z., Chase T.N., Monsma, F.J., and Sibley, D.R. (1990). D_1 and D_2 dopamine receptor-regulated gene expression of striatonigral and striatopallidal neurons. Science 250, 1429–1432.

Graybiel, A.M. (1990). Neurotransmitters and neuromodulators in the basal ganglia. Trends Neurosci 13, 244–254.

Groves, P.M. (1983). A theory of the functional organization of the neostriatum and the neostriatal control of voluntary movement. Brain Res Rev 5, 109–132.

Jaeger, D., Kita, H., and Wilson, C.J. (1994). Surround inhibition among projection neurons is weak or nonexistent in the rat neostriatum. J Neurophysiol 72, 2555–2558.

Kawaguchi, Y., Wilson, C.J., and Emson, P.C. (1990). Projection subtypes of rat neostriatal matrix cells revealed by intracellular injection of biocytin. J Neurosci 10, 3421–3438.

Kawaguchi, Y., Wilson, C.J., Augood, S.J., and Emson, P.C. (1995). Striatal interneurons: chemical, physiological and morphological characterization. Trends Neurosci 18, 527–535.

Kawaguchi, Y. (1997). Neostriatal cell subtypes and their functional role. Neurosci Res 27, 1–8.

Kemp, J.M., and Powell, T.P.S. (1971). The structure of the caudate nucleus of the cat: light and electron microscopy. Philos Trans Roy Soc Lond B262, 383–401.

Kita, H. (1993). GABAergic circuits of the striatum. In "Progress in Brain Research 99" (G.W. Arbuthnott and P.C. Emson, eds.), pp. 51–72, Elsevier Science, Amsterdam.

Kita, H. (1996). Glutamatergic and GABAergic postsynaptic responses of striatal spiny neurons to intrastriatal and cortical stimulation recorded in slice preparations. Neurosci 70, 925–940.

Kita., H., Kosaka, T., and Heizmann, C.W. (1990). Parvalbumin immunoreactive neurons in the rat neostriatum: a light and electron microscopic study. Brain Res 536, 1–15.

Lohse, M.J., Klotz, K.N., Lindenborn-Fotinos, J., Reddington, M., Schwabe, U., and Olsson, R.A. (1987). 8-Cyclopentyl-1,3-dipropylxanthine (DPCPX)—a selective high affinity antagonist radioligand for A_1 adenosine receptors. Naunyn-Schmiedeberg's Arch Pharmacol 336, 204–210.

Loopuijt, L.D., and van der Kooy, D. (1985). Organization of the striatum: collateralization of its efferent axons. Brain Res 348, 86–99.

Lovinger, D.M., and Choi, S. (1995). Activation of adenosine A_1 receptors initiates short-term synaptic depression in rat striatum. Neurosci Lett 199, 9–12.

Melenka, R.C. and Kocsis, J.D. (1988). Presynaptic inhibition of carbachol and adenosine on cortical synaptic transmission. J Neurosci 8, 3750–3756.

Miller, W.C., and DeLong, M.R. (1988). Parkinsonian symptomatology: an anatomical and physiological analysis. Ann NY Acad Sci 515, 287–302.

Mitchell, I.J., Clark, C.E., Boyce, S., Robertson, R.G., Peggs, D., Sambrook, M.A., and Crossman, A.R. (1989). Neural mechanisms underlying parkinsonian symptoms based upon regional uptake of 2-deoxyglucose in monkeys exposed to 1-methyl-4-phenyl-1,2,3,6-tetrahydropyridine. Neurosci 32, 213–226.

Mori, A., Shindou, T., Ichimura, M., Nonaka, H., and Kase, H. (1996). The role of adenosine A_{2A} receptors in regulating GABAergic synaptic transmission in striatal medium spiny neurons. *J Neurosci* **16**, 605–611.

Mori, A., Takahashi, T., Miyashita, Y., and Kasai, H. (1994a). Two distinct glutamatergic synaptic inputs to striatal medium spiny neurones of neonatal rats and paired-pulse depression. *J Physiol (Lond)* **476**, 217–228.

Mori, A., Takahashi, T., Miyashita, Y., and Kasai, H. (1994b). Quantal properties of H-type glutamatergic synaptic input to the striatal medium spiny neurons. *Brain Res* **654**, 177–179.

Nini, A., Feingold, A., Slovin, H., and Bergman, H. (1995). Neurons in the globus pallidus do not show correlated activity in the normal monkeys, but phase-locked oscillations appear in the MPTP models of parkinsonism. *J Neurophysiol* **74**, 1800–1805.

Norenberg, W., Wirkner, K., Assmann, H., Richter, M., and Illes, P. (1998). Adenosine A_{2A} receptors inhibit the conductance of NMDA receptor channels in rat neostriatal neurons. *Amino Acids* **14**, 33–39.

Norenberg, W., Wirkner, K., and Illes, P. (1997). Effects of adenosine and some of its structural analogues on the conductance of NMDA receptor channels in subset of rat neostriatal neurons. *Br J Pharmacol* **122**, 71–80.

Obeso, J.A., Rodriguez, M.C., and DeLong, M.R. (1997). Basal ganglia pathophysiology: a critical review. In "Advances in Neurology" (J.A. Obeso, M.R. DeLong, and C.D. Marsden, eds.), Vol. 74, pp. 3–18, Lippincott-Raven, Philadelphia.

Paskevich, P.A., Evans, H.K., and Domesick, V.B. (1991). Morphological assessment of neuronal aggregates in the striatum of the rat. *J Comp Neurol* **305**, 361–369.

Raz, A., Feingold, A., Zelanskaya, V., Vaadia, E., and Bergman, H. (1996). Neuronal synchronization of tonically active neurons in the striatum of neuronal and parkinsonian primates. *J Neurophysiol* **76**, 2083–2088.

Rosin, D.L., Botkin, S., and Lindin, J. (1997). Ultrastructual localization of adenosine A_{2A} receptor immunoreactivity in rat striatum. *Soc Neurosci Abstr* **23**, 1494.

Rosin, D.L., Robeva A., Woodard R.L., Guyenet P.G., Linden J. (1998). Immunohistochemical localization of adenosine A_{2A} receptors in the rat central nervous system. *J. Comp Neurol* **401**, 163–186.

Schiffmann, S.N., Jacobs, O., and Vanderhaeghen, J.-J. (1991a). Striatal restricted adenosine A_2 receptor (RDC8) is expressed by enkephalin but not by substance P neurons: an *in situ* hybridization histochemistry study. *J Neurochem* **57**, 1062–1067.

Schiffmann, S.N., Libert, F., Vassart, G., and Vanderhaeghen, J.-J. (1991b). Distribution of adenosine A_2 receptor mRNA in the human brain. *Neurosci Lett* **130**, 177–181.

Smith, Y., Bevan, M.D., Shink, E., and Bolam, J.P. (1998). Microcircuitry of the direct and indirect pathways of the basal ganglia *Neurosci* **86**, 353–387.

Stern, E.A., Jaeger, D., and Wilson, C.J. (1998). Membrane potential synchrony of simultaneously recorded striatal spiny neurons *in vivo*. *Nature* **394**, 475–478.

Surmeier, D.J., Eberwine, J., Wilson, C.J., Cao, Y., Stefani, A., and Kitai, S.T. (1992). Dopamine receptor subtypes colocalize in rat striatonigral neurons. *Proc Natl Acad Sci USA* **89**, 10178–10182.

Suzuki, F., Shimada, J., Mizumoto, H., Karasawa, A., Kubo, K., Nonaka, H., Ishii, A., and Kawakita, T. (1992). Adenosine A_1 antagonists. 2. Structure–activity relationships on diuretic activities and protective effects against acute renal failure. *J Med Chem* **35**, 3066–3075.

Tremblay, L., Filion, M., and Bedard, P.J. (1989). Responses of pallidal neurons to striatal stimulation in monkeys with MPTP-induced parkinsonism. *Brain Res* **498**, 17–33.

Trivedi, B.K., Bridges, A.J., Patt, W.C., Priebe, S.R., and Bruns, R.F. (1989). N^6-Bicycloalkyladenosine with unusually high potency and selectivity for adenosine A_1 receptor. *J Med Chem* **32**, 8–11.

Trussel, L.O., and Jackson, M.B. (1985). Adenosine-activated potassium conductance in cultured striatal neurons. *Proc Natl Acad Sci USA* **82**, 4857–4861.

Uchimura, N., and North R.A. (1991). Baclofen and adenosine inhibit synaptic potentials mediated by aminobutyric acid and glutamate release in rat nucleus accumbens. *J Pharmacol Exp Ther* **258**, 663–668.

Wichmann, T., and DeLong, M.R. (1993). Pathophysiology of parkinsonan motor abnormalities. In "Advances in Neurology," (H. Narabayashi, T. Nagatu, N. Yanagisawa, and Y. Mizuno, Eds.), Vol. 60, pp. 53–61, Raven Press, New York.

Wilson, C.J. (1990). Basal ganglia, In "The Synaptic Organization of the Brain" (G.W. Shepherd, Ed) pp. 279–316, Oxford University Press, New York.

Wilson, C.J., Chang, H.T. and Kitai, S.T. (1990). Firing patterns and synaptic potentials of identified giant aspiny interneurons in the rat neostriatum. *J Neurosci* **10**, 508–519.

CHAPTER 7

Regulation of Neurotransmitter Release in Basal Ganglia by Adenosine Receptor Agonists and Antagonists *in Vitro* and *in Vivo*

PETER J. RICHARDSON
Department of Pharmacology, University of Cambridge, Cambridge, United Kingdom

MASAKO KUROKAWA
Kyowa Hakko Kogyo Co., Ltd., Pharmaceutical Research Laboratories, Nagaizumi-cho, Sunto-gun, Shizuoka, Japan

I. INTRODUCTION

The control of neurotransmitter release is a fundamental property of neuromodulators such as adenosine, and one that can be used to localize receptors as well as increase our overall understanding of adenosine action. In combination with other techniques, including electrophysiology (see Chapter 6), receptor autoradiography, and *in situ* hybridization (see Chapter 2), the fundamental mechanisms by which adenosine and its receptors control motor behavior can be elucidated.

Adenosine is usually regarded as a neuroprotecting agent and/or a retaliatory metabolite (Newby, 1984). However, adenosine receptor ligands have profound and diverse effects on transmitter release in the central nervous system (CNS), which suggest additional roles for this nucleoside in the control of neuronal activity. The ubiquitous distribution of adenosine and our poor understanding of the processes that control its extracelluar concentrations have complicated investigations into the physiological roles of this nucleoside. Thus, although resting extracellular concentrations are believed to be approximately 40 nM (e.g., Ballarin *et al.*, 1991) and large increases are seen under ischemic conditions, little is known of the fine control of extracelluar adenosine levels and, thus, of adenosine receptor activity. There are two major sources of extracelluar adenosine: it is a product of ectophosphohydrolase enzymes present on the surface of many cells that break down presynaptically released ATP (e.g., Cunha *et al.*, 1994; Richardson and Brown, 1987a), and it is released from a number of cells via reversal of adenosine transporters, under conditions of metabolic stress or intense stimulation (Cunha *et al.*, 1996a; Lloyd *et al.*, 1993; Mitchell *et al.*, 1993; Richardson and Brown, 1987a). The relative contribution of these two sources of adenosine is hard to assess *in situ*, although in brain slices, adenosine derived from released adenosine triphosphate (ATP) appears to be important at high rates of stimulation (Cunha *et al.*, 1996; See Section III,C). Of interest in the context of adenosine and potential therapies of Parkinson's disease is the observation that, in the rat striatum, lesioning of the nigrostriatal pathway has no effect on extracelluar adenosine concentrations (Herrera-Marschitz *et al.*, 1994). This is despite the observation from numerous studies that the adenosine A_{2A} receptor has profound effects on gene expression in such lesioned striata but little effect when dopamine levels are normal (see Chapter 8).

II. METHODOLOGY

In general, release of transmitter from CNS tissue preparations *in vitro* is evoked by electrical stimulation, elevated potassium concentrations, or sodium channel binding toxins such as veratridine. Obviously, the nature of the stimulus can influence the effectiveness of adenosine receptor agonists because the ability of the receptor to affect release will depend on the second messenger/effector systems involved, and these may be bypassed by (for instance) depolarization mediated by elevated potassium concentrations. In most preparations, the pools of transmitter are radiolabeled by prior incubation with a labeled metabolic percussor (e.g., ^{3}[H]-choline) or the transmitter itself (e.g., ^{3}[H]-γ-amino butyric acid [GABA]). The ability of selective agonists and antagonist to affect the evoked release of radiolabel can then be investigated. There are three main preparations used to assess receptor influence on transmitter release. The first involves the use of isolated nerve terminals (synaptosomes), which can be used to study the effects of (presynaptic) nerve terminal receptors on transmitter release. The second is brain slices where the effect of receptors on different parts of neurons and the interplay between neurons have to be considered when assessing the results because glial and neuronal interconnections are largely maintained. The most serious problem with both of these *in vitro* techniques is the variable nature of the release process in different slices or batches of synaptosomes, so appropriate controls are required in each experiment. The dual (or multiple) stimulus protocol is widely used, in which every slice or batch of synaptosomes first receives a depolarizing stimulus (e.g., elevated potassium concentrations or electrical stimulation) and then, after a recovery period, is restimulated in the presence of the appropriate ligand. The ratio of the amount of transmitter released by the two depolarizing stimuli, when compared with a control that only received the depolarizing stimuli, gives an indication of the effect of the ligand (e.g., Brown *et al.*, 1990; Jin *et al.*, 1993; Kirk and Richardson, 1994; Richardson *et al.*, 1987; Fig. 1). The slice preparation can also be used successfully to assess the release of endogenous neurotransmitters detected electrophysiologically by assessing their actions on neurons within the slice (Mori *et al.*, 1996; see Chapter 6). Finally, *in vivo* intrastriatal dialysis has been widely used to estimate the transmitter concentration in the intercellular space of the living brain. This probably estimates transmitter overflow from active synapses and, thus, can be used as a measure of the activity of transmitters in a given brain region, in either the presence or the absence of specific stimuli. Each approach has its advantages and disadvantages. For example, the use of synaptosomes restricts the investigation to the nerve terminal but simplifies the analysis because there is no need to consider the effect of other

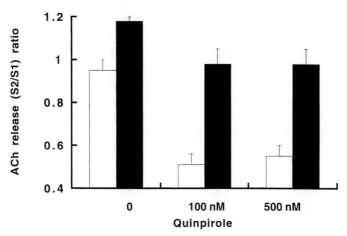

FIGURE 1   CGS 21680 reverses the dopamine receptor-mediated inhibition of ACh release. The release of ^{3}H-ACh from perfused striatal synaptosomes was evoked with 15 mM KCl in a dual superfusion experiment (as described in Gubitz *et al.*, 1996) and the amount of radioactivity released by the second stimulus (S2) expressed as a ratio of that released by the first stimulus (S1). Inclusion of CGS 21680 (0.1 nM, black bars) in S2 increased the release by approximately 20%. The dopamine receptor agonist quinpirole (white bars) inhibited the release of by approximately 40%, an effect almost completely reversed by CGS 21680.

transmitters on the nerve terminals being studied (Kurokawa *et al.*, 1994). The slice preparation permits analysis of the effect of the receptor on transmitter release wherever it is expressed on the nerve but can suffer from complications arising from variable access to deep layers of the slice and from interactions among the many structures present within the slice. In both synaptosomal preparations and slices, different populations of nerve terminals releasing the same transmitter are likely to be present, which also complicates the analysis. Intracerebral microdialysis is used to determine whether receptor ligands have measurable effects on transmitter release *in vivo* but, as with some synaptosome preparations and slices, it can be difficult to determine on which cells and/or nerve terminals the drug is acting.

Early studies on the ability of adenosine to affect transmitter release demonstrated an inhibition of acetylcholine (ACh) release from the neuromuscular junction (Ginsborg and Hirst, 1972; Ribeiro and Walker, 1975). Most of the early studies (reviewed by Phillis and Wu, 1981) of adenosine receptor effects on central neurons were performed on rat brain slices and synaptosomes, and adenosine was shown to inhibit the release of ACh, dopamine, norepinephrine, serotonin, GABA, and glutamate (Dolphin and Prestwich, 1985; Harms *et al.*, 1978; 1979; Hollins and Stone, 1980; Michaelis *et al.*, 1979). Since the advent of receptor specific ligands for the A_1 and A_{2A} receptors (see Chapter 3) and the cloning of the adenosine receptors, it has become easier to determine the receptors responsible for the observed actions of adenosine. In the basal ganglia, most attention has focused on the actions of the A_1 and $_{2A}$ receptors, which are expressed at moderate (A_1) to high (A_{2A}) levels in the striatum (see Chapter 2). A number of effects ascribed to A_2 receptors are probably mediated by the A_{2B} receptor, but in the absence of specific ligands, there is little known of the role of this receptor in the control of neurotransmitter release. Similarly, selective ligands for the A_3 receptor have only recently been produced and, as yet, there is little information about the role of this receptor in basal ganglia neurons.

III. THE ADENOSINE A_1 RECEPTOR IN THE BASAL GANGLIA

A. LOCALIZATION OF THE A_1 RECEPTOR

The localization of adenosine receptors in the basal ganglia was originally determined using neurotoxins such as kainic acid, which revealed the A_1 receptor to be present on both intrinsic striatal neurons and corticostriatal nerve terminals (Alexander and Reddington, 1989; Goodman and Snyder, 1982;

Wojcik and Neff, 1983). Studies of neurotransmitter release showed the A_1 receptor to be present on the dopaminergic nerve terminals of the nigrostriatal neurons (Harms *et al.*, 1979), glutamatergic terminals of the corticostriatal pathway (Malenka and Kocsis, 1988), and the nerve terminals of the striatal cholinergic interneurons (Richardson and Brown, 1987a). Immunohistochemistry has confirmed these results showing that in the striatum and globus pallidus approximately 40% of the intrinsic neurons express the A_1 reeptor (Rivkees *et al.*, 1995). Adenosine A_1 receptor mRNA has also been shown to be present in the striatum by *in situ* hybridization and RT-PCR (see Chapter 2; Dixon *et al.*, 1996; Ferré *et al.*, 1996). The results of these approaches have been largely consistent and suggest that this receptor is expressed in multiple sites in the striatum, including intrinsic GABAergic and cholinergic neurons as well as on the terminals of the major afferent pathways.

B. MECHANISM OF ACTION OF THE ADENOSINE A_1 RECEPTOR

The A_1 receptor couples preferentially to Gi and Go G-proteins, causing inhibition of adenylyl cyclase in a pertussis toxin-sensitive manner. Although the precise secondary messenger and effector systems employed by the A_1 receptor are likely to vary in different cells, other effector systems controlled by this receptor include opening of K^+ channels and inhibition of Ca^{2+} channels (reviewed by Palmer and Stiles, 1995). However, in general, adenosine A_1 receptor-mediated control of transmitter release is seldom affected by K^+ channel blockers, such as tetraethylammonium, 4-aminopyridine (Cass and Zahniser, 1991), and glibenclamide (Calabresi *et al.*, 1997), suggesting that the control of potassium channels is not a major effector system of the neuronal adenosine A_1 receptor. In contrast, there is abundant evidence that the A_1 receptor inhibits Ca^{2+} channel activity in various parts of the brain. More than one type of voltage sensitive Ca^{2+} channel is regulated by this receptor, including L-, N-, P-, and perhaps Q-type channels (Mei *et al.*, 1996; Mogul *et al.*, 1993; Umemiya and Berger, 1994; Wu and Sggau, 1994). In addition to these mechanisms of action, both inhibition and stimulation of phospholipase C by the A_1 receptor have been observed, although its relevance to the action of this receptor in the CNS is unclear (Palmer and Stiles, 1995).

C. A_1 RECEPTOR MODULATION OF ACh RELEASE

The A_1 receptor has been shown to inhibit veratridine evoked release of acetylcholine from striatal synaptosomes (Brown *et al.*, 1990; Kirk and

Richardson, 1994). Similarly, A_1 receptor selective agonists inhibit electrically evoked release of acetylcholine from striatal slices (Jin *et al.*, 1993), consistent with the detection of mRNA encoding this receptor in the large (i.e., cholinergic) neurons of the rat striatum (Dixon *et al.*, 1996). It is possible that *in situ* much of the adenosine controlling acetylcholine release in the striatum is derived from extracelluar ATP because the striatal cholinergic nerve terminal releases ATP on depolarization (Richardson and Brown, 1987b). This ATP is then broken down on the surface of these nerve endings, resulting in the production of sufficient adenosine to inhibit further transmitter release via an action at the A_1 receptor (Richardson *et al.*, 1987). The role of this feedback is not clear, because under condition of high transmitter release, the ATP breakdown pathway would be inhibited by subsequently released ATP (James and Richardson, 1993). This suggests that the feedback may only operate under conditions of low to moderate stimulation or, alternatively, that adenosine is only produced in bursts after transmitter release has ceased. Because these nerve terminals also bear adenosine A_{2A} receptors (Brown *et al.*, 1990; see Section IV,C), the role of this feedback *in situ* may be quite complex. In the striatum, the stimulation dependence of the balance between feedback inhibition (via the A_1 receptor) and stimulation (via the A_{2A} receptor) has not been clarified, although it has in similar situations described by Correia de Sá *et al.* (1996) at the rat diaphragm neuromuscular junction and by Cunha *et al.* (1996b) in the hippocampus. In all three situation, it appears that ATP released upon stimulation from the nerve terminal is degraded to adenosine, which subsequently feeds back on presynaptic receptors. The contribution of such ATP-derived adenosine appears to outweight that of directly released adenosine in some experimental situations, such as the immunopurfied cholinergic nerve terminal (Richardson *et al.*, 1987) and the neuromuscular junction (Cunha *et al.*, 1996a), although it is often difficult to assess the relative importance *in situ* of directly released adenosine and ATP-derived adenosine.

D. A_1 RECEPTOR MODULATION OF GABA RELEASE

The A_1 receptor is expressed in a subpopulation of the medium spiny output neurons of the striatum, including neurons expressing either tachykinins or enkephalin (Ferré *et al.*, 1996). This receptor has been shown to inhibit GABA release in the cerebral cortex (Hollins and Stone, 19980), the nucleus accumbens (Uchimura and North, 1991), and the substantia nigra (Wu *et al.*, 1995). However, in striatal synaptosome preparations, the A_1 receptor agonist *R*-phenylisopropyladenosine (*R*-PIA) failed to inhibit potassium (15 mM)-evoked GABA release from nerve terminals (Kirk and Richardson, 1994). In addition, adenosine A_1 receptor agonists had no effect on synaptically evoked GABA release in striatal slices (Mori *et al.*, 1996). *In vivo* extracelluar GABA levels (as measured by microdialysis) in the striatum were, however, reduced by the A_1 receptor agonist cyclopentyladenosine (CPA), although this effect may have been mediated in part by inhibition of glutamate release from corticostriatal nerve terminals (Ferré *et al.*, 1996). These authors also observed that intrastriatal infusion of the A_1-selective agonist CPA counteracted the stimulatory effects of dopamine D_1 receptor agonists (infused into the striatum) on entopeduncular GABA concentrations, suggesting that the striatal A_1 receptor serves at least in part to control the striato-Gpi/entopeduncular pathway. This observation is part of the evidence suggesting that there is a site of adensine–dopamine interaction in the striato-Gpi/entopeduncular neurons (of the direct pathway; see Chapter 1), some of which express both A_1 and D_1 receptors (Ferré *et al.*, 1997). In addition, A_1 receptors are also present in the globus pallidus and substantia nigra, although probably primarily on GABAergic nerve terminals in these areas (e.g., Mayfield *et al.*, 1993, 1996).

E. A_1 Receptor Modulation of Dopamine Release

Other neurotransmitter systems affected by the A_1 receptor in the basal ganglia include the nigrostriatal nerve terminals, where electrically stimulated release of dopamine in striatal slices is inhibited by adenosine receptor agonists, in a manner inhibited by the A_1-selective antagonist DPCPX (Jin *et al.*, 1993; Lupica *et al.*, 1990). Similar effects have been seen *in vivo*, where adenosine agonists reduce extracelluar dopamine concentrations (Zetterstrom and Fillenz, 1990). Other *in vivo* dialysis studies suggest that both A_1 and A_2 receptors may be present on striatal dopaminergic nerve terminals but that the inhibitory effect of the A_1 receptor predominates (Okada *et al.*, 1996a). High extracelluar Mg^{2+} concentrations potentiate the action of the A_1 receptor, consistent with an inhibitory effect of this receptor on Ca^{2+} channels (Okada *et al.*, 1996b). The precise location and subtype of the A_2 receptor mediating the stimulatory effects on dopamine release remain to be determined (see Section IV,E).

F. A_1 Receptor Modulation of Glutamate Release

Glutamate release is inhibited by adenosine A_1 receptors from a variety of CNS synapses, including those of the corticostriatal pathway (Lovinger and

Choi, 1995; Malenka and Kocsis, 1988). Corticostriatal glutamatergic transmission is also inhibited under condition of aglycemia, an effect mediated by endogenous adenosine action on the release of glutamate from these nerve terminals (Calabresi *et al.*, 1997). *In vivo*, extracelluar levels of glutamate in the striatum are increased by the nonselective A_1/A_2 receptor antagonist 8-phenyltheophylline, probably by blockade of the A_1 receptor on the corticostriatal nerve terminals (Corsi *et al.*, 1997). This inhibitory action of adenosine A_1 receptors on excitatory transmission is seen in many areas of the brain and may contribute to the neuroprotectant properties of adenosine receptor agonists (Ramkumar *et al.*, 1995; Rudolphi *et al.*, 1992).

IV. THE ADENOSINE A_2 RECEPTORS IN THE BASAL GANGLIA

The existence of two A_2 receptors was first recognized on the basis of differences in their sensitivity to adenosine and the apparent inability of the A_{2B} receptor to stimulate adenylyl cyclase in broken membrane preparations (see Bruns *et al.*, 1987). However, prior to the advent of A_{2A} receptor selective ligands and the cloning of the A_{2A} and A_{2B} receptors, it was often difficult to distinguish between the effects of these adenosine receptors.

A. LOCALIZATION OF THE A_2 RECEPTORS

The use of selective neurotoxins and A_2 receptor stimulation of adenylyl cyclase suggested that most A_2 receptors are expressed in intrinsic striatal neurons (Wojcik and Neff, 1983). Lee and Reddington (1986) then showed the presence of another non-A_1 binding site distributed throughout the brain, which was consistent with the proposal of Daly *et al.* (1983), who suggested that a low-affinity A_2 receptor (A_{2B}) was distributed throughout the brain, whereas the other (the A_{2A}) was restricted to the basal ganglia. The receptor identified by Wojcik and Neff (1983) probably corresponded to the A_{2A} receptor because autoradiography using ^{3}H-CGS 21680 showed the A_{2A} receptor to be restricted to the caudate putamen, nucleus accumbens, and olfactory tubercle (Jarvis *et al.*, 1989). After cloning of these two receptors, such a distribution was confirmed, the A_{2B} receptor mRNA being detectable throughout the brain but in insufficient quantities to allow its precise localization to be determined (Dixon *et al.*, 1996; Stehle *et al.*, 1992). In contrast, the A_{2A} receptor was localized to the striatopallidal neurons of the basal ganglia (Augood and Emson, 1994; Dixon *et al.*, 1996; Pollack *et al.*, 1993; Schiffmann *et al.*, 1991) and to the striatal cholinergic interneurons

(Dixon *et al.*, 1996; see Chapter 2). Due to the concentration of the A_{2A} receptor in the basal ganglia and the lack of ligands selective for the A_{2B} receptor, most studies of transmitter release have focused on the A_{2A} receptor.

B. Mechanism of Action of the A_2 Receptors

A_2 receptors are positively coupled to adenylyl cyclase via G_s G-proteins (e.g., Marala and Mustafa, 1993), although in most binding studies guanine nucleotides only cause a small shift in the affinity of the A_{2A} receptor for the selective agonist CGS 21680. The reasons for this relative insensitivity are not clear although both proteolysis of the receptor and divalent cations have been implicated in the control of the affinity of this receptor (see Sebastião and Ribeiro, 1996). A_{2A} receptors have been reported to both increase (ACh, glutamate) and decrease (GABA) the release of neurotransmitters. The mechanism by which the A_{2A} receptor both stimulates and inhibits neurotransmitter release have not been clarified, although the former probably involves stimulation of voltage-sensitive Ca^{2+} channel activity (see Section IV,C), as seen in other areas of the brain (Mogul *et al.*, 1993; Umemiya and Berger, 1994).

C. A_{2A} Receptor Modulation of ACh Release

The first indication that the A_{2A} receptor controls striatal ACh release was in 1987 (Richardson and Brown, 1987b), when both adenosine and the nonselective agonist 2-chloroadenosine showed a reduced ability to inhibit veratridine-stimulated ACh release at high concentrations. This could have been explained by the presence of both inhibitory A_1 receptors and stimulatory A_2 receptors on these nerve terminals. Given the high concentration of the A_{2A} receptor in the striatum, these observations suggested the possibility that A_{2A} receptor antagonists could be used as striatal specific anticholinergic agents for the therapy of Parkinson's disease (Brown, 1988). This idea was reinforced in behavioral experiments in which A_2 receptor agonists counteracted apomorphine-induced turning in unilaterally lesioned (nigrostratiatal pathway) rats (Brown *et al.*, 1991), in a manner blocked by the muscarinic antagonist atropine (Vellucci *et al.*, 1993). Subsequently, the presence of both A_1 and A_{2A} receptors on striatal cholinergic nerve terminals was confirmed (Brown *et al.*, 1987, 1990; Kirkpatrick and Richardson, 1993; Kurokawa *et al.*, 1994).

A dual signaling system was shown to be employed by the A_{2A} receptor in the striatal cholinergic nerve terminal by Gubitz *et al.* (1996), where both intracellular signaling pathways activate Ca^{2+} channels. One intracellular pathway involved cAMP and protein kinase A activation of P-type voltage-sensitive Ca^{2+} channels; the other involved protein kinase C-mediated activation of N-type Ca^{2+} channels. These pathways interact such that the protein kinase A pathwy dominates, and the protein kinase C pathway can only be detected when protein kinase A is inhibited (Gubitz et al., 1996). It is probable that phospholipase C is involved in the protein kinase C pathways because other G_S-linked receptors have been shown to stimulate this enzyme in cloned cell lines, particularly when they are expressed at high levels (Zhu et al., 1994).

These observations suggested that the A_{2A} receptor stimulation of acetylcholine release via protein kinase C can bypass other modulators that act by inhibition of adenylyl cyclase (e.g., adenosine via the A_1 receptor and dopamine via the D_2 receptor). Indeed, the nonselective A_1/A_2 receptor agonist 5'-ethocarboxamidoadenosine (NECA) increase ACh release via the A_2 receptor rather than inhibiting release via the A_1 receptor (Kirkpatrick and Richardson, 1993). Similarly, the A_{2A} receptor overrides the ability of the dopamine D_2 receptor agonist quinpirole to inhibit ACh release (Jin et al., 1993; see Fig. 1). However, other mechanisms may also be involved in the predominant effect of the A_{2A} receptor because selective agonists have been shown to cause the appearance of a low-affinity state of the A_1 receptor (for agonists) in nerve terminals, an effect mediated by protein kinase C (Dixon et al., 1997). The A_{2A} receptor, by a direct intramembrane interaction, also reduced the affinity of the dopamine D_2 receptor for agonists (Ferré et al., 1991), so there are probably multiple routes by which this receptor can override the influence of at least some other transmitter receptors in these nerve terminals (Fig. 2). There have been reports that the A_{2A} receptor only increases ACh release in electrically stimulated striatal slices when dopamine D_2 receptor agonists are present (Jin and Fredholm, 1997; Jin et al., 1993). The reasons for the discrepancy with the results obtained by using synaptosomal preparations are unclear, although it is unlikely that the structure of the slice is the cause because K^+ (15 mM)-stimulated release of ACh is increased by CGS 21680 in rat striatal slices, in a manner unaffected by GABA receptor antagonists (Richardson et al., unpublished observations). It is also unlikely that dopamine is influencing the release of ACh in synaptosomal preparations because in some experiments the cholinergic nerve terminals were affinity purified (e.g., Brown et al., 1990) and in others there has been no cross-talk among the different synaptosomes in the systems used (Kurokawa et al., 1994).

The effect of A_{2A} receptor stimulation on ACh release has also been investigated in situ by intrastriatal microdialysis. Administration (i.c.v.) of the agonist CGS 21680 into the striatum caused an increase in extracelluar ACh concentrations even in the presence of the GABA receptor antagonists bicu-

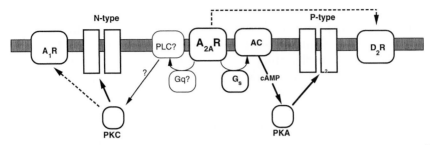

FIGURE 2 Actions of the A_{2A} receptor in the striatal cholinergic nerve terminal. A summary of the known actions of the A_{2A} receptor in the striatal cholinergic nerve terminal. The link between the A_{2A} receptor and PKC activation remains to be investigated. The direct intramembrane interaction between the A_{2A} receptor and the dopamine D_2 receptor (Ferré et al., 1991) is indicated. Dashed lines are inhibitory influences, solid lines excitatory. The inhibitory effect of PKA on the PKC-mediated stimulation of the N-type Ca^{2+} channel (Gubitz et al., 1996) is not indicated.

culline and 2-hydroxysaclofen (Kurokawa et al., 1996; Fig. 3). Therefore, this was not an indirect effect due to a modulation of GABA release (see Section IV,D), although it is apparent that blockade of GABA receptors substantially increases the release of ACh. The magnitude of the increase in ACh release

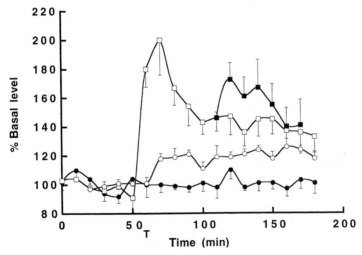

FIGURE 3 CGS 21680 potentiation of extracelluar ACh in the striatum *in vivo*. CGS 21680 (10 μg, ic.v.) increases the extracelluar concentration of ACh in the presence (■) and absence (◑) of the GABA receptor antagonist bicuculline (30 μM in dialysis probe) and 2-hydroxysaclofen (100 μM), as determined by intrastriatal dialysis. GABA antagonists were continually present from time 60 (■, ◲) and, under these conditions, the GABA agonist muscimol had no effect on striatal ACh levels. The data are percentages of the baseline value, which was 6.4 ± 0.7 pmol per 20 μl collected every 10 min (Kurokawa et al., 1996).

induced by CGS 21680 was similar in the presence and absence of bicuculline and 2-hydroxysaclofen, although it was maintained for much longer in the absence of these GABA receptor antagonists (Kurokawa *et al.*, 1996). Of particular interest in this study was the observation that CGS 21680 had a greater effect on ACh concentration in the absence of dopamine (i.e., after reserpine treatment of lesion of the nigrostriatal pathway), which is consistent with the proposal that A_{2A} receptor antagonists may be helpful in the amelioration of Parkinson's disease (Kurokawa *et al.*, 1996).

D. A_{2A} RECEPTOR MODULATION OF GABA RELEASE

The release of GABA from KCl depolarized rat striatal synaptosomes is inhibited by CGS 21680 (Kirk and Richardson, 1994; Kurokawa *et al.*, 1994). This effect was only seen with low (15 mM) concentrations of KCl and not with high concentrations (30 mM), showing that the effector system employed was sensitive to strong depolarization. CGS 21680 also inhibited synaptically evoked GABA release in striatal slices, presumably from the recurrent collaterals of striatopallidal neurons (Mori *et al.*, 1996; see Chapter 6). In synaptosomal preparations, no evidence was found for cAMP mediating this effect, indeed elevated cAMP levels reversed the inhibition seen upon stimulation of the A_{2A} receptor. Inhibitors of both protein kinase C and N-type Ca^{2+} channels mimicked the effect of A_{2A} receptor agonists, suggesting that the receptor may be operating via protein kinase C (Kirk and Richardson, 1995). However, in slices, Mori *et al.* (1996) obtained evidence that A_{2A} receptor-mediated control of GABA release was mediated by elevations in cAMP. Therefore, either the A_{2A} receptor employs two intracellular signaling pathways in the control of GABA release (see Section IV,C) or the presence of multiple populations of GABAergic nerve terminals in striatal synaptosomal preparations (efferent recurrent collaterals, different interneurons) obscured the involvement of cAMP in the control of the A_{2A} receptor regulated (striatopallidal) nerve terminals.

In contrast to these results, Mayfield *et al.* (1993, 1996) reported that A_{2A} receptor agonists increased GABA release in slices of the globus pallidus, and Ferré *et al.* (1993) showed that intrastriatal administration of CGS 21680 counteracts the inhibitory effects of dopamine D_2 agonists on pallidal GABA levels. There are a number of possible reasons for this discrepancy between observed increase or decreased in pallidal GABA release. First, Sebastião and Ribeiro (1996) suggested that endogenous dopamine in pallidal slices would reduce GABA release via dopamine D_2 receptors. Application of A_{2A} receptor agonists could antagonise this, perhaps by a direct intramembrane action

(Ferré *et al.*, 1991), resulting in more release of GABA. However, since Mori *et al.* (1996) observed a decrease in GABA release with CGS 21680 in striatal slices, which presumably also contained endogenous dopamine, this explanation is unlikely. An alternative suggestion is that inhibition of GABA release by the A_{2A} receptor reduced the inhibitory tone on cell and nerve terminals in these slices. Relief of this inhibitory tone would then cause the release of more GABA (Richardson *et al.*, 1998). Such a suggestion remains to be tested.

E. A_2 Receptor Modulation of Dopamine Release

In the guinea pig, A_2 (either A_{2A} or A_{2B} or both) receptors were shown to increase dopamine release from striatal preparations (Ebstein and Daly, 1982), in a manner inhibited by elevated Ca^{2+} concentrations, suggesting the possible modulation of Ca^{2+} channel activity reminiscent of that seen by Mogul *et al.* (1993) and Gubitz *et al.* (1996). Administration of CGS 21680 *in vivo* failed to affect extracelluar levels of dopamine, suggesting that the principal A_2 receptor on the striatal dopaminergic nerve terminals in the A_{2B} (Okada *et al.*, 1996a). Other A_2 receptor-mediated effects on the nigrostriatal dopamine system include a stimulation of dopamine synthesis (Chowdhury and Fillenz, 1991), probably by stimulation of tyrosine hydroxylase (Choksi *et al.*, 1997; Onali *et al.*, 1988).

F. A_2 Receptor Modulation of Glutamate Release

The ability of A_{2A} receptor agonists to increase glutamate release has been observed in a number of brain regions (e.g., the ischemic cerebral cortex) (O'Regan *et al.*, 1992), although the precise subtype involved is unknown, and in the hippocampus, where an A_{2A} receptor may be involved (Caciagli *et al.*, 1995). Similarly, in the striatum CGS 21680, the A_{2A} receptor agonist, has been reported to increase extracelluar levels of glutamate *in vivo* (Popoli *et al.*, 1995). The relationship between the A_{2A} receptor and glutamate function in the striatum requires further study because it has been shown that rotation behavior induced by unilateral intrastriatal injection of the metabotropic glutamate receptor agonists requires a functional A_{2A} receptor. This has been interpreted as mGluR (type I) receptors potentiating the effects of adenosine A_{2A} receptor stimulation on the striatopallidal neurons and/or the cholinergic interneurons (Kearney and Albin, 1995; Kearney et al., 1997).

Overall, adenosine controls the release of a number of transmitters in the striatum, and it appears, more often than not, that both inhibitory and excitatory adenosine receptors are present on the same nerves and nerve terminals. This obviously allows for a greater range of control by adenosine, both in terms of the magnitude and direction of the modulation, as well as the concentration range over which the neurons are sensitive to adenosine.

V. RELEVANCE OF THE A_{2A} RECEPTOR TO THE THERAPY OF PARKINSON'S DISEASE

Our understanding of the cellular mechanisms of striatal A_{2A} receptor action can be summarized (bearing in mind the discrepancies mentioned here) as the inhibition of GABA release (in both the striatum and pallidum) from nerve terminals of striatopallidal neurons and an increase in the release of acetylcholine from striatal cholinergic interneurons. We suggested that the adenosine A_{2A} receptor-mediated inhibition of striatal GABA release reduces feedback inhibition by striatopallidal recurrent collateral axons. Consequently, blockade of this receptor would result in increased feedback inhibition of the striatopallidal neurons (Richardson et al., 1997; see Chapter 8). Because the increase in proenkephalin expression seen in animal models of Parkinson's disease (Augood et al., 1989) is associated with increased activity of these neurons (Mitchell et al., 1989), this model is consistent with the reduction in striatal proenkephalin expression caused by A_{2A} receptor antagonists (see Chapter 8). There are, however, a number of questions that still need to be answered. For instance, the striatonigral neurons are also regulated by striatopallidal recurrent collaterals (Yung et al., 1996), as may be the interneurons; thus, pharmacological intervention at the A_{2A} receptor could affect both striatal output pathways. There is evidence for this in Chapter 8, where A_{2A} receptor antagonists affect the expression of Substance P in striato-Gpi/nigral neurons. The effect of the A_{2A} receptor on the pallidal nerve terminals needs to be clarified, and the reasons for the discrepancies between the effects of agonists on GABA release from synaptosomes and pallidal slices needs to be explained. If the A_{2A} receptor inhibits GABA release from the pallidal nerve terminals, this will affect the excitability of pallidal neurons, and an A_{2A} receptor antagonist could therefore be expected to increase GABA action in the external pallidum. According to the direct/indirect pathway model of the basal ganglia (Albin *et al.*, 1989), this would not result in an antiparkinsonian effect. However, it is now widely recognized that this model is simplistic and that the Gpe and subthalamic nucleus do not act as simple relay stations (Parent and Hazrati, 1995). To understand the actions of A_{2A} receptor antagonists in the Gpe, it is essential to identify the neurons receiving the (A_{2A} receptor-sensitive) GABAergic input from the striatiopallidal neurons.

The reduction in ACh release caused by A_{2A} receptor antagonists may also help to restore the balance between dopamine and ACh in the dopamine-depleted striatum. The importance of the A_{2A} receptor in controlling striatal ACh release is the subject of some debate (Richardson *et al.*, 1998; Svenningsson and Fredholm, 1998), which cannot be resolved at the present time. Of some interest is the observation that the A_{2A} receptor overrides the inhibitory effects of adenosine A_1 and dopamine D_2 receptor agonists in the cholinergic interneuron. Consequently, the administration of A_{2A} antagonists would unmask tonic activity at both of these receptors, resulting in a reduction in ACh action in the striatum. As mentioned in Section IV,D, there is evidence that cholinergic mechanisms are involved in the A_{2A} receptor-mediated control of motor behavior, and it has been suggested that ACh serves to maintain striatal output neurons in an excitable or quiescent state (Atkins *et al.*, 1990). It is therefore possible that in the absence of dopamine (i.e., in Parkinson's disease) the ability of ACh to maintain such states of the striatal output neurons is enhanced. The administration of A_{2A} receptor antagonists, by reducing the release of ACh, may reduce the influence of ACh on striatal output neuron firing rates.

In conclusion, the adenosine A_1 and A_{2A} receptors have numerous effects on neurotransmitter release in the striatum, which are consistent with the control of the striatopallidal pathway in particular. However, there are a number of lines of evidence suggesting that modulation of A_{2A} receptor activity can also affect the striato-Gpi/nigral pathway (see Chapter 8), suggesting that ligands binding to this receptor may have other more indirect effects. In this context, it is interesting to note that the cholinergic interneuron is able to control the activity of both striatopallidal and striato-Gpi/nigral neurons, and so may serve as an important focus of adenosine-mediated control of the striatum. However, because recurrent collateral axons of the striatopallidal neurons may directly influence striato-Gpi/nigral neurons, it is also probable that a major site of action of this receptor is the striato-pallidal neurons. Analysis of the relative importance of the A_{2A} receptors expressed on these two neurons in rectifying in rectifying the imbalance of striatal activity seen in Parkinson's disease will greatly increase our understanding of this area of the brain.

REFERENCES

Albin, R.L., Young, A.B., and Penney, J.B. (1989). The functional anatomy of basal ganglia disorders. *Trends Neurosci* **12**, 366–375.

Alexander, S.P., and Reddington, M. (1989). The cellular-localization of adenosine receptors in rat neostriatum. *Neurosci* **28**, 645–651.

Atkins, P.T., Surmeier, D.J., and Kitai, S.T. (1990). Muscarinic modulation of a transient K^+ conductance in rat neostriatal neurons. *Nature* **344**, 240–242.

Augood, S.J., and Emson, P.C. (1994). Adenosine A_{2A} receptor messenger-RNA is expressed by enkephalin cells but not by somatostatin cells in rat striatum—a coexpression study. *Mol Brain Res* **22**, 204–210.

Augood, S.J., Emson, P.C., Mitchell, I.J., Boyce, S., Clarke, S.E., and Crossman, A.R. (1989). Cellular-localization of enkephalin gene-expression in MPTP-treated cynomolgus monkeys. *Mol Brain Res* **6**, 85–92.

Ballarin, M., Fredholm, B.B., Ambrosio, S., and Mahy, N. (1991). Extracelluar levels of adenosine and its metabolites in the striatum of awake rats: inhibition of uptake and metabolism. *Acta Physiol Scand* **142**, 97–103.

Brown, S.J. (1988). *Purinergic Modulation of Cholinergic Synaptosomes.* Ph.D. thesis, University of Cambridge, Cambridge, England.

Brown, S.J., Reddington, M., and Richardson, P.J. (1987). Adenosine receptors and their modulation of neurotransmitter release at the cholinergic nerve terminal. *J Neurochem* **48**, S92.

Brown, S.J., James, S., Reddington, M., and Richardson, P.J. (1990). Both A_1 and A_{2A} purine receptors regulate striatal acetylcholine release. *J Neurochem* **55**, 31–38.

Brown, S.J., Gill, R., Evenden, J., Iversen, S.D., and Richardson, P.J. (1991). Striatal A_2 receptor regulates apomorphine induced turing in rats with unilateral dopamine denervation. *Psychopharmacol* **103**, 78–82.

Bruns, R.F., Lu, G.H., and Pugsley, T.A. (1987). Adenosine receptor subtypes: binding studies. In "Topics and Perspectives in Adenosine Research" (Gerlach, E., and Becker, B.F., eds.), pp. 59–73, Springer-Verlag, Berlin.

Caciagli, F., Di Iorio, P., Ciccarelli, R., Ballerini, P., Giuliani, P., Shinozaki, H., and Nicoletti, F. (1995). Class II of metabotropic glutamate receptors modulate the evoked release of adenosine and glutamate from rat hippocampal slices. *Pharmacol Res* **31**(suppl), 167.

Calabresi, P., Centonze, D., Pisani, A., and Bernardi, G. (1997). Endogenous adenosine mediates the presynaptic inhibition induced by aglycaemia at corticostriatal synapses. *J Neurosci* **17**, 4509–4516.

Cass, W.A., and Zahniser, N.R. (1991). Potassium channel blockers inhibit D_2 dopamine, but not A_1 adenosine, receptor-mediated inhibition of striatal dopamine release. *J Neurochem* **57**, 147–152.

Choksi, N.Y., Hussain, A., and Booth, R.G. (1997). 2-Phenylaminoadenosine stimulates dopamine synthesis in rat forebrain *in vitro* and *in vivo* via adenosine A_2 receptors. *Brain Res* **761**, 151–155.

Chowdhury, M., and Fillenz, M. (1991). Presynaptic adenosine A_2 and NMDA receptors regulate dopamine synthesis in rat striatal synaptosomes. *J Neurochem* **56**, 1783–1788.

Correia de Sá, P., Timoteo, M.A., and Ribeiro, J.A. (1996). Presynaptic A_1 inhibitory/A_{2A} facilitatory adenosine receptor activation balance depends on the motor stimulation paradigm at the rat hemidiaphragm. *J Neurophysiol* **76**, 3910–3919.

Corsi, C., Pazzagli, M., Bianchi, L., DellaCorte, L., Pepeu, G., and Pedata, F. (1997). *In vivo* amino acid release from the striatum of aging rats: adenosine modulation. *Neurobiol Aging* **18**, 243–250.

Cunha, R.A., Sebastião A.M., and Ribeiro, J.A. (1994). Purinergic modulation of the evoked release of 3H-acetylcholine from the hippocampus and cerebral cortex of the rat; role of the ectonucleotidases. *Eur J Neurosci* **6**, 33–42.

Cunha, R.A., Vizi, E.S., Ribeiro, J.A., and Sebastião, A.M. (1996a). Preferential release of ATP and its extracelluar catabolism as a source of adenosine upon high but not low frequency stimulation of rat hippocampal slices. *J Neurochem* **67**, 2180–2187.

Cunha, R.A., correia de Sá, P., Sebastião, A.M., and Ribeiro, J.A. (1996b). Adenosine receptors at rat hippocampal and neuromuscular synapses. *Br J Pharmacol* **119**, 253–260.

Daly, J.W., Butts-Lamb, P., and Padgett, W. (1983). Subclasses of adenosine receptors in the central nervous system. Interaction with caffeine and related methyl xanthines. *Cell Mol Neurobiol* **3**, 69–80.

Dixon, A.K., Gubitsz, A.K., Sirinathsinghji, D.J.S., Richardson, P.J., and Freeman, T.C. (1996). Tissue distribution of adenosine receptor messanger-RNAs in the rat. *Br J Pharmacol* **118**, 1461–1468.

Dixon, A.K., Widdowson, L., and Richardson, P.J. (1997). Desensitisation of the adenosine A_1 receptor by the A_{2A} receptor in the rat striatum. *J Neurochem* **69**, 315–321.

Dolphin, A.C., and Prestwich, S.A. (1985). Pertussis toxin reverses adenosine inhibition of neuronal glutamate release. *Nature* **316**, 148–150.

Ebstein, R.P., and Daly, J.W. (1982). Release of norepinephrine and dopamine from brain vesicular preparations: effects of adenosine analogues. *Cell Mol Neurobisol* **2**, 193–204.

Ferré, S., von Euler, G., Johansson, B., Fredholm, B.B., and Fuxe, K. (1991). Stimulation of high-affinity adenosine-A_2 receptors decreases the affinity of dopamine D_2 receptors in rat striatal membranes. *Proc Natl Acad Sci USA* **88**, 7237–7241.

Ferré, S., O'Connor, W.T., Fuxe, K., and Ungerstedt, U. (1993). The striopallidal neuron—a main locus for adenosine dopamine interactions in the brain. *J Neurosci* **13**, 5402–5406.

Ferré, S., O'Connor, W.T., Svenningsson, P., Bjorklund, L., Lindberg, J., Tinner, B., Stromberg, I., Goldstein, M., Qgren, S.O., Ungerstedt, U., Fredholm, B.B., and Fuxe, K. (1996). Dopamine D_1 receptor-mediated facilitation of GABAergic neurotransmission in the rat strioentopedunclar pathway and its modulation by adenosine A_1 receptor-mediated mechanisms. *Eur J Neurosci* **8**, 1545–1553.

Ferré, S., Fredholm, B.B., Morelli, M., Popoli, P., and Fuxe, K. (1997). Adenosine dopamine receptor–receptor interactions as an integrative mechanism in the basal ganglia. *Trends Neurosci* **20**, 482–487.

Ginsborg, B.L., and Hirst, G.D.S. (1972). The effect of adenosine on the release of transmitter from the phrenic nerve of the rat. *J Physiol (Lond)* **224**, 629–645.

Goodman, R.R., and Snyder, S.H. (1982). Autoradiographic localization of adenosine receptors in rat brain using ^{3}H-cyclohexyladenosine. *J Neurosci* **2**, 1230–1242.

Gubitz, A.K., Widdowson, L., Kurokawa, M., Kirkpatrick, K.A., and Richardson, P.J. (1996). Dual signalling by the adenosine A_{2A} receptor involves activation of both N- and P-type calcium channels by different G proteins and protein kinases in the same striatal nerve terminals. *J Neurochem* **67**, 374–381.

Harms, H.H., Wardeh, G., and Mulder, A.H. (1978). Adenosine modulates depolarzation-induced release of 3H-noradrenaline from slices of rat brain cortex. *Eur J Pharmacol* **49**, 305–308.

Harms, H.H., Wardeh, G., and Mulder, A.H. (1979). Effects of adenosine on depolarization-induced release of various radiolablelled neurotransmitters from slices of rat corpus striatum. *Neuropharmacol* **18**, 577–580.

Herrera-Marschitz, M., Luthman, J., and Ferré, S. (1994). Unilateral neonatal intracerebroventricular 6-hydroxydopamine administration in rats: II. Effects on extracelluar monoamine, acetylcholine and adenosine levels monitored with *in vivo* microdialysis. *Psychopharmacol* **116**, 451–456.

Hollins, C., and Stone, T.W. (1980). Adenosine inhibition of γ-aminobutyric acid release from slices of rat cerebral cortex. *Br J Pharmacol* **69**, 107–112.

James, S., and Richardson, P.J. (1993). Production of adenosijne from extracelluar ATP at the striatal cholinergic synapse. *J Neurochem* **60**, 219–227.

Jarvis, M.F., Schultz, R., Hutchison, A.J., Do, U.H., Sills, M.A., and Williams, M. (1989). [^{3}H]-CGS 21680, a selective A$_2$ adenosine receptor agonist directly labels A$_2$ receptors in rat brain tissue. *J Pharmacol Exp Ther* **251**, 888–893.

Jin, S.Y., and Fredholm, B.B. (1997). Adenosine A$_{2A}$ receptor stimulation increases release of acetylcholine from rat hipocampus but not striatum, and does not affect catecholamine release. *Naunyn-Schmiedeberg's Arch Pharmacol* **355**, 48–56.

Jin, S.Y., Johansson, B., and Fredholm, B.B. (1993). Effects of adenosine-A$_1$ and adenosine-A$_2$ receptor activation on electrically-evoked dopamine and acetylcholine-release from rat striatal slices. *J Pharmacol Exp Ther* **267**, 801–808.

Kearney, J.A.F., and Albin, R.L. (1995). Adenosine A$_2$ receptor mediated modulation of contralateral rotation induced by metabotropic glutamate receptor activation. *Eur J Pharmacol* **287**, 115–120.

Kearney, J.A.F., Frey, K.A., and Albin, R.L. (1997). Metabotropic glutamate agonist-induced rotation: a pharmacological, FOS immunohistochemical, and [C-14]-2-deoxyglucose autoradiographic study. *J Neurosci* **17**, 4415–4425.

Kirk, I.P., and Richardson, P.J. (1994). Adenosine A$_{2A}$ receptor mediated modulation of striatal [^{3}H]-GABA and [^{3}H]-ACh release. *J Neurochem* **62**, 960–966.

Kirk, I.P., and Richardson, P.J. (1995). Inhibition of striatal GABA release by the adenosine A$_{2A}$ receptor is not mediated by increases in cyclic AMP. *J Neurochem* **64**, 2801–2809.

Kirkpatrick, K.A., and Richardson, P.J (1993). Adenosine receptor mediated modulation of acetylcholine release from rat striatal synaptosomes. *Br J Pharmacol* **110**, 949–954.

Kurokawa, M., Kirk, I.P., Kirkpatrick, K.A., Kase, H., and Richardson, P.J. (1994). Inhibition by KF17837 of adenosine A$_{2A}$ receptor-mediated modulation of striatal GABA and ACh release. *Br J Pharmacol* **113**, 43–48.

Kurokawa, M., Koga, K., Kase, H., Nakamura, J., and Kuwans, Y. (1996). Adenosine A$_{2A}$ receptor-mediated modulation of striatal acetylcholine-release in-vivo. *J Neurochem* **66**, 1882–1888.

Lee, K.S., and Reddington, M. (1986). Autoradiographic evidence for multiple CNS binding sites for adenosine derivatives. *Neurosci* **19**, 535–549.

Lovinger, D.M., and Choi, S. (1995). Activation of adenosine-A$_1$-receptors initiates short-term synaptic depression in rat striatum. *Neurosci Lett* **199**, 9–12.

Lupica, C.R., Cass, W.A., Zahniser, N.R., and Dunwiddie, T.V. (1990). Effects of the selective adenosine-A$_2$ receptor agonist CGS 21680 on in vitro electrophysiology, camp formation and dopmaine release in rat hippocampus and striatum. *J Pharmacol Exp Ther* **252**, 1134–1141.

Malenka, R.C., and Kocsis, J.D. (1988). Presynaptic actions of carbachol and adenosine on corticostriatal transmission in vitro. *J Neurosci* **8**, 3750–3756.

Marala, R.B., and Mustafa, S.J. (1993). Direct evidence for the coupling of A$_2$ adenosine receptor to stimulatory guanine nucleotide binding protein in bovine brain striatum. *J Pharmacol Exp Ther* **266**, 294–300.

Mayfield, R.D., Suzuki, F., and Zahniser, N.R. (1993). Adenosine A$_{2A}$ receptor modulation of electrically evoked endogenous GABA release from slices of rat globus-pallidus, *J Neurochem* **60**, 2334–2337.

Mayfield, R.D., Larson, G., Orona, R.A., and Zahniser, N.R. (1996). Opposing actions of adenosine A$_{2A}$ and dopamine D$_2$ receptor activation on GABA release in the basal ganglia: evidence for an A$_{2A}$/D$_2$ receptor interaction in globus pallidus. *Synapse* **22**, 132–138.

Mei, Y.A., Lefoll, F., Vaudry, H., and Cazine, L. (1996). Adenosine inhibits L-type and N-type calcium channels in pituitary melanotrophs—evidence for the involvement of a G-protein in calcium-channel gating. *J Neuroendocrinol* **8**, 85–91.

Michaelis, M.L., Michaelis, E.K., and Myers, S.L. (1979). Adenosine modulation of synaptosomal dopamine release. *Life Sci* **24**, 2083–2092.

Mitchell I. J., Clarke, C.E., Boyce, S., Robertson, R.G., Peggs, D., Sambrook, M.A., and Crossman, A.R. (1989). Neural mechanisms underlying parkinsonian symptoms based upon regional uptake of 2-deoxyglucose in monkeys exposed to 1-methyl-4-phenyl-1,2,3,6-tetrahydropyridine. *Neurosci* **32**, 213–226.

Mogul, D.J., Adams, M.E., and Fox A.P. (1993). Differential activation of adenosine receptors decreases N-type but potentiates P-type Ca^{2+} current in hippocampal CA3 neurons. *Neuron* **10**, 327–334.

Mori, A., Shinodou, T., Ichimura, M., Nonaka, H., and Kase, H. (1996). The role of adenosine A_{2A} receptors in regulating GABAergic synaptic transmission in striatal medium spiny neurons. *J Neurosci* **16**, 605–611.

Okada, M., Mizuno, K., and Kaneko, S. (1996a). Adenosine A_1 and A_2 receptors modulate extracelluar dopamine levels in rat striatum. *Neurosci Lett* **212**, 53–56.

Okada, M., Mizuno, K., Okuyama, M., and Kaneko, S. (1996b). Magnesium-ion augmentation of inhibitory effects of adenosine on dopamine release in the rat striatum. *Psych Clin Neurosci* **50**, 147–156.

Onali, P., Olianas, M.C., and Bunse, B. (1988). Evedence that adenosine A_2 and dopamine autoreceptors antagonistically regulate tyrosine hydroxylase activity in rat striatal synaptosomes. *Brain Res* **456**, 302–309.

O'Regan, M.H., Simpson, R.E., Perkins, L.M., and Phillis, J.W. (1992). The selective A_2 adenosine receptor agonist CGS 21680 enhances excitatory amino acid release from the ischaemic rat cerebral cortex. *Neurosci Lett* **138**, 169–172.

Palmer, T.M., and Stiles, G.L. (1995). Adenosine receptors. *Neuropharmacol* **34**, 683–694.

Parent, A., and Hazrati, L.N. (1995). Functional-anatomy of the basal ganglia. 2. The place of subthalamic nucleus and external pallidum in basal ganglia circuitry. *Brain Res Rev* **20**, 128–154.

Phillis, J.W., and Wu, P.H. (1981). The role of adenosine and its nucleotides in central synaptic transmission. *Prog Neurobiol* **16**, 187–239.

Pollack, A.E., Harrison, M.B., Wooten, G.F., and Fink, J.S. (1993). Differential localization of A_{2A} adenosine receptor messenger-RNA with D_1 and D_2 dopamine-receptor messenger-RNA in striatal output pathways following a selective lesion of striatonigral neurons. *Brain Res* **631**, 161–166.

Popoli, P., Betto, P., Reggio, R., and Ricciarello, G. (1995). Adenosine A_{2A} receptor stimulation enhances striatal extracelluar glutamate levels in rats. *Eur J Pharmacol* **287**, 215–219.

Ramkumar, V., Nic, Z., Rybak, L.P., and Maggirwar, S.B. (1995). Adenosine, antioxidant enzymes and cytoprotection. *Trends Pharmacol Sci* **16**, 283–285.

Ribeiro, J.A., and Walker, J. (1975). The effect of adenosine triphosphate and adenosine diphosphate on transmission at the rat and frog neuromuscular junctions. *Br J Pharmacol* **54**, 213–218.

Richardson, P.J., and Brown, S.J. (1987a). ATP release from affinity purified rat cholinergic nerve terminals. *J Neurochem* **48**, 622–630.

Richardson, P.J., and Brown, S.J. (1987b). Adenosine and ATP at the cholinergic nerve terminal. In "Cellular and Molecular Basis of Cholinergic Function" (Dowdall, M.J., and Hawthorne, J.N., eds.), pp. 436–443, Ellis Horwood, Chichester, UK.

Richardson, P.J., Brown, S.J., Balyes, E.M., and Luzio, J.P (1987). Ectoenzymes control adenosine modulation of immunoisolated cholinergic synapses. *Nature* **327**, 232–234.

Richardson, P.J., Kase, H., and Jenner, P.G. (1997). Adenosine A_{2A} receptor antagonists as new agents for the treatment of Parkinson's disease. *Trends Pharmacol Sci* **18**, 338–344.

Richardson, P.J., Kase, H., and Jenner, P.G. (1998). Adenosine A_{2A} receptors: where are they? what do they do?-reply. *Trends Pharmacol Sci* **19**, 47–48.

Rivkees, S.A., Price, S.L., and Zhou, F.C. (1995). Immunohistochemical detection of A_1 adenosine receptors in rat-brain with emphasis on localization in the hippocampal-formation, cerbral-cortex, cerbellum, and basal ganglia. *Brain Res* **677**, 193–203.

Rudolphi, K.A., Schubert, P., Parkinson, F.E., and Fredholm, B.B. (1992). Neuroprotective role of adenosine in cerebral ischaemia. *Trends Pharmacol Sci* **13**, 439–445.

Schiffmann, S.N., Jacobs, O., and Vanderhaegen, J.J. (1991). Striatal restricted adenosine A_2 receptor (RDC8) is expressed by enkephalin, but not by substance P neurons: an *in situ* hybridisation histochemistry study. *J Neurochem* **57**, 1062–1067.

Sebastião, A.M., and Ribeiro, J.A. (1996). Adenosine A_2 receptor-mediated excitatory actions on the nervous system. *Prog Neurobiol* **48**, 167–189.

Stehle, J.H., Rivkees, S.A., Lee, J.J., Weaver, D.R., Deeds, J.D., and Reppert, S.M. (1992). Molecular cloning and expression of the cDNA for a novel A_2 adenosine receptor subtype. *Mol Endocrinol* **6**, 384–393.

Svenningsson, P., and Fredholm, B.B. (1998). Adenosine A_{2A} receptors: where are they? what do they do? *Trends Pharmacol Sci* **19**, 47–48.

Uchimura, N., and North, R.A. (1991). Baclofen and adenosine inhibit synaptic potentials mediated by gamma-aminobutyric-acid and glutamate release in rat nucleus-accumbens. *J Pharmacol Exp Ther* **258**, 663–668.

Umemiya, M., and Berger, A.J. (1994). Activation of adenosine A_1 and A_2 receptors differentially modulates calcium channels and glycinergic synaptic transmission in rat brainstem. *Neuron* **13**, 1439–1446.

Vellucci, S.V., Sirinathsinghji, D.J.S., and Richardson, P.J. (1993). Adenosine A_2 receptor regulation of apomorphine induced turning in rats with unilateral striatal dopamine denervation. *Psychopharmacol* **111**, 383–388.

Wojcik, W.J., and Neff, N.H. (1983). Differential location of adenosine A_1 and A_2 receptors in striatum. *Neurosci Lett* **41**, 55–60.

Wu, L.G., and Saggau, P. (1994). Adenosine inhibits evoked synaptic transmission primarily by reducing presynaptic calcium influx in area CA1 of hippocampus. *Neuron* **12**, 1139–1148.

Wu, Y.N., Mercuri, NB., and Johnson, S.W. (1995). Presynaptic inhibition of gamma-aminobutyric acid B-mediated synaptic current by adenosine recorded *in-vitro* in midbrain dopamine neurons. *J Pharmacol Exp Ther* **273**, 576–581.

Young, K.K.L., Smith, A.D., Levey, A.I., and Bolam, J.P (1996). Synaptic connections between spiny neurons of the direct and indirect pathways in the neostriatum of the rat—evidence from dopamine-receptor and neuropeptide immunostaining. *Eur J Neurosci* **8**, 861–869.

Zetterstrom, T., and Fillenz, M. (1990). Adenosine agonists can both inhibit and enhance *in vivo* striatal dopamine release. *Eur J Pharmacol* **180**, 137–143.

Zhu, X., Gilbert, S., Birnbaumer, M., and Birnbaumer, L. (1994). Dual signaling potential is common among Gs-coupled receptors and dependent on receptor density. *Mol Pharmacol* **46**, 460–469.

CHAPTER 8

Control of Gene Expression in Basal Ganglia by Adenosine Receptors

ALISTAIR K. DIXON

Parke Davis Neuroscience Research Center, Cambridge University Forvie Site, Cambridge, United Kingdom

PETER J. RICHARDSON

Department of Pharmacology, University of Cambridge, Cambridge, United Kingdom

I. INTRODUCTION

Medium-size spiny neurons of the straitum are organized into two parallel, histochemically distinct efferent systems. Neurons with axons extending to the internal segment of the globus palliudus (Gpi) and substantia nigra pars reticulata preferentially express substance P (SP) and dynorphin, and form the striato-Gpi/nigral pathway. Neurons extending to the ipsilateral globus pallidus preferentially express enkephalin and form the striatopallidal pathway (see Figure in Chapter 1 and Chapters 6 and 9). It is generally accepted that D_1 and D_2 dopamine receptors are largely segregated in these two efferent populations, with D_1 receptors predominantly expressed by striato-Gpi/nigral neurons and D_2 receptors expressed by striatopallidal neurons (Gerfen *et al.*, 1990; Le Moine *et al.*, 1990a, 1991; also see Surmeier *et al.*, 1993).

Adenosine A_{2A} receptor mRNA is abundantly expressed in the rat striatum, specifically in those output neurons containing dopamine D_2 receptor and enkephalin, but apparently not in dopamine D_1 receptor and SP-containing neurons (see Chapter 2; Fink *et al.*, 1992; Pollack *et al.*, 1993; Schiffmann and Vanderhaeghen, 1993; Schiffmann *et al.*, 1991). The distribution of the A_1 receptor is not so distinct, with the receptor being expressed in both of the major output pathways of the striatum as well as in cholinergic interneurons (see Chapter 2; Dixon *et al.*, 1996; Ferré *et al.*, 1996; Rivkees *et al.*, 1995).

A. NEUROPEPTIDE GENE EXPRESSION

The control of neuronal activity and, ultimately, neuropeptide gene expression in the striatum is influenced by the complex interplay among many neurotransmitter systems and their receptors, of which dopamine is one of the most important. Dopaminergic afferents from the midbrain cell groups in the ventral tegmental area and substantia nigra modulate the expression of striatal peptides. However, the expression of striatal enkephalin and SP are differentially regulated by the mesostriatal dopaminergic system. For example, removal of the striatal dopamine input by lesioning of the nigrostriatal tract (with 6-hydroxydopamine) produces an increase in enkephalin immunoreactivity and mRNA expression and a decrease in SP immunoreactivity and mRNA content in the rat striatum (Gerfen *et al.*, 1991; Normand *et al.*, 1988; Voorn *et al.*, 1987; Young *et al.*, 1986). In addition, it has been demonstrated that the 6-hydroxydopamine lesion-induced increase in striatal preproenkephalin mRNA can be attenuated by treatment with dopamine D_2 receptor-specific agonists, whereas D_1-receptor-specific agonist treatment either augmented the lesion-induced increase or had no effect (Pollack and Wooten, 1992). The lesion-induced decrease in SP mRNA levels was reversed by intermittent treatment with the D_1-selective agonist SKF-38393 (Gerfen *et al.*, 1990). Similarly, chronic antagonism of striatal dopamine receptors results in alterations in the expression of striatal peptides. In the rat-selective D_2 receptor, blockade leads to an increase in striatal proenkephalin gene expression, whereas selective D_1 receptor antagonism results in a decrease (Morris and Hunt, 1991). Also, D_2 receptor stimulation decreases striatal proenkephalin mRNA levels, whereas D_1 receptor stimulation prevents the effects of D_1 receptor blockade (Angulo, 1992). Overall, data from both lesioning studies and receptor antagonist and agonist treatments suggest that the D_2 receptor inhibits the synthesis of mRNA encoding the enkephalin peptides. The D_1 receptor may also (directly or indirectly) modulate striatal proenkephalin mRNA abundance.

The effects of dopamine agonists and antagonists on the activity of the striatal tachykinin peptides, such as SP, are not so clear cut. Chronic treatment with haloperidol, a neuroleptic antagonist of both D_1 and D_2

receptors, decreases the amount of striatal SP, whereas sulpiride, a neuroleptic that binds preferentially to D_2 receptors, increases SP mRNA levels (Jaber et al., 1994). This observation may also be influenced by differences among the interactions of these drugs with nondopamine receptors. However, the atypical neuroleptic, clozapine, has no effect on SP mRNA levels (Angulo et al., 1990).

These alterations in levels of peptide gene expression correlate directly with alterations in striatal neuronal activity because lesioning of the dopamine input results in an increase in striatopallidal neuronal activity and a decrease in striato-Gpi/nigral neuronal activity, as measured by 2-deoxyglucose uptake (Mitchell et al., 1989; Trugman and Wooten, 1987). Therefore, measurement of neuropeptide gene expression in specific cell types can be used to assess the level of neuronal activity in selected pathways.

Another important influence on striatal neuropeptide gene expression is mediated by acetylcholine (ACh). For example, chronic systemic treatment with the muscarinic antagonist scopolamine partially attenuates the increase in striatal proenkephalin mRNA levels induced by both 6-hydroxydopamine lesion and D_2 receptor blockade (Pollack and Wooten, 1992), suggesting that at least some of the effects of dopamine receptor blockade on proenkephalin expression are mediated through the cholinergic interneuron. Similarly, the increase in c-fos expression caused by dopamine depletion is partly blocked by muscarinic antagonists (Morelli et al., 1995). However, the role of the cholinergic interneuron in the control of SP expression is less clear, with scopolamine reported either to have no effect on the changes induced by D_2 receptor blockade (Pollack and Wooten, 1992) or to reverse the effects of nigrostriatal lesions (Nisenbaum et al., 1994). The role of striatal ACh in the control of gene expression is further complicated by the report that the effects of systemic scopolamine may not mediate at the level of the striatum (Nisenbaum et al., 1994).

B. IMMEDIATE EARLY GENE EXPRESSION

The expression of immediate early genes (IEGs) such as c-fos is rapidly and transiently activated in the nervous system in response to a variety of stimuli, including cAMP, inositol trisphosphate formation, and calcium influx (Ginty et al., 1992; Morgan and Curran, 1989). Consequently, the induction of c-fos expression has been used as an anatomical marker of neuronal activity in many systems (Sagar et al., 1988). Both D_1 receptor agonists (Robertson et al., 1989) and D_2 receptor antagonists (Sirinathsinghji et al., 1994) induce c-fos expression in the striatum. Reserpine-induced dopamine depletion and haloperidol both increase c-fos expression in striatopallidal neurons, an effect attenuated by systemic administration of adenosine A_{2A} receptor antagonists (Boegman and Vincent, 1996; Pollack and Fink, 1995). This is consistent with the ability of the adenosine A_{2A} receptor agonist CGS 21680 to increase c-fos expression in the nucleus accumbens (Pinna et al., 1997) and in the dopamine-depleted dorsal striatum (Fenu et al., 1997; Morelli et al., 1995). In addition, a link between the striatal adenosine A_{2A} receptor and the dopamine D_1 receptor has been identified using levels of c-fos expression as a marker of neuronal activity. In unilaterally 6-hydroxy-dopamine-lesioned rats, the administration of the A_{2A} receptor antagonist, SCH 58261, and CGS15943A potentiated turning behavior and striatal expression of c-fos induced by the dopamine D_1 receptor agonist SKF-38393 (Pinna et al., 1996) This was most likely an indirect interaction (i.e., mediated by the local neural network) between the A_{2A} and D_1 receptors, which are largely expressed on different neurons, with the dopamine D_1 receptor-dependent increase in c-fos expression occurring in striato-Gpi/ nigral neurons. Thus, the differential regulation of neuropeptide gene expression by dopamine receptors is reflected in a differential ability to regulate c-fos expression. In striatopallidal neurons, c-fos expression is induced by D_2 receptor antagonists, whereas in striato-Gpi/nigral neurons c-fos expression is induced by D_1 receptor agonists. Other IEGs whose expression is known to be decreased by adenosine A_{2A} receptor antagonists include NGF1-α, NGF1-β, and jun β (Svenningsson et al., 1995, 1997). It therefore appears that the control of IEG expression in the striatum is under the tonic control of both adenosine and dopamine.

The consequences and nature of interactions between adenosine and dopamine systems in the basal ganglia are of particular interest because dopaminergic regulation of striatal efferent pathways is central to the planning and execution of correct movement and posture. Akinesia, which accompanies Parkinson's disease, has been related to increased striatopallidal activity (Albin et al., 1989). Therefore, we have investigated how adenosine might act via A_1 and A_{2A} receptors to influence the activity of neurons that form striatal efferent pathways as measured by changes in the expression of the neuropeptides proenkephalin and SP. Effects of adenosine antagonists on striatal peptide mRNA levels were investigated in the dopamine-depleted striatum and following chronic D_2 receptor blockade. The effect of the partially selective A_2 antagonist CGS15943A on striatal proenkephalin mRNA levels was investigated in rats that had received unilateral 6-hydroxy-dopamine lesions. In addition, the effects of the A_{2A}-selective antagonist KF17837 and the A_1-selective antagonist DPCPX on striatal proenkephalin and SP mRNA levels were investigated in rats chronically treated with the selective D_2 receptor antagonist eticlopride. For this purpose, the technique of quantitative in situ hybridization was employed.

II. EFFECT OF CGS15943A ON
PROENKEPHALIN mRNA LEVELS
IN DOPAMINE-DEPLETED STRIATUM

The first study investigated the effect of the partially selective adenosine A_2 receptor antagonist CGS15943A on proenkephalin mRNA levels in the dopamine-depleted striatum. Rats unilaterally depleted in dopamine by a 6-hydroxydopamine-induced lesion of the left nigrostriatal pathway subsequently received chronic saline or CGS15943A treatments. Only rats displaying significant apomorphine-induced contralateral rotation behavior were selected for subsequent treatments. However, the extent of the lesion was also checked by *in situ* hybridization with a tyrosine hydroxylase mRNA-specific probe applied at the level of the substantia nigra. Only those animals that exhibited more than 95% (unilateral) destruction of the substantia nigra as determined by tyrosine hydroxylase mRNA expression (Fig. 1B) were included in subsequent quantification of neuropeptide mRNA levels in the striatum. Figure 1A is representative of tyrosine hydroxylase mRNA expression at the level of the substantia nigra in sham-lesioned animals; only those animals exhibiting bilaterally intact substantia nigra were included in subsequent analysis.

Brain sections, representative of the treatment groups analyzed, following *in situ* hybridization with an [S^{35}]-labeled oligonucleotide probe complimentary to proenkephalin mRNA are presented in Figure 1C–F. It can be seen that the increase in proenkephalin labeling induced by 6-hydroxydopamine lesioning (Fig. 1D) is markedly attenuated by chronic CGS15943A treatment (Fig. 1F). A decrease in striatal proenkephalin labeling following CGS15943A treatment in the sham-lesioned animals (Fig. 1E) compared with the striatum of the saline-treated sham-lesioned animals (Fig. 1C) is also discernible.

Average optical densities measured over the striatum of animals in each treatment group ($n = 4$) are presented graphically in Figures 2 and 3. In the saline-treated animals, the level of striatal proenkephalin mRNA expression, as determined by average optical density, was 53% greater than that in the unlesioned striatum (see Fig. 2). Following chronic CGS15943A treatment, the level of striatal proenkephalin mRNA expression was only 13% higher than that in the unlesioned striatum. However, because CGS15943A caused a 15% ($p < 0.001$) reduction in proenkephalin expression in the unlesioned striatum, this adenosine receptor antagonist was only partially able to reduce the increase caused by the lesion (to 36% compared with the unlesioned CGS15943A-treated striatum; see Fig. 2). Levels of proenkephalin mRNA expression did not significantly differ among sham-lesioned and unlesioned striata within both the saline- and CGS15943A-treated groups (see Fig. 3). The significant ($p < 0.001$) 15% decrease in proenkephalin mRNA expression

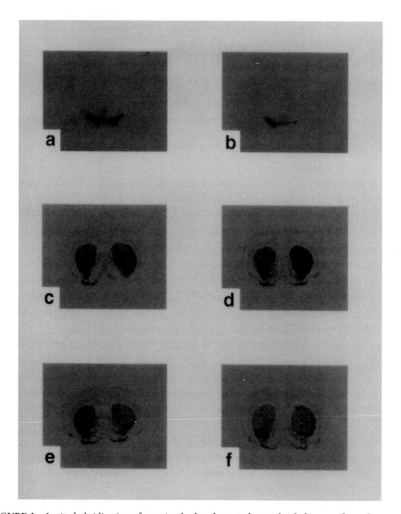

FIGURE 1 *In situ* hybridization of tyrosine hydoxylase- and proenkephalin-specific probes. **a** and **b** are representative X-ray autoradiographs generated by hybridization of an ^{35}S-labeled antisense probe specific to rat tyrosine hydroxylase mRNA. **a** represents a section at the level of the substantia nigra in a sham-lesioned animal; **b**, a section at the corresponding level from an animal that has previously received a 6-hydroxydopamine lesion to the right substantia nigra. **c** represents proenkephalin mRNA expression in the striatum following a sham lesion to the right nigrostriatal tract and subsequent saline treatment. **d** represents right-side 6-hydroxydopamine-lesioned animals treated with saline; **e**, sham-lesioned animals treated with CGS15943A; and **f**, 6-hydroxydopamine-lesioned animals subsequently treated with CGS15943A. Drug administrations were as follows: 6-hydroxydopamine 8 μg in 4 μl 0.2% ascorbate/0.9% saline over a 5-minute period, AP + 3.0 mm from the interaural line; L + 1.2 mm; V − 7.3 mm below the dura, with the incisor bar 2.3 mm below the interaural line. CGS15943A ip 0.1 mg/kg twice per day.

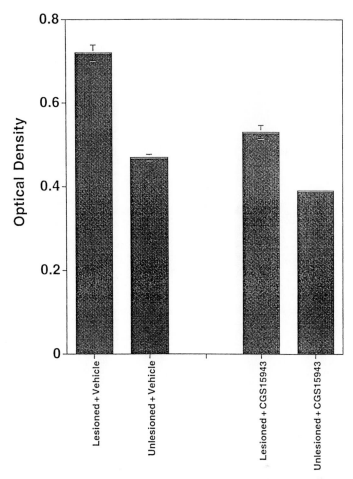

FIGURE 2 Proenkephalin expression in the striatum (nigrostriatal lesions). Histograms representing relative proenkephalin mRNA levels, as average optical density across the striatum, in 6-hydroxydopamine-lesioned animals. Statistical analysis using ANOVA, followed by a two-tailed student's t-test, demonstrated a significant ($p < 0.001$) reduction in proenkephalin mRNA levels in the lesioned striatum of CGS15943A-treated animals ($n = 4$) in comparison with levels in the lesioned striatum of saline-treated animals ($n = 4$). There was also a significant ($p < 0.05$) reduction in the proenkephalin levels in the intact striatum of CGS15943A-treated animals in comparison with saline-treated animals. Error bars represent $\pm$ SEM.

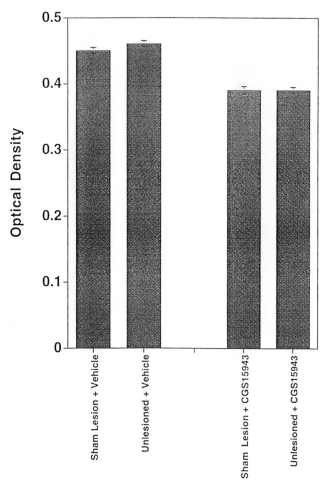

FIGURE 3 Proenkephalin expression in the striatum (sham lesions). Histograms representing relative proenkephalin mRNA levels, as average optical density across the striatum, in sham-lesioned animals. Statistical analysis using ANOVA, followed by a two-tailed student's t-test, demonstrated a significant ($p < 0.05$) reduction in proenkephalin mRNA levels in the striata of CGS15943A-treated animals ($n = 5$) in comparison with saline-treated animals ($n = 4$). Error bars represent $\pm$ SEM.

observed in the CGS15943A-treated, unlesioned (and sham-lesioned) striatum, compared with the unlesioned saline-treated striatum, shows that this antagonist-blocked adenosine receptor stimulated proenkephalin expression in both the presence and absence of significant levels of extracellular dopamine.

III. EFFECT OF A$_2$ AND A$_1$ ADENOSINE
RECEPTOR ANTAGONISM ON LEVELS OF
STRIATAL PEPTIDE GENE EXPRESSION

The second study investigated the influence of the A$_{2A}$ and A$_1$ adenosine receptor specific antagonists, KF17837 and DPCPX, on levels of striatal proenkephalin and SP mRNA expression, respectively, following chronic D$_2$ dopamine receptor antagonism.

Autoradiographs of representative brain sections, showing the level of proenkephalin mRNA expression following all treatment regimes, are presented in Figure 4. On a purely qualitative basis, the alterations in proenkephalin mRNA expression are immediately evident. Chronic treatment with KF17837 and DPCPX alone or combination appear to have no effect, compared with levels of mRNA expression in control. However, chronic eticlopride and eticlopride + DPCPX treatment both resulted in a marked increase in proenkephalin mRNA expression. It can also be seen that in each case KF17837 attenuated this increase when used in combination with both treatment regimes.

Again, these results were examined quantitatively, with average optical densities measured over the striatum of animals in each treatment group ($n =$ 4, six sections per animal). Results of this analysis are presented in Figure 5. There was no significant change in proenkephalin mRNA expression, with respect to control, following treatment with KF17837, DPCPX, or KF17837 plus DPCPX (see Fig. 5). However, chronic eticlopride treatment induced a significant ($p < 0.001$) 67% increase. Yet chronic eticlopride treatment in combination with KF17837 only resulted in a significant ($p < 0.001$) 26.5% increase, representing a 63% reduction in eticlopride-induced proenkephalin mRNA upregulation. Chronic eticlopride plus DPCPX also resulted in a significant ($p < 0.001$) 62% increase; again, the inclusion of KF17837 attenuated this increase. Chronic eticlopride with KF17837 and DPCPX treatment resulted in a significant ($p < 0.001$) 26% increase, representing a 59% reduction in the eticlopride plus DPCPX-induced increase in proenkephalin mRNA expression.

Striatal levels of SP mRNA expression were also assessed in these animals. Representative X-ray autoradiographs following *in situ* hybridization with a [S^{35}] labeled oligonucleotide probe complementary to SP mRNA are presented in Figure 6. The only discernible qualitative change at this stage is a marked reduction in SP mRNA expression, with respect to control, following chronic eticlopride plus DPCPX treatment.

This X-ray autoradiographic data then underwent quantitative analysis, as described previously, the results of which are presented in Figure 7. SP mRNA

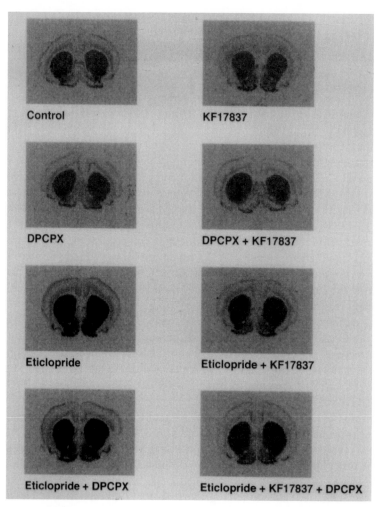

FIGURE 4 Proenkephalin expression (eticlopride treatment). X-ray autoradiographs generated by hybridization of an ^{35}S-labeled antisense oligonucleotide probe specific to rat proenkephalin mRNA. Representative sections are presented, illustrating levels of proenkephalin mRNA in the striata of animals from each treatment group indicated. Drug administration was for 15 days: eticlopride (ip), 5 mg/kg, once per day; KF17837 (po) once per day, 2 mg/kg in 0.3% Tween; DPCPX (ip), 2 mg/kg.

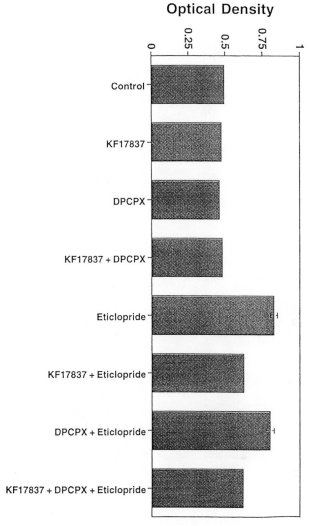

FIGURE 5 Proenkephalin expression in the striatum (eticlopride treatment). Histograms representing relative proenkephalin mRNA levels, as average optical density across the striatum, in animals from each treatment group indicated ($n = 4$). Error bars represent + SEM; in some instances, these are too small to be observed. Significant differences were seen among striata treated with eticlopride alone and those treated with eticlopride plus KF17837 in the presence or absence of DPCPX ($p < 0.001$).

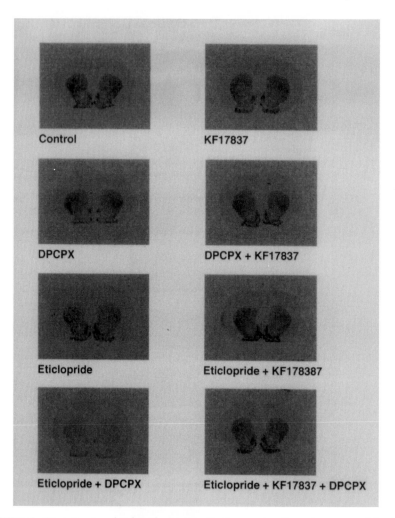

FIGURE 6   SP expression (eticlopride treatment). X-ray autoradiographs generated by hybridization of an ^{35}S-labeled antisense oligonucleotide probe specific to rat SP mRNA. Representative sections are presented, illustrating levels of SP mRNA in the striata of animals from each
treatment group indicated.

expression was not significantly altered in relation to control levels, following
chrnoic KF17837, DPCPX, or KF17837 plus DPCPX treatment (see Fig. 7).
Chronic eticlopride treatment resulted in a slight but significant ($p < 0.05$) 7%
decrease in SP mRNA expression. However, chronic eticlopride plus KF17837
resulted in no significant change in SP mRNA expression levels. A particularly

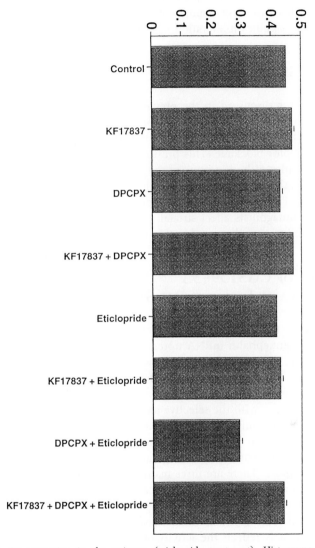

FIGURE 7 SP expression in the striatum (eticlopride treatment). Histograms representing relative SP mRNA levels, as average optical density across the striatum, in animals from each treatment group indicated ($n = 4$). Error bars represent + SEM; in some instances, these are too small to be observed. Significant differences were seen among untreated striata and those treated with eticlopride alone ($p < 0.05$) and eticlopride plus DPCPX ($p < 0.001$). Administration of KF17837 in the presence of eticlopride and DPCPX caused a significant increase in SP expression ($p < 0.001$).

marked 35% ($p < 0.001$) decrease in SP mRNA expression was observed following chronic eticlopride plus DPCPX treatment. Yet the inclusion of KF17837 in this treatment regime completely reversed this downregulation, resulting in no significant alteration in levels of striatal SP mRNA expression.

IV. DISCUSSION

The experiments discussed in the previous section clearly demonstrate that A_{2A} receptor antagonists are able to restore normal levels of neuropeptide expression in the striatum under conditions of dopamine depletion and dopamine receptor blockade. This presumably reflects a normalization in the neuronal activities of both groups of output pathways and is consistent with the hypothesis that A_{2A} receptor antagonists could help to ameliorate some of the systems of Parkinson's disease. The precise mechanisms by which adenosine receptor antagonists affect striatal neuronal activity are not so clear cut, but the possibilities are discussed in this section.

A. EFFECT OF CGS15943A
IN UNILATERALLY LESIONED RAT STRIATUM

The observation that CGS15943A, a selective A_2 receptor antagonist, reversed the striatal proenkephalin mRNA upregulation induced by dopamine depletion may reflect the molecular events underlying previously observed adenosine/dopamine complementarity. The effects of CGS15943A were most likely mediated through its actions at the adenosine A_{2A} receptor subtype, and similar effects were seen with the selective anatgonist KF17837. It appears that in the absence of dopamine D_2 receptor activation, the upregulation of proenkephalin expression requires a functional A_{2A} receptor, so the degree of proenkephalin expression may be regulated by the competing influences of these two receptors. There are three main possibilities that could account for the A_{2A} receptor-mediated control of the expression of proenkephalin mRNA: a direct effect on the soma of the striatopallidal neurons, control of feedback inhibition, and ACh modulation of these neurons. Because proenkephalin expression probably reflects the activity of these neurons, the possible roles of the A_{2A} receptor in the control of other neurons need to be considered.

The adenosine A_{2A} receptor regulates the release of at least two striatal neurotransmitters, γ-aminobutyric acid (GABA) and ACh, both of which have been documented to control the activity of striatal medium spiny output neurons (see Chapter 7). The A_{2A} receptor reduces GABAergic inhibition of the efferent neurons by inhibiting GABA release from striatal nerve terminals.

This effect is probably exerted on the terminals of the recurrent collaterals of the striatopallidal projection neurons (see Chapter 7; Kirk and Richardson, 1994; Mori et al., 1996), although it is conceivable that other GABAergic neurons may also be involved. Nevertheless, antagonism of striatal A_{2A} receptors would tend to decrease striatopallidal activity and thus reduce the expression of proenkephalin mRNA. An alternative mechanism that may also contribute to the A_{2A} receptor mediated control of proenkephalin mRNA expression involves the striatal cholinergic interneurons, which have been implicated in D_2 receptor control of striatal proenkephalin mRNA levels (Pollack and Wooten, 1992). Despite their small numbers, the activity of these neurons is of profound importance to the adequate performance of extrapyramidal motor behavior. It has been recognized for some time that dopamine D_2 receptor agonists inhibit, and antagonists stimulate, striatal ACh release—these receptors being expressed on the cholinergic interneurons (Le Moine et al., 1990b; Wong et al., 1983). Thus D_2 receptor blockade would increase ACh release, which would maintain striatopallidal output neurons in an excitable state (see Chapter 7; Richardson et al., 1997) increasing their firing activity and expression of proenkephalin. Such a model is consistent with the ability of muscarinic agonists to stimulate c-fos expression in striatopallidal neurons (Bernard et al., 1993), of physostigmine to increase, and of scopolamine to decrease, striatal preproenkephalin mRNA (Lucas and Harlan, 1995). In addition, several studies have demonstrated the ability of the A_{2A} receptor to stimulate ACh release from striatal synaptosomes and slices (Brown et al., 1990; Jin et al., 1993; Kirk and Richardson, 1994), a process possibly mediated by both protein kinases A and C (see Chapter 7; Gubitz et al., 1996). Therefore, a degree of the adenosine A_{2A} receptor-mediated control of striatal proenkephalin gene expression may be via ACh, with A_{2A} receptor antagonists reducing the elevated striatal ACh levels caused by D_2 receptor blockade.

It is not possible to determine the relative importance of these three routes by which the A_{2A} receptor controls striatopallidal neuronal activity, although the ACh-mediated mecanism is likely to be significant because it has been noted that atropine antagonizes the behavioral effects of A_{2A} receptor agonists in rat (Vellucci et al., 1993).

A similar experiment to the one carried out here was performed by Schiffmann and Vanderhaeghen (1993), using the nonselective adenosine antagonist caffeine. The effect of caffeine on proenkephalin expression in the lesioned striatum was qualitatively the same as those observed in this study. However, chronic administration of this drug increased enkephalin mRNA in the intact striatum, as opposed to the decrease caused by CGS15943A observed here. They suggest that this phenomenon can be explained by depletion of dopamine caused by a blockade of presynaptic A_{2B} receptors located on nigrostriatal terminals, even though caffeine acts at most adenosine receptors. Furthermore, the major metabolite of caffeine, paraxanthine, has been reported to be a dopamine D_1 receptor agonist (Ferré *et al.*, 1990), and because dopamine D_1 receptor agonist treatment induces an increase in proenkephalin mRNA levels in the intact striatum (Pollack and Wooten, 1992) the reported increase may have been due to the action of paraxanthine at the dopamine D_1 receptor. The difference in the results obtained in this study may also reflect the more selective nature of CGS15943A in comparison with caffeine. CGS15943A antagonism of A_{2A} receptors in the intact striatum would result in increased inhibition (GABAergic) or decreased stimulation (cholinergic) of the striatopallidal output pathway, consistent with the decrease in striatal proenkephalin gene expression.

B. Effect of KF17837 in Striatum of Rats Treated with Eticlopride

Further studies were carried out to assess the contribution and influence of adenosine A_1 and A_{2A} receptors over striatal peptide gene expression, following chronic dopamine D_2 receptor blockade. This approach was adopted, as opposed to 6-hydroxydopamine nigrostriatal lesioning, because it was of interest to establish how adenosine A_{2A} antagonists influence striatal neuronal activity in both models of Parkinson's disease. In addition, the role of the dopamine D_2 receptor could be specifically assessed using the selective antagonist eticlopride. Rats received chronic systemic treatment with the specific adenosine A_1, A_{2A}, and dopamine D_2 receptor antagonists DPCPX, KF17837, and eticlopride in all possible combinations, and the resultant alterations in striatal proenkephalin and SP gene expression were determined.

KF17837 administered alone, at a dose known to reduce the catalepsy induced by haloperidol (see Chapter 4; Kanda *et al.*, 1994), had no effect on levels of striatal proenkephalin gene expression, suggesting that there is no tonic A_{2A} receptor effect on gene expression. This is in contrast to the previously observed effects of the A_{2A} receptor antagonist CGS15943A in the intact striatum of unilaterally 6-hydroxydopamine-lesioned rats. The reasons for this are unclear, although it may be a consequence of the nonselective nature of this antagonist.

The adenosine A_1 receptor antagonist DPCPX also had no significant effect on striatal proenkephalin gene expression when administered with or without the A_{2A} receptor-selective antagonist KF17837, suggesting no tonic A_1 receptor-mediated control of this gene. This is despite the fact that this receptor is expressed in approximately 40% of all striatal neurons (Rivkees *et al.*, 1995), including those expressing proenkephalin (Ferré *et al.*, 1996). DPCPX administration also had no significant effect on the eticlopride-induced increase in striatal proenkephalin gene expression or its attenuation by KF17837, further emphasizing the lack of influence of the A_1 receptor in these experiments.

The increase in striatal proenkephalin gene expression seen with eticlopride is consistent with the findings of Pollack and Wooten (1992) and was attenuated by KF17837. This was similar to the effect of CGS15943A in the dopamine denervated striatum, although the effect was quantitatively greater. This may be due to differences in experimental design, or this finding could reflect the increased selectivity of KF17837 over CGS15943A for the A_{2A} receptor. The KF17837-induced reduction in (eticlopride-stimulated) proenkephalin gene expression was only partial, possibly as a consequence of the techniques employed and of the experimental design, or this may reflect the influence of other striatal neuronal pathways in the control of striatopallidal neuronal activity.

Alterations in striatal SP mRNA levels were investigated to assess the regulatory effect of adenosine A_1 and A_{2A} receptors on the activity of neurons that constitute the direct striato-Gpi/nigral pathway. Treatment with the adenosine A_1 and A_{2A} receptor antagonists DPCPX and KF17837, alone or in combination, had no effect on levels of striatal SP expression. Thus specific blockade of these adenosine receptors results in no alteration, as detected by changes in gene expression, in the activity of striato-Gpi/nigral neurons. It has been observed that caffeine causes a decrease in levels of SP mRNA in the intact striatum (Schiffmann and Vanderhaegen, 1993). However, it appears that such effects may not be mediated via the blockade of adenosine A_1 or A_{2A} receptors; the nonspecific actions of caffeine make it difficult to postulate as to the nature of pathways that may be involved in such observations.

Chronic administration of eticlopride did decrease striatal SP mRNA levels. This small but significant effect of dopamine D_2 receptor blockade is again consistent with the observations of Pollack and Wooten (1992). The eticlopride-mediated effects presented in this chapter also support the hypothesis that dopamine differentially regulates proenkephalin- and SP-expressing neurons in the striatum (Reimer *et al.*, 1992), as D_2 receptor blockade decreased SP mRNA but increased proenkephalin mRNA. Because dopamine D_1 and D_2 receptors are largely segregated in the two populations of striatal efferent neurons (Gerfen, 1992), it appears that dopamine D_2 receptor-mediated modulation of striatopallidal neuronal activity occurs via an indirect mechanism. However, a direct effect on D_2 receptors expressed on striato-Gpi/nigral neurons is possible because the segregation of these receptors into the two histochemically distinct efferent systems may not be absolute (Surmeier *et al.*, 1993).

The effect of chronic dopamine D_2 receptor blockade on levels of striatal SP was markedly enhanced by coadministration of DPCPX. Indeed DPCPX and eticlopride appear to have an almost synergistic relationship, together effecting a 35% reduction in levels of SP mRNA. This effect may arise from both receptors coupling via Gi to similar intracellular second messengers and effector systems (e.g., inhibition adenylyl cyclase activity) (Onali et al., 1985; Palmer and Stiles, 1995). Interestingly, both dopamine D_2 and adenosine A_1 receptors are expressed by cholinergic interneurons in the striatum (Dixon et al., 1996; MacLennan et al., 1994), where they inhibit the release of ACh (Brown et al., 1990). Consequently, blockade of both receptors would increase striatal ACh tone and decrease SP expression (Lucas and Harlan, 1995; Wang and McGinty, 1996). This would be consistent with the ability of muscarinic antagonists to induce c-fos expression in striato-Gpi/nigral neurons (Bernard et al., 1993) because fos has been implicated in changes in SP expression (Svenningsson et al., 1997). In addition, increases in ACh tone would inhibit dopamine release from nigrostriatal afferents (via presynaptic muscarinic receptors; Stoof et al., 1992), leading to a reduction in the dopaminergic drive to the striato-Gpi/nigral neurons.

The eticlopride- and eticlopride plus DPCPX-induced decreases in striatal SP mRNA levels were both reversed by specific adenosine A_{2A} receptor antagonism, effected by chronic KF17837 treatment. Several factors may be important in the mediation of this effect, although it is most likely to be an indirect effect because there are few if any striato-Gpi/nigral neurons expressing A_{2A} receptor mRNA (Pollack et al., 1993). Because the A_{2A} receptor is located primarily on the enkephalinergic and cholinergic neurons, it is likely that the effect of A_{2A} receptor blockade on SP expression occurs via one (or both) of these neurons. Furthermore, because muscarinic agonists decrease and antagonists increase SP expression (Bernard et al., 1993; Wang and McGinty, 1996), reduced ACh concentrations caused by blockade of the A_{2A} receptor would be expected to restore normal levels of expression. It is therefore conceivable that the changes in expression observed in these experiments were mediated, at least in part, by dopamine and adenosine effects on the striatal cholinergic interneurons. One alternative mechanism that needs to be considered is that blockade of the A_{2A} receptor would increase dopamine D_2 receptor action due to relief of the direct intramembrane inhibition of the latter receptor (Ferré et al., 1991). However, because eticlopride was administered to block D_2 receptors in these experiments, this seems unlikely. It should also be recognized that systemic administration of these drugs means that some of the observed changes in expression may be due to action at nonstriatal sites.

In conclusion, the results presented in this chapter demonstrate that blockade of adenosine A_{2A} receptors in several distinct neuronal populations helps to restore the balance of striatal function. This blockade serves to increase the inhibition of both striatopallidal and cholinergic interneurons, while increasing the activity of striato-Gpi/nigral neurons following striatal dopamine depletion or chronic D_2 receptor blockade. At the molecular level, these findings taken in conjunction with other studies highlight the potential importance of A_{2A} antagonists as antiparkinsonian drugs.

REFERENCES

Albin, R.L., Young, A.B., and Penney, J.B. (1989). The functional anatomy of basal ganglia disorders. *Trends Neurosci* **12**(10), 366–375.

Angulo, J.A., Cadet, J.L., Woolley, C.S., Suber, F., and McEwen, B.S. (1990). Effect of chronic typical and atypical neuroleptic treatment on proenkephalin mRNA levels in the striatum and nucleus accumbens of the rat. *J Neurochem* **54**, 1889–1894.

Angulo, J.A. (1992). Involvement of dopamine D_1 and D_2 receptors in the regulation of proenkephalin messenger-RNA abundance in the striatum and accumbens of the rat. *J Neurochem* **58**, 1104–1109.

Bernard, V., Dumartin, B., Lamy, E., and Bloch, B. (1993). Fos immunoreactivity after stimulation or inhibition of muscarinic receptors indicates anatomical specificity for cholinergic control of striatal efferent neurons and cortical-neurons in the rat. *Eur J Neurosci* **5**, 1218–1225.

Boegman, R.J., and Vincent, S.R. (1996). Involvement of adenosine and glutamate receptors in the induction of c-fos in the striatum by haloperidol. *Synapse* **22**, 70–77.

Brown, S.J., James, S., Reddington, M., and Richardson, P.J. (1990). Both A_1 and A_{2A} purine receptors regulate striatal acetylcoline release. *J Neurochem.* **55**, 31–38.

Dixon, A.K., Gubitz, A.K., Sirinathsinghji, D.J.S., Richardson, P.J., and Freeman, T.C. (1996). Tissue distribution of adenosine receptor messanger-RNAs in the rat. *Br J Pharmacol* **118**, 1461–1468.

Fenu, S., Pinna, A., Ongini, E., and Morelli, M. (1997). Adenosine A_{2A} receptor antagonism potentiates L-DOPA-induced turning behaviour and c-fos expression in 6-hydroxydopamine-lesioned rats. *Eur J Pharmacol* **321**, 143–147.

Ferré, S., Guix, J., Salles, A., Badia, P., Parra, F., Jane, M., Herrera-Marschitz, M., Ungerstedt, U., and Cacas, M. (1990). Paraxanthine displaces the binding of [^{3}H] SCH 23390 from rat striatal membranes. *Eur J Pharm* **179**, 295.

Ferré, S., von Euler, G., Jonsson, B., Fredholm, B.B., and Fuxe, K. (1991). Simulation of high affinity adenosine A_2 receptors decreases the affinity of dopamine D_2 receptors in rat striatal membranes. *Proc Natl Acad Sci USA* **88**, 7238–7241.

Ferré, S., O'Connor, W.T., Svenningsson, P., Bjorklund, L., Lindberg, J., Tinner, B., Stromberg, I., Goldstein, M., Qgren, S.O., Ungerstedt, U., Fredholm, B.B., and Fuxe, K. (1996). Dopamine D_1 receptor-mediated facilitation of GABAergic neurotransmission in the rat strioentopeduncular pathway and its modulation by adenosine A_1 receptor-mediated mechanisms. *Eur J Neurosci* **8**, 1545–1553.

Fink, J.S., Weaver, D.R, Rivkees, S.A., Peterfreund, R.A., Pollack, A.E., Adler, E.M., and Reppert, S.M. (1992). Molecular cloning of the rat A_2 adenosine receptor: selective co-expression with D_2 dopamine receptors in rat striatum. *Mol Brain Res* **14**, 186–195.

Gerfen, C.R., Engber, T.M., Mahan, L.C., Susel, Z., Chase, T.N., Monsma, F.J., Jr., and Sibley, D.R. (1990). D_1 and D_2 dopamine-receptor regulated gene expression of striato-Gpi/nigral and striatopallidal neurons. *Science* **250**, 1429–1432.

Gerfen, C.R., McGinty, J.F., and Young, S.W., III. (1991). Dopamine differentially regulates dynorphin, substance P, and enkephalin expression in striatal neurons: *in situ* hybridization histochemical analysis. *J Neurosci* **11**, 1016–1031.

Ginty, D.D., Bading, H., and Greenberg, M.E. (1992). Trans-synaptic regulation of gene expression. *Curr Opinion Neurobiol* **2**, 312–316.

Gubitz, A.K., Widdoson, L., Kurokawa, M., Kirkpatrick, K.A., and Richardson, P.J. (1996). Dual signalling by the adenosine A_{2A} receptor involves activation of both N- and P-type calcium channels by different G proteins and protein kinases in the same striatal nerve terminals. *J Neurochem* **67**, 374–381.

Jaber, M., Tison, F., Fournier, M.C., and Bloch, B. (1994). Differential influence of haloperidol and sulpiride on dopamine receptors and peptide mRNA levels in the rat striatum and pituitary. *Mol Brain Res* **23**, 14–20.

Jin, S., Johansson, B., and Fredholm, B.B. (1993). Effects of adenosine A_1 and A_2 receptor activation on electrically evoked dopamine and acetylcholine release from rat striatal slices. *J Pharmacol Exp Ther* **267**, 801–808.

Kanda, T., Shiozaki, S., Shimada, J., Suzuki, F., and Nakamura, J. (1994). KF17837: a novel selective adenosine A_{2A} receptor antagonist with anticataleptic activity. *Eur J Pharmacol* **256**, 263–268.

Kirk, I.P., and Richardson, P.J. (1994). Adenosine A_{2A} receptor-mediated modulation of striatal [^{3}H]-GABA and [^{3}H]-ACh release. *J Neurochem* **62**, 960–966.

Le Moine, C., Normand, E., Guitteny, A.F., Fouque, B., Teoule, R., and Bloch, B. (1990a). Dopamine receptor gene expression by enkephalin neurons in the rat forebrain. *Proc Natl Acad Sci USA* **87**, 230–234.

Le Moine, C., Tison, F., and Bloch, B. (1990b). D_2 dopamine receptor gene expression by cholinergic neurons in the rat striatum. *Neurosci Lett* **117**, 248–252.

Le Moine C., Normand, E., and Bloch, B. (1991). Phenotypical characterisation of the rat striatal neurons expressing the D_1 dopamine receptor gene. *Proc Natl Acad Sci USA* **88**, 4205–4209.

Lucas, L.R., and Harlan, R.E. (1995). Cholinergic regulation of tachykinin- and enkephalin-gene expression in the rat striatum. *Mol Brain Res* **30**, 181–195.

MacLennan, A.J., Lee, N., Vincent, S.R., and Walker, D.W. (1994). D_2 dopamine receptor messenger-RNA distribution in cholinergic and somatostatinergic cells of the rat caudateputamen and nucleus-accumbens. *Neurosci Lett* **180**, 214–218.

Mitchell, I.J., Clarke, C.E., Boyce, S., Robertson, R.G., Peggs, D., Sambrook, M.A., and Crossman, A.R. (1989). Neural mechanisms underlying parkinsonian symptoms based upon regonal uptake of 2-deoxyglucose in monkeys exposed to 1-methyl-4-phenyl-1,2,3,6-tetrahydropyridine. *Neurosci* **32**, 213–226.

Morelli, M., Pinna, A., Wardas, J., and Di Chiara, G. (1995). Adenosine A_2 receptors stimulate c-fos expression in striatal neurons of 6-hydroxydopamine-lesioned rats. *Neurosci* **67**, 49–55.

Morgan, J.I., and Curran, T. (1989). Stimulus-transcription coupling in neurons: role of central immediate-early genes. *Trends Neurosci* **12**, 495–563.

Mori, A., Shindou, T., Ichimura, M., Nonaka, H., and Kase, H. (1996). The role of adenosine A_{2A} receptors in regulating GABAergic synaptic transmission in striatal medium spiny neurons. *J Neurosci* **16**, 605–611.

Morris, B.J., and Hunt, S.P. (1991). Proenkephalin mRNA levels in rat striatum are increased and decreased, respectively, by selective D_2 and D_1 dopamine receptor antagonists. *Neurosci Lett* **125**, 201–204.

Nisenbaum, L.K., Kitai, S.T., and Gerfen, C.R. (1994). Dopaminergic and muscarinic regulation of striatal enkephalin and substance P messenger RNAs following striatal dopamine denervation: effects of systemic and central administration of quinpirole and scopolamine. *Neurosci* **63**, 435–449.

Normand E., Popovici T., Onteniente B., Fellman D., Piatier-Tonneau D., Auffray C., and Bloch B. (1988). Dopaminergic neurons of the sbstantia nigra modulate preproenkephalin A gene expression in rat striatal neurons. *Brain Res* **439**, 39–46.

Onali, P., Olianas, M.C., and Gessa, G.L. (1985). Characterisation of dopamine-receptors mediating inhibition of adenylate cyclase activity in rat brain striatal membranes. *Mol Pharmacol* 28, 138–145.

Palmer, T.M., and Stiles G.L. (1995). Adenosine receptors. *Neuropharmacol* 34, 683–694.

Pinna, A., diChiara, G., Wardas, J., and Morelli, M. (1996). Blockade of A_{2A} adenosine receptors positively modulates turning behaviour and c-Fos expression induced D_1 agonists in dopamine-dnervated rats. *Eur J Neurosci* 8, 1176–1181.

Pinna, A., Wardas, J., Cristalli, G., and Morelli, M. (1997). Adenosine A_{2A} receptor agonists increase Fos-like immunoreactivity in mesolimbic areas. *Brain Res* 759, 41–49.

Pollack, A.E., and Wooten, G. (1992). D_2 dopaminergic regulation of striatal preproenkephalin mRNA levels is mediated in part through cholinergic interneurons. *Mol Brain Res* 13, 35–41.

Pollack, A.E., and Fink, J.S. (1995). Adenosine antagonists potentiate D_2 dopamine-dependent activation of Fos in the striatopallidal pathway. *Neurosci* 68, 721–728.

Pollack, A.E., Harrison, M. B., Wooten, G.F., and Fink, J.S. (1993). Differential localization of A_{2A} adenosine receptor mRNA with D_1 and D_2 dopamine receptor mRNA in striatal output pathways following selective lesions of striato-Gpi/nigral neurons. *Brain Res* 631, 161–166.

Reimer, S., Sirinatsinghji, D.J.S., Nikolorakis, K.E., and Hollt, V. (1992). Differential dopaminergic regulation of proenkephalin mRNAs in the basal ganglia of rats. *Mol Brain Res* 12, 259–266.

Richardson, P.J., Kase, H., and Jenner, P.G. (1997). Adenosine A_{2A} receptor antagonists as new agents for the treatment of Parkinson's disease. *Trends Pharmacol Sci* 18, 338–344.

Rivkees, S.A., Price, S.L., and Zhou, F.C. (1995). Immunohistochemical detection of A_1 adenosine receptors in rat-brain with emphasis on localization in the hippocampal-formation, cerebral-cortex, cerebellum, and basal ganglia. *Brain Res* 677, 193–203.

Robertson, H.A., Peterson, M.R., Murphy, K., and Robertson, G.S. (1989). D_1-dopamine receptor agonists selectively activate striatal c-fos independent of rotational behaviour. *Brain Res* 503, 346–349.

Sagar, S.M., Sharp, F.R., and Curran, T. (1988). Expression of c-fos protein in brain: metabolic mapping at the cellular level. *Science* 240, 1328–1331.

Schiffmann, S.N., Jacobs, O., and Vanderhaegen, J.J. (1991). Striatal restricted adenosine A_2 receptor (RDC8) is expressed by enkephalin, but not by substance P neurons: an *in situ* hybridisation histochemistry study. *J Neurochem* 57, 1062–1067.

Schiffmann, S.N., and Vanderhaegen, J.J. (1993). Adenosine A_2 receptors regulate the gene expression of striatopallidal and striato-Gpi/nigral neurons. *J Neurosci* 13, 1087.

Sirinathsinghji, D.J., Schuligoi, R., Heavens, R.P., Dixon, A., Iversen, S.D., and Hill, R.G. (1994). Temporal changes in the messenger RNA levels of cellular immediate early genes and neurotransmitter/receptor genes in the rat neostriatum and substantia nigra after acute treatment with eticlopride, a dopamine D_2 receptor antagonist. *Neurosci* 62, 407–423.

Stoof, J.C., Drukarch, B., DeBoer, P., Westerink, B.H.C., and Groenewegen, H.J. (1992). Regulation of the activity of striatal cholinergic neurons by dopamine. *Neurosci* 47, 755–770.

Surmeier, D.J., Reiner, A., Levine, M.S. and Ariano, M.A. (1993). Are neostriatal dopamine receptors co-localized? *Trends Neurosci* 16, 299–305.

Svenningsson, P., Strom, A., Johansson, B., and Fredholm, B.B. (1995). Increased expression of c-jun, junb, ap-1, and preproenkephalin messenger-RNA in rat striatum following a single injection of caffeine. *J Neurosci* 15, 3583–3593.

Svenningsson, P., Georgieva, J., Kontny, E., Heilig, M., and Fredholm, B.B. (1997). Involvement of a c-fos-dependent mechanism in caffeine-induced expression of the preprotachykinin A and neurotensin/neuromedin N genes in rat striatum. *Eur J Neurosci* 9, 2135–2141.

Trugman, J.M., and Wooten, G.F. (1987). Selective D_1 and D_2 dopamine agonists differentially alter basal ganglia glucose utilization in rats with unilateral 6-hydroxydopamine substantia nigra lesions. *J Neurosci* 7, 2927–2935.

Vellucci, S.V., Sirinathsinghji, D.J.S., and Richardson, P.J. (1993). Adenosine A_2 receptor regulation of apomorphine induced turning in rats with unilateral straital dopamine denervation. *Psychopharmacol* 111, 383–388.

Voorn, P., Roest, G., and Groenewegen, H.J. (1987). Increase of enkephalin and decrease of substance P immunoreactivity in the dorsal and ventral striatum of the rat midbrain 6-hydroxydopamine lesions. *Brain Res* 412, 391–396.

Wang, J.Q., and McGinty, J.F. (1996). Muscarinic receptors regulate striatal gene expression in normal and amphetamine treated rats. *Neurosci* 75, 43–56.

Wong, D.T., Bymaster, F.P., Reid L.R., Fuller, R.W., Perry K.W., and Korfeld, E.C. (1983). Effect of a stereospecific D-2 dopamine agonist on acetylcholine concentration in the corpus striatum of rat brain. *J. Neural Transm* 58, 55–67.

Young, W.S., III, Bonner, T.I., and Brann, M.R. (1986). Mesencephalic dopaminergic neurons regulate the expression of neuropeptide mRNAs in the rat forebrain. *Proc Natl Acad Sci USA* 83, 9827–9831.

CHAPTER 9

Knockout Mice in the Study of Dopaminergic Diseases

SHIRO AOYAMA AND HIROSHI KASE

Pharmaceutical Research Institute, Kyowa Hakko Kogyo Co., Ltd., Shizuoka, Japan

JA-HYUN BAIK

Medical Research Center (Molecular Biology Section), College of Medicine, Yonsei University, Seoul, South Korea

EMILIANA BORRELLI

Institut de Génetique et de Biologie Moléculaire et Cellulaire, C.U. de Strasbourg, France

I. INTRODUCTION

Dopamine regulates a variety of physiological functions, including movement, reward mechanisms, cognition and hormone release. Four dopaminergic pathways have been described: 1) the nigrostriatal, 2) mesolimbic, 3) mesocortical, and 4) tuberoinfundibular. Dopamine is synthesized by neurons of mesencephalic nuclei; its release activates membrane receptors of the seven transmembrane domain G-protein coupled family. Afterward it is rapidly recaptured by the dopamine transporter and degraded by specific enzymes. Progress in molecular neurobiology has enhanced our knowledge about the physiological role of most dopamine receptors as well as of other components of the dopaminergic system.

Interestingly, D_2 receptor-deficient mice present a strong locomotor phenotype with analogies to human Parkinson's disease symptoms. These data strongly suggest a key role of D_2Rs in the control of locomotor function and underline the possibility that the locomotor deficits observed in Parkinson's disease might be mainly dependent on the lack of activation of these receptors. In this respect, it is important to mention the role of adenosine in

Adenosine Antagonists and Parkinson's Disease
Copyright © 2000 by Academic Press. All rights of reproduction in any form reserved.

the control of locomotor function in the striatum. In particular, it is interesting to study the role of the adenosine A_{2A} receptor *in vivo*. This receptor is expressed in striatal neurons, which belong to the indirect pathway and as such colocalize with the D_2 receptor. Understanding the relationship between the A_{2A} and D_2 receptors may lead to the development of novel therapies for diseases affecting the dopaminergic pathway. Genetically altered mutant mice in which members of the dopamine or adenosine receptor families have been deleted represent excellent models to investigate the role of these receptors *in vivo*. They also represent tools for the development of drugs aimed at the treatment of dopaminergic dysfunctions.

Understanding the physiology of the dopaminergic system has an important bearing on many brain disorders in humans. For example, Hornykiewicz (1966) found that in postmortem brains of patients with Parkinson's disease the content of dopamine, norepinephrine, and serotonin was low. Of the three biogenic amines, dopamine was the most drastically reduced, and this was the first observation that showed an association between a deficiency in dopamine and a brain disease. This discovery stimulated further research into alterations of dopaminergic transmission in other neurological and psychiatric illnesses, such as depression, schizophrenia, and dementia.

In the brain, dopamine (DA) is synthesized by mesencephalic neurons in the substantia nigra (SN) and ventral tegmental area (VTA) (Alexander and Crutcher, 1990; Graybiel, 1990). SN and VTA are integral parts of the complex neural network that constitutes the basal ganglia. Dopaminergic neurons arise from these nuclei and project to the striatum, cortex, limbic system, and hypothalamus. Through these pathways, dopamine affects many physiological functions, such as the control of movement and hormone secretion, as well as motivated and emotional behaviors (Jackson and Westlind-Daniesson, 1994).

In particular, the nigrostriatal pathway is composed of neurons that project from the SN to the striatum. This pathway is specifically involved in the control of movement and sensorimotor coordination, and it is the degeneration of these neurons that leads to Parkinson's disease (Hornykiewicz, 1966; Seeman and Niznik, 1990). Parkinson's disease is characterized by the incapacity to initiate voluntary movements, and its primary symptoms are akinesia, bradykinesia, and resting tremor. Other dopaminergic pathways include 1) the mesolimbic–mesocortical pathways that influence learning, memory, and motivated behaviors, including activities related to reward; and 2) the hypothalamic tuberoinfundibular pathway, which participates in the control of the synthesis and release of pituitary hormones.

DA interacts with membrane receptors belonging to the large family of seven transmembrane domain (7TM) G-protein coupled receptors. Their activation leads to the formation or inhibition of intracellular second messengers. To date, five different DA receptors have been cloned from different species.

Based on their structural and pharmacological properties, a general subdivision into two groups has been made: the D_1-like receptors, which stimulate intracellular cAMP levels, comprising D_1 receptors (Dearry et al., 1990; Zhou et al., 1990) and D_5 receptors (Grandy et al., 1991; Sunahara et al., 1991), and the D_2-like receptors, which inhibit intracellular cAMP levels, comprising D_2 (Bunzow et al., 1988; Dal Toso et al., 1989), D_3 (Sokoloff et al., 1990), and D_4 (Van Tol et al., 1991) receptors. D_2-like receptors, in addition, may also couple to other cellular effectors such as phosphinositide hydrolysis (Picetti et al., 1997). The study of the anatomical distribution of D_1 and D_2-like receptors has shown overlapping patterns of expression. D_1 receptors and D_2 receptors are the most abundantly expressed, while D_3, D_4, and D_5 receptors have a more restricted pattern of expression. Pharmacologically, it is possible to discriminate between D_1-like and D_2-like receptors. Indeed, D_1 receptors bind the benzazepine antagonist SCH-23390, whereas D_2 receptor recognizes with high affinity the butyrophenones, spiperone, and haloperidol. Nevertheless, ligands with appreciable selectivity able to discriminate within the D_1 and D_2-like subfamilies remain to be discovered.

D_1 and D_2 receptors are strongly expressed in the striatum by medium spiny neurons. Striatal D_1 and D_2 receptors seem to be confined to different subsets of neurons (Gerfen, 1992; Hersch et al., 1995; Yung et al., 1995), such that striatonigral neurons bear D_1 receptors, whereas striatopallidal neurons express D_2 receptors. However, neurons expressing both receptors have also been described (Ariano et al., 1997; Meador-Woodruff et al., 1991). The coordinated activity of striatonigral and striatopallidal output neurons is needed to produce coordinated voluntary movements.

Targeted mutagenesis of specific genes in vivo, by homologous recombination, offers a means of estimating the physiological effects of gene products. Using this technique, null mice for components of the dopaminergic systems have been generated, providing animal models to evaluate, in a more selective and precise manner, the role of these proteins in dopaminergic transmission (Accili et al., 1996; Baik et al., 1995; Drago et al., 1994; Giros et al., 1996; Xu et al., 1994; Zhou and Palmiter, 1995).

In this chapter, we summarize these findings, focusing on the phenotype of knockout mice for different dopamine receptors and the impact they have on our understanding of the dopaminergic system.

II. D_2-LIKE RECEPTORS

A. DOPAMINE D_2 RECEPTOR

The cloning of the first member of the dopaminergic receptor family was achieved by low-stringency screening of a rat brain cDNA library, using as a

TABLE 1   The different dopamine receptor subtypes

	D1	D5	D2	D3	D4
Structure					
Amino acids					
human	446	477	414/443 (D2S/D2L)	400	387
rat, mouse	446	475	415/444 (D2S/D2L)	446	385
mRNA (Kb)	4.2	3.0-3.7	2.9	8.3	5.3
Human chromosomal localization	5q 35.1	4p 15.1-16.1	11q 22-23	3q 13.3	11p
Signalling pathway	↑ cAMP ↑ IP3	↑ cAMP	↓ cAMP ↑ K channel	↓ cAMP	↓ cAMP
mRNA distribution	caudate-putamen nucleus accumbens olfactory tubercle	hippocampus lateral mammillary nucleus parafascicular nucleus	caudate-putamen nucleus accumbens olfactory tubercle pituitary	olfactory tubercle nucleus accumbens islands of Calleja	frontal cortex medulla midbrain
Selective agonist	SKF 38393	SKF 38393	quinpirole	7-OH-DPAT	apomorphine
Selective antagonist	SCH 23390	SCH 23390	spiperone	UH 232	clozapine

probe the β_2-adrenergic receptor coding sequence (Bunzow *et al.*, 1988). A cDNA encoding a putative receptor with a predicted length of 415 amino acids (aa) was isolated. The expression of this cDNA in mouse fibroblast cells was found to display pharmacological features typical of the native striatal dopamine D_2 receptor. The human homologue of the rat D_2 receptor was subsequently cloned encoding a protein that is 96% identical to the rat receptor, with one amino acid deletion (Dal Toso *et al.*, 1989). Table 1 shows a schematic representation of D_2 receptor topology. Interestingly, the D_2 receptor presents a long third intracytoplasmic loop, typical of receptors that inhibit adenylyl cyclase (AC) activity. Northern blots and *in situ* hybridization analysis showed that the D_2 receptor is highly expressed in the caudate-putamen, nucleus accumbens, and olfactory tubercles. Importantly, D_2 receptor mRNAs were also highly expressed in the dopaminergic cell bodies of neurons within the SN pars compacta and VTA, suggestive of an autoreceptor role for D_2 receptor.

The cloned D_2 receptor causes inhibition of AC through coupling to inhibitory G-proteins (Gi) (Cote *et al.*, 1983). However, this receptor is also negatively coupled to phosphoinositide (PI) hydrolysis and Ca^{2+} mobilization (Picetti *et al.*, 1997). Inhibition of PI hydrolysis could account for the decrease of Ca^{2+} levels observed in pituitary cells after DA administration (Vallar and Meldolesi, 1989).

B. Two Isoforms of D$_2$ Receptor

Two different isoforms of the dopamine D$_2$ receptor exist *in vivo*, named D2L and D2S. These isoforms are derived by alternative splicing of the sixth exon of the gene (Dal Toso *et al.*, 1989; Giros *et al.*, 1990). D$_{2L}$ is the longer isoform composed by 444 aa in rat (Chio *et al.*, 1990; Monsma *et al.*, 1990) and mouse (Montmayeur *et al.*, 1991) and 443 in human (Dal Toso *et al.*, 1989; Giros *et al.*, 1989; Grandy *et al.*, 1989; Selbie *et al.*, 1989). In contrast, D$_{2S}$ is composed of 415 aa in rat (Bunzow *et al.*, 1988) and mouse (Montmayeur *et al.*, 1991) and 414 in human (Dal Toso *et al.*, 1989; Giros *et al.*, 1989). D$_{2L}$ differs from D$_{2S}$ only by a 29-aa insertion in the putative third intracellular loop of the receptor. Interestingly, both isoforms are colocalized in the same cells and in all the regions where D$_2$ receptors are expressed. The two isoforms also share the same pharmacological profile (Dal Toso *et al.*, 1989; Giros *et al.*, 1989; Monsma *et al.*, 1990; Montmayeur *et al.*, 1991). The larger isoform is predominantly expressed in brain, although the ratio of the two isoforms can vary in some locations (Montmayeur *et al.*, 1991).

We have shown that D$_{2L}$ and D$_{2S}$ differ in their ability to inhibit AC when transfected in cells which do not contain the $\alpha_i 2$-subunit of the inhibitory G-protein (Gα_i2; Montmayeur and Borrelli, 1991). It appears that the 29-aa insert confers a selectivity on the D$_{2L}$ receptor for Gα_i2, because in the presence of this G-protein subunit greater inhibition of AC is observed (Montmayeur *et al.*, 1993). However, even in the absence of Gα_i2, this receptor is able to interact, although less efficiently, with other G-proteins. Guiramand *et al.*, (1995) generated aa mutations in the D$_{2L}$ insert to identify the residues conferring the Gα_i2 coupling specificity. Interestingly, the conversion of aspartate 249 into valine resulted in a mutated receptor that was no longer dependent on Gα_i2 to efficiently inhibit AC. This demonstrates a key role of the 29-aa insertion in the selection of the G-protein with which D$_2$ receptor isoforms interact. These data suggest that the differential G-protein coupling characteristics that exist between the two isoforms underly functional differences in the regulation of the signaling pathways activated by D$_{2L}$ and D$_{2S}$ *in vivo*.

C. D$_3$ Receptor

The D$_3$ receptor is 52% homologous to the D$_2$ receptor at the aa level (Sokoloff *et al.*, 1990). The D$_3$ gene is localized on chromosome 3 in the human genome. The D$_3$ coding region, as for the D$_2$ receptor gene, is interrupted by multiple introns, and recently two, apparently nonfunctional, RNA splice variants of the rat D$_3$ receptor gene have been identified (Giros *et al.*, 1991). Dopamine itself and most dopamine receptor agonists (except bromocriptine) bind with a much higher affinity to D_3 receptors than to the D_2 receptors (Gingrich and Caron, 1993). In contrast, the affinity of D_3 receptors for antagonists, such as haloperidol, remoxipride, $(-)$-sulpride, clozapine, and spiperone, is lower than that of D_2 receptors (Gingrich and Caron, 1993; Malmberg *et al.*, 1993). Two exceptions, AJ76 and UH232, were found to have greater affinity for the D_3 receptor than for the D_2 receptor, and have been described as selective D_3 autoreceptor antagonists (Sokoloff *et al.*, 1990). The highest level of D_3 mRNA expression is in the islands of Calleja, the olfactory tubercle, a few septal nuclei, the hypothalamus, and distinct regions of the thalamus (Levesque *et al.*, 1992). This pattern of localization in limbic regions suggests that the D_3 receptor may mediate dopaminergic control of cognition and emotion (Sokoloff *et al.*, 1990). Interestingly, a selective loss of dopamine D_3-type receptor mRNA expression in parietal and motor cortices of patients with chronic schizophrenia has been reported (Schmauss *et al.*, 1993).

The D_3 receptor is also expressed by dopaminergic neurons, indicating that it may serve an autoreceptor function with the D_2 receptor. Such a role for the D_3 receptor would be consistent with its high apparent affinity for dopamine, which at very low concentrations reduces the firing of dopaminergic neurons (Starke *et al.*, 1989). However, this function of the D_3 receptor remains unproven.

When stably expressed in CHO cells, D_3 receptors mediate inhibition of cAMP accumulation and can stimulate DNA synthesis and cell proliferation (Chio *et al.*, 1994). This latter effect is dependent on the stimulation of a pertussis toxin-sensitive G-protein, but independent of intracellular changes in cAMP levels.

D. D_4 RECEPTOR

The D_4 receptor cDNA was cloned by low-stringency screening of a human neuroblastoma cell cDNA library using the rat D_2 receptor cDNA as a probe (Van Tol *et al.*, 1991). The D_4 receptor gene also contains introns in its coding region (Van Tol *et al.*, 1991) and is localized on chromosome 11p15.5 (Gelernter *et al.*, 1992). The D_4 receptor shows an overall homology with D_2 and D_3 receptors of 41% and 39%, respectively; its structural characteristics are described in Table 1. The D_4 receptor displays a similar or lower pharmacological affinity for dopamine receptor antagonists and agonists as compared with D_2 and D_3 receptors. However, the atypical antipsychotic clozapine, and its congener octoclothepin, exhibited about 10-fold higher affinity for the D_4 receptor than for the D_2 receptor (Van Tol *et al.*, 1991). Interestingly, the dissociation constant for clozapine measured *in vitro* is similar to the concentration of clozapine measured in the blood of individuals administered with this drug during antipsychotic therapy. This suggests that D_4 receptor may be the primary target of the antipsychotic action of clozapine, although it also binds to muscarinic acetylcholine and 5-HT2 receptors. The expression and distribution of the D_4 receptor is lower and much more restricted than that of the D_2 receptor. Highest expression is found in the frontal cortex, midbrain, amygdala, and medulla, with lower levels observed in the striatum and olfactory tubercles (O'Malley et al., 1992). D_4 receptor activation inhibits cAMP accumulation in CHO cells and potentiates ATP-stimulated [^{3}H] archidonic acid (AA) release. AA release is known to occur through a protein kinase C-dependent pathway, thus providing indirect evidence that D_4 receptors might also lead to the activation of the protein kinase C pathway (Chio et al., 1994).

Several polymorphic variants of D_4 receptor have been found in humans, which differ by the number of repeat units (composed of 16 aa), located in the third cytoplasmic loop region of the receptor (Van Tol et al., 1992). To date, 27 different haplotypes that code for 20 different receptor variants have been identified, and these polymorphic variants display slightly different pharmacological properties (Asghari et al., 1994). An increased number of D_4 receptors was reported in schizophrenic patients, which suggested a role for these receptors in human psychosis (Seeman et al., 1993). Exon III polymorphism of the D_4 receptor gene has been associated with the novelty-seeking behavior, one of the human personality traits (Benjamin et al., 1996; Ebstein et al., 1996), and the number of exon III repeats seems to affect the binding of ligands to D_4 receptor (Giros et al., 1991).

III. D_1-LIKE RECEPTORS

A. D_1 RECEPTOR

The human and rat D_1 receptor sequences differ considerably from those of the dopamine D_2-like receptor subfamily (Dearry et al., 1990; Monsma et al., 1990; Sunahara et al., 1990; Zhou et al., 1990). In contrast to the D_2-like subfamily, D_1-like receptors are encoded by intronless genes and also have short third cytoplasmic loops with long C-termini (Sunahara et al., 1990), which are typical characteristics of receptors that activate AC. The C-terminal region of dopamine D_1-like receptors is about seven times longer than that of dopamine D_2-like receptors (see Table 1). This segment is rich in serines and threonines, which may provide substrates for phosphorylation. The human D_1 receptor is localized on chromosome 5. Expression of the cloned rat and human D_1 receptors in various mammalian cells has shown Kd values for the antagonist [^{3}H] SCH 23390 of 0.2 nM–0.63 nM (Dearry *et al.*, 1990; Monsma *et al.*, 1990; Sunahara *et al.*, 1990; Zhou *et al.*, 1990) consistent with the values reported for the native striatal receptor.

D_1 receptor protein and mRNA are expressed in the caudate-putamen, nucleus accumbens, and olfactory tubercle, and also in the cerebral cortex, limbic region, hypothalamus, and thalamus (Dearry *et al.*, 1990; Monsma *et al.*, 1990; Sunahara *et al.*, 1990; Zhou *et al.*, 1990). The D_1 receptor is linked to the stimulation of AC, but coupling to other second messenger pathways also occurs (e.g., activation of PI hydrolysis) (Undie *et al.*, 1994) and inhibition of AA release in rat striatal cells (Schinelli *et al.*, 1994).

B. D_5 RECEPTOR

The second member of the D_1-like receptor subfamily is the D_5 or D_{1B} receptor (Grandy *et al.*, 1991; Sunahara *et al.*, 1991). The human D_5 receptor cDNA encodes a putative 477-aa protein with high homology to the D_1 receptor. Overall, the percentage of homology is about 50% between the D_1 and D_5 receptors, reaching 80% within the membrane-spanning regions. The D_5 receptor gene lacks introns and two pseudogenes for this receptor have been identified in the human genome (Grandy *et al.*, 1991). Both pseudogenes contain insertions and deletions in the coding region that result in in-frame stop codons leading to truncated, nonfunctional receptors. The human D_5 receptor gene is located at 4p15.1–p15.33, centromeric to the location of the Huntington's disease locus (Eubanks *et al.*, 1992). Northern blots and *in situ* hybridization analysis revealed that the receptor is neuron specific, localized primarily within limbic region of the brain; no messenger RNA was detected in other tissues (Grandy *et al.*, 1991; Sunahara *et al.*, 1991). The D_5 receptor is also known to be positively coupled to AC activity.

IV. DOPAMINE D_1 AND D_2 RECEPTOR INTERACTIONS IN BASAL GANGLIA

The basal ganglia is the major brain system through which the cerebral cortex influences motor function. Five large subcortical nuclei constitute the basal ganglia: the caudate nucleus, putamen (together, these two nuclei are called the neostriatum or striatum), globus pallidus, subthalamic nucleus, and substantia nigra. Processing of cortical input in the striatum is modulated by dopaminergic input from the substantia nigra. There are two major output pathways from the striatum (Fig. 1). The direct pathway is the striatal projection to the internal segment of the globus pallidus and substantia nigra pars reticulata, which then projects to the thalamus. The in-

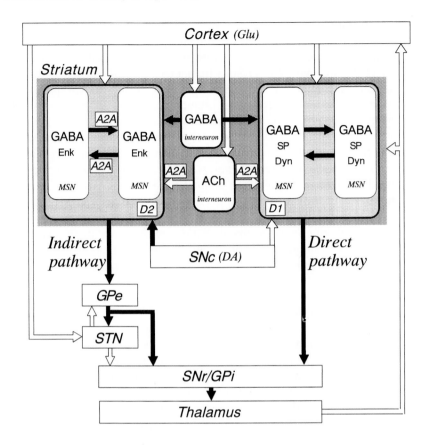

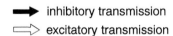

FIGURE 1   Diagram of the neural connection of basal ganglia

direct pathway projects from the striatum to the external segment of the globus pallidus, which then projects to the subthalamic nucleus. The subthalamic nucleus in turn projects back to both pallidal segments and the substantia nigra. This functional neostriatal unit consists of medium-size spiny neurons. These neurons use the inhibitory neurotransmitter, γ-aminobutyric acid (GABA) (Alexander and Crutcher, 1990). Neurons bearing D_1 receptors constitute the direct striatonigral output pathway. These neurons also express dynorphin and substance P (Gerfen et al., 1990), whereas neurons bearing D_2 receptors constitute the indirect striatopallidal pathway and express enkephalin.

The significance of D_1 and D_2 receptor-specific regulation of striatonigral and striatopallidal pathways is related to their opposing effects on GABAergic neurons and their regulation of the expression of colocalized neuropeptides (see Fig. 1). Normal movement results from a coordinated balance of cortical and thalamic excitation of the striatonigral and striatopallidal pathways, which regulate the tonic activity of substantia nigra pars reticulata neurons. The dopaminergic projection from the substantia nigra has dual effects on neurons in the neostriatum. Dopamine excites the striatonigral pathway while it inhibits the striatopallidal pathway. A reduction of the dopaminergic input to the striatum results in increased expression of enkephalin and a decrease in substance P (Gerfen *et al.*, 1990; see Chapter 8). Alterations in the activity of the components of the direct and indirect pathways can disrupt this balance, which can lead either to the production of involuntary movements or to akinesia or bradykinesia as occurs in Parkinson's disease. In this context, mice lacking dopamine receptors offer a great opportunity to assess the specific role of each receptor subtype in these functional interactions.

V. DOPAMINE AND ADENOSINE

Dopaminergic neurotransmission is not the only system involved in the control of motor funtion in the striatum. Another key regulator of basal ganglia activity is adenosine. Adenosine's activity is produced through its binding to adenosine receptors, which similar to dopaminergic receptors, belong to the seven transmembrane domain G-protein coupled receptor family. In the brain, four different adenosine receptors have been identified, the A_1, A_{2A}, A_{2B}, and A_3 receptors (Fredholm *et al.*, 1994). A_1 and A_3 receptors are negatively coupled to AC, whereas A_{2A} and A_{2B} receptors are positively coupled to it (see Chapter 5). Adenosine receptors are found in the central nervous system (CNS) as well as in the periphery (see Chapter 2). The A_1 receptors have a diffuse expression throughout the brain; in the striatum they are present on both medium spiny neurons and on cholinergic interneurons (Alexander and Reddington, 1989; Dixon *et al.*, 1996; Rivkees *et al.*, 1995). A_{2B} receptors are mainly present in the periphery but have also been reported in brain (Stehle *et al.*, 1992). A_3 receptors are expressed throughout the CNS and many peripheral tissues (Dixon *et al.*, 1996).

Interestingly, adenosine agonists have been shown to alter locomotion and in particular to modulate the activity of dopamine (Ferré *et al.*, 1992). The A_{2A} receptor is particularly interesting in this regard, because it is expressed in the striatum, nucleus accumbens, olfactory tubercle, and the globus pallidus (Jarvis and Williams, 1989; Parkinson and Fredholm, 1990). One interesting feature of this receptor is its colocalization with dopamine D_2

receptors (Fink *et al.*, 1992). The A_{2A} receptor is in fact expressed on the GABAergic neurons of the indirect pathway. Indeed, the adenosine A_{2A} receptor exerts opposing effect on D_2 receptor-mediated signal transduction (Yang *et al.*, 1995), gene expression (Boegman and Vincent, 1996: Morelli *et al.*, 1995), neurotransmitter release (Mayfield *et al.*, 1996), and behavioral responses (Ferré *et al.*, 1992). An important observation is the ability of A_{2A} receptors to control the expression of enkephalin in the striatal neurons of the indirect pathway. Dopamine depletion leads to an increase in preproenkephalin gene expression (Augood *et al.*, 1989), and adenosine A_{2A} receptor antagonists reverse this effect (Richardson *et al.*, 1997; see Chapter 8). Adenosine antagonist-induced motor activation was also inhibited by treatments that causes acute dopamine depletion or by blockade of D_1 or D_2 receptors (Ferré *et al.*, 1992). Furthermore, adenosine receptor agonists inhibit, and adenosine receptor antagonists potentiate, the motor activating effects of dopamine agonists (Ferré *et al.*, 1992). Antagonistic intramembrane A_{2A}–D_2 interaction (Ferré *et al.*, 1991, 1992, 1993, 1994a, 1994b) and antagonistic A_{2A}–D_2 interaction in adenylate cyclase signal transduction were proposed as mechanisms responsible for the motor effects of adenosine receptor agonists and antagonists (Ferré *et al.*, 1997).

In addition, adenosine receptor stimulation directly regulates neurotransmission. For example, presynaptic A_{2A} receptors localized on collateral axons of striatal GABAergic neurons directly exert an inhibitory modulation of GABA release in the striatum (Mori *et al.*, 1996; see Chapter 6). The ability of adenosine A_{2A}-selective agonists to inhibit GABA release in striatal synaptosomes further supports adenosine A_{2A}-mediated direct regulation of GABAergic feedback inhibition (Kurokawa *et al.*, 1994; see Chapter 7). Hence, because inhibition of GABA release onto striatopallidal neurons is likely to increase their activity, antagonists of adenosine A_{2A} receptors should improve hypokinetic movement disorders such as Parkinson's disease (Richardson *et al.*, 1997). As described later in this chapter, adenosine A_{2A} receptor knockout mice do not respond to the A_{2A} agonist CGS21680, which reduces locomotor activity in wild-type mice, and show a reduction of the expression of enkephalin (Ledent *et al.*, 1997). These results further support a direct regulation of the locomotor activity and the expression of enkephalin. Conversely, D_2 receptor knockout mice should provide information on the regulatory role of the adenosine A_{2A} receptor in the striatum.

The ability of A_{2A} receptor antagonists to alter motor function may have relevance to the treatment of Parkinson's disease. Adenosine A_{2A} receptor antagonists may be able to reestablish the physiological functioning and balance of striatal neurons in parkinsonian patients. Understanding the mechanisms of action of adenosine A_{2A} antagonists in terms of A_{2A}–D_2

interaction and/or A_{2A} direct action would be critical in determining whether A_{2A} antagonist can be used as monotherapy and/or as an adjunct to levodopa or dopamine agonist therapy in treating Parkinson's disease.

Dopamine and adenosine receptor-deficient mutant mice have been generated (Accili *et al.*, 1996; Baik *et al.*, 1995; Drago *et al.*, 1994; Ledent *et al.*, 1997; Rubinstein *et al.*, 1997; Xu *et al.*, 1994, 1997; Table 2), allowing discrimination of function of each receptor *in vivo*.

VI. D_2 RECEPTOR-DEFICIENT MICE

We generated D_2 receptor knockout mice (Baik *et al.*, 1995), which showed a striking impairment of motor behavior. These mice have slower movements and an abnormal posture and gait, with splayed hind legs when compared with normal animals. When these phenotypes were studied using locomotor behavioral tests, such as the open field, ring test, and rotarod test, the homozygous D_2 receptor-deficient mice showed severe impairments (Table 2). Rearing, a component of stereotyped behavior, was also absent in D_2 receptor-deficient mice.

D_2 receptor-deficient mice show a slight reduction of their body weight resulting from a 10–15% reduction in water and food intake (see Table 2) showing an involvement of the D_2 receptor in the control of feeding behavior. Interestingly, we showed that no compensation (in levels of expression) by other members of the D_2-like receptor subfamily or of D_1-like receptors occurred in these animals. The D_2 receptor deficiency led to a strong elevation of enkephalin levels in the striatum of D_2 receptor-deficient mice, and we also observed a slight decrease of substance P expression, whereas the level of expression of dynorphin seemed to be unaltered (Baik *et al.*, 1995). Strikingly, these findings are reminiscent of the modifications observed in the striatum of 6-hydroxydopamine (6-OHDA)-lesioned animals (Gerfen *et al.*, 1990). In the D_2 receptor-deficient mice, an increase in cortical expression of glutamic acid decarboxylase (GAD) was observed. Because chronic administration of D_2 receptor antagonists causes activation of striatopallidal GABA pathways (Ogren and Fuxe, 1988) and induces increase in striatal GAD mRNA levels (Laprade and Soghomonian, 1995), we suggest that the increased GAD expression in the cortex of D_2 receptor-deficient mice might represent a compensatory mechanism to overcome the increased stimulation of the striatopallidal pathway. This hypothesis awaits confirmation.

Reduced fertility was observed in the breeding of homozygous D_2 receptor-deficient mice indicating alterations of the hypothalamic-pituitary-gonadal axis. We have determined that D_2 receptor-deficient mice have very high

TABLE 2 Comparison of the phenotypes between different dopamine/adenosine receptor null mice

	D₁ receptor null mice (xu et al., 1994a,b; Drago et al., 1994)	D₂ receptor null mice (Baik et al., 1995)	D₃ receptor null mice (Accili et al., 1996)	D₄ receptor null mice (Rubinstein et al., 1997)	A₂ₐ receptor null mice (Ledent et al., 1997)
General phenotypes	viable 30% reduction in body weight no gross abnormalities (Xu et al.) poorly groomed coat and huntched posture (Drago et al.) fertile	viable 15% reduction in body weight reduction in water and food intake reduced fertility	viable no gross developmental deficit fertile	viable normal growth fertile	viable normal appearance higher body mass fertile increased blood pressure and heart rate increased platelet aggregation
Pharmacology	SCH23982 binding—absent SCH23390 binding—absent spiroperidol binding—unaltered	spiperone binding-absent SCH23390 binding-unaltered	iodosulpride binding-absent in the presence of domperidone	spiperone binding-unaltered SCH23390 binding-unaltered	CGS21680 binding- absent
Behavior	normal righting, placing and grasp reflex normal coordination no akinesic behavior normal locomotor activity (Drago et al.) mild hyperlocomotion (Xu et al.) reduced rearing (Drago et al.)	abnormal posture and gait severe locomotor impairment reduced rearing less coordinated cataleptic behavior	normal gait increased locomotor activity increased rearing normal coordination	reduced spontaneous locomotion reduced rearing more coordinated more responsive to ethanol, cocaine and amphetamine less sensitive to clozapine	reduced exploratory behaviour increased anxiety strong depressant by caffeine more aggressive (male) slower response to acute pain stimuli
Neuropeptide/ transmitter regulations	substance P- reduced dynorphin- reduced enkephalin- unaltered	substance P- slightly reduced dynorphin- unaltered enkephalin- increased GAD- increased TH- unaltered		DOPAC- increased	substance P- reduced enkephalin- reduced
Hormonal regulations	no altered parathyroid function normal growth hormone level	increased level of prolactin decreased size of testes and ovaries			

levels of circulating prolactin, which may be the cause of fertility problems (Saiardi *et al.*, 1997). In addition, large hyperplasia are found in the pituitaries of D_2 receptor-deficient mice. These finding suggest a role for D_2 receptor not only in the regulation of prolactin synthesis and release, but also on the control of pituitary cell proliferation.

The phenotypic changes observed in D_2 receptor-deficient animals support an essential role for these receptors in the dopaminergic control of physiological function connected to movement and the regulation of hormone secretion.

VII. ADENOSINE A_{2A} RECEPTOR-DEFICIENT MICE

Adenosine A_{2A} receptor-deficient mice that are viable and fertile have been obtained (Ledent *et al.*, 1997). A_{2A} receptor-deficient mice do not respond to CGS21680, confirming the knockout and the specificity of this ligand for the A_{2A} receptor. Interestingly, the exploratory activity of A_{2A} receptor mutants is reduced, suggesting alterations in basal ganglia function. Indeed, the nonselective adenosine antagonist caffeine, which stimulates locomotion in normal animals, provokes a reduction of exploratory activity in A_{2A} receptor-deficient mice. These results may be due to the activation of other adenosine receptor subtypes in the absence of the A_{2A} receptor. Another feature of animals lacking A_{2A} receptors is that they are more aggressive as established in the resident–intruder test. In agreement with the involvement of adenosine in nociception, blood pressure, and platelets aggregation, absence of A_{2A} receptors leads to animals that respond slowly to pain and have higher blood pressure, heart rate, and platelet aggregation. Thus, these animals represent a unique tool to study the effect of different drugs to modulate these functions in a model system in which the A_{2A} receptor is absent.

Because A_{2A} receptors occur on striatal enkephalinergic neurons also expressing D_2 receptors, A_{2A} receptor knockout mice show a reduction of the expression of enkephalin. Interestingly, this phenotype is exactly the opposite of that found in D_2 receptor-deficient mice, where the expression of enkephalin is upregulated. This indicates that both A_{2A} and D_2 receptors can directly regulate the expression of this peptide, probably through the modulation of the cAMP pathway. These findings also support the antagonistic action of adenosine and dopamine receptors in striatal neurons, which belong to the indirect output pathway.

VIII. ANIMAL MODELS OF NEUROPATHOLOGIES: D_2 RECEPTOR-DEFICIENT MICE AND PARKINSON'S DISEASE

Parkinson's disease is primarily due to degeneration of the dopaminergic neurons in the substantia nigra, destruction of the nigrostriatal pathway, and the consequent decrease in striatal dopamine content. Interestingly, genetic ablation of D_2 receptor results in parkinsonian-like locomotor phenotype. Although we are aware that the mechanisms underlying motor dysfunction in Parkinson's disease and D_2 receptor-deficient mice symptoms are not the same, the similarity of the locomotor phenotype is intriguing. It suggests that lack of dopamine in Parkinson's disease might particularly affect the function of striatal D_2 receptors and that D_2 receptor has a key function in motor skills control. Indeed, the observations that D_2 receptor-deficient mice have impaired locomotion is consistent not only with akinesia in Parkinson's disease, but also with hypoactivity resulting from antagonist blockade of dopamine receptors. Importantly, D_1 receptor knockout mice display either normal (Drago *et al.*, 1994) or a mild hyperactivity (Xu *et al.*, 1994), in contrast with D_2 receptor-deficient mice (Baik *et al.*, 1995). Moreover, in dopamine-deficient mice, a significant improvement of locomotion and stereotypy was obtained when they were treated with low doses of D_2 receptor agonist, indicating that D_1 receptor stimulation is not required for D_2 receptor-mediated behaviors. Thus, we believe that careful characterization of D_2 receptor-deficient mice will help our understanding of the mechanisms responsible for the movement disorders of Parkinson's disease. These mice might also be used to test novel drug therapies for restoring locomotor activity.

We have started experiments aimed at studying whether the administration of a novel adenosine A_{2A} selective antagonist, KW-6002, might restore motor activity in D_2 receptor-deficient mice. The results obtained so far strongly support A_{2A} antagonists as a potential alternative therapy for Parkinson's disease. Indeed, preliminary experiments show that blockade of A_{2A} receptors in D_2 receptor-null mice reestablish locomotor activity and the coordination of movement. In addition, A_{2A} receptor antagonists reverse the elevation of enkephalin levels. This means that A_{2A} receptors, in the absence of D_2 receptors, can regulate locomotor activity, coordination of movement, and peptide gene expression, although they do not exclude a contribution of the intramembrane $A_{2A}-D_2$ receptor interaction in intact systems. These results therefore are encouraging for the use of A_{2A} antagonists in the treatment of Parkinson's disease as a potential nondopaminergic approach to treatment.

The generation of knockout mice lacking specific neuronal receptors and their exploitation for testing different pharmacological agents is only just beginning. We believe that these mutants represent important tools for analyzing not only their involvement in the control of different physiological functions, but also as a testbed for novel pharmacological therapies *in vivo*.

REFERENCES

Accili, D., Fishburn, C.S., Drago, J., Steiner, H., Lachowicz, J.E., Park, B.-H., Gauda, E.B., Lee, E.J., Cool, M.H., Sibley, D.R., Gerfen, C.R., Westphal, H., and Fuchs, S. (1996). A targeted mutation of the D_3 dopamine receptor gene is associated with hyperactivity in mice. *Proc Natl Acad Sci USA* 93, 1945–1949.

Alexander, G.E., and Crutcher, M.D. (1990). Functional architecture of basal ganglia circuits: neural substrates of parallel processing. *Trends Neurosci* 13, 266–272.

Alexander, S.P., and Reddington, M. (1989). The cellular localization of adenosine receptors in rat neostriatum. *Neurosci* 28, 645–651.

Ariano, M.A., Larson, E.R., Noblett, K.L., Sibley, D.R., and Levine, M.S. (1997). Coexpression of striatal dopamine receptor subtypes and excitatory amino acid subunits. *Synapse* 26, 400–414.

Asghari, V., Schoots, O., van Kats, S., Ohara, K., Jovanovic, V., Guan, H.-C., Bunzow, J.R., Petronis, A., and Van Tol, H.H. (1994). Dopamine D_4 receptor repeat: analysis of different native and mutant forms of the human and rat genes. *Mol Pharmacol* 46, 364–373.

Augood, S.J., Emson, P.C., Mitchell, I.J., Boyce, S., Clarke, C.E., and Crossman, A.R. (1989). Cellular localisation of enkephalin gene expression in MPTP-treated cynomolgus monkeys. *Brain Res Mol Brain Res* 6, 85–92.

Baik, J.-H., Picetti, R., Saiardi, A., Thiriet, G., Dierich, A., Depaulis, A., Le Meur, M., and Borrelli, E. (1995). Parkinsonian-like locomotor impairment in mice lacking dopamine D_2 receptors. *Nature* 377, 424–428.

Benjamin, J., Li, L., Patterson, C., Greenberg, B.J., Murphy, D.L., and Hamer, D.H. (1996). Population and familial association between the D_4 dopamine receptor gene and measures of novelty seeking. *Nature Genet* 12, 81–84.

Boegman, R.J., and Vincent, S.R. (1996). Involvement of adenosine and glutamate receptors in the induction of c-fos in the striatum by haloperidol. *Synapse* 22, 70–77.

Bunzow, J.R., Van Tol, H.H., Grandy, D.K., Albert, P., Salon, J., Christie, M., Machida, C.A., Neve, K.A., and Civelli, O. (1988). Cloning and expression of a rat D_2 dopamine receptor. *Nature* 336, 783–787.

Chio, C.L., Hess, G.F., Graham, R.S., and Huff, R.M. (1990). A second molecular form of D_2 dopamine receptor in rat and bovine caudate nucleus. *Nature* 343, 266–269.

Chio, C.L., Lajiness, M.E., and Huff, R.M. (1994). Activation of heterologously expressed D_3 dopamine receptors: Comparison with D_2 dopamine receptors. *Mol Pharmacol* 45, 51–60.

Cote, T.E., Frey, E.A., Grewe, C.W., and Kebabian, J.W. (1983). Evidence that the D_2 dopamine receptor in the intermediate lobe of the rat pituitary gland is associated with an inhibitory guanyl nucleotide component. *J Neuro Trans Suppl* 18, 139–147.

Dal Toso, R., Sommer, B., Ewert, M., Herb, A., Pritchett, D.B., Bach, A., Shivers, B.D., and Seeburg, PH. (1989). The dopamine D_2 receptor: two molecular forms generated by alternative splicing. *EMBO J* 8, 4025–4034.

Dearry, A., Gingrich, J.A., Falardeau, P., Fremeau, R.T., Jr., Bates, M.D., and Caron, M.G. (1990). Molecular cloning and expression of the gene for a human D_1 dopamine receptor. *Nature* 347, 72–75.

Dixon, A.K., Gubitz, A.K., Sirinathsinghji, D.J., Richardson, P.J., and Freeman, T.C. (1996). Tissue distribution of adenosine receptor mRNAs in the rat. *Br J Pharmacol* 118, 1461–1468.

Drago, J., Gerfen, C.R., Lachowicz, J.E., Steiner, H., Hollon, T.R., Love, P.E., Ooi, G.T., Grinberg, A., Lee, E.J., Huang, S.P., Bartlett, P.F., Jose, P.A., Sibley, D.R., and Westphal, H. (1994). Altered striatal function in a mutant mouse lacking D_{1A} dopamine receptor. *Proc Natl Acad Sci USA* 91, 12564–12568.

Ebstein, R.P., Novick, O., Umansky, R., Priel, B., Osher, Y., Blaine, D., Bennet, E.R., Nemanov, L., Katz, M., and Belmarker, R.H. (1996). Dopamine D_4 receptor (D_4DR) exon III polymorphism associated with the human personality trait of novelty seeking. *Nature Genet* 12, 78–80.

Eubanks, J.H., Altherr, M., Wagner-McPherson, C., McPherson, J.D., Wasmuth, J.J., and Evans, G.A. (1992). Localization of the D_5 dopamine receptor gene to human chromosome 4p15.1–p15.3, centromeric to the Huntington's disease locus. *Genomics* 12, 510–516.

Ferré, S., von Euler, G., Johansson, B., Fredholm, B.B., and Fuxe, K. (1991). Stimulation of high-affinity adenosine A_2 receptors decreases the affinity of dopamine D_2 receptors in rat striatal membranes. *Proc Natl Acad Sci USA* 88, 7238–7241.

Ferré, S., and Fuxe, K. (1992). Dopamine denervation leads to an increase in the intramembrane interaction between adenosine A_2 and dopamine D_2 receptors in the neostriatum. *Brain Res* 594, 124–130.

Ferré, S., Fuxe, K., von Euler, G., Johansson, B., and Fredholm, B.B. (1992). Adenosine–dopamine interactions in the brain. *Neurosci* 51, 501–512.

Ferré, S., Snaprud, P., and Fuxe, K. (1993). Opposing actions of an adenosine A_2 receptor agonist and a GTP analogue on the regulation of dopamine D_2 receptors in rat neostriatal membranes. *Eur J Pharmacol* 244, 311–315.

Ferré, S., Schwarcz, R., Li, X.M., Snaprud, P., Ogren, S.O., and Fuxe, K. (1994a). Chronic haloperidol treatment leads to an increase in the intramembrane interaction between adenosine A_2 and dopamine D_2 receptors in the neostriatum. *Psychopharmacol (Berl)* 116, 279–284.

Ferré, S., O'Connor, W. T., Snaprud, P., Ungerstedt, U., and Fuxe, K. (1994b). Antagonistic interaction between adenosine A_{2A} receptors and dopamine D_2 receptors in the ventral striopallidal system. Implications for the treatment of schizophrenia. *Neurosci* 63, 765–773.

Ferré, S., Fredholm, B.B., Morelli M., Popoli, P., and Fuxe, K. (1997). Adenosine–dopamine receptor–receptor interactions as an integrative mechanism in the basal ganglia. *Trends Neurosci* 20, 482–487.

Fink, J.S., Weaver, D.R., Rivkees, S.A., Peterfreund, R.A., Pollack, A.E., Adler, E.M., and Reppert, S.M. (1992). Molecular cloning of the rat A_2 adenosine receptor: selective co-expression with D_2 dopamine receptors in rat striatum. *Brain Res Mol Brain Res* 14, 186–195.

Fredholm, B.B., Abbracchio, M.P., Burnstock, G., Daly, J.W., Harden, T.K., Jacobson, K.A., Leff, P., and Williams, M. (1994). Nomenclature and classification of purinoceptors. *Pharmacol Rev* 46, 143–156.

Gelernter, J., Kennedy, J.L., Van Tol, H.H., Civelli, O., and Kidd, K.K. (1992). The D_4 dopamine receptor (DRD_4) maps to distal 11p close to HRAS. *Genomics* 13, 208–210.

Gerfen, C.R., Engber, T.M., Mahan, L.C., Susel, Z., Chase, T.N., Monsma, F.J., Jr., and Sibley, D.R. (1990). D_1 and D_2 dopamine receptor-regulated gene expression of striatonigral and striatopallidal neurons. *Science* 250, 1429–1432.

Gerfen, C.R. (1992). The neostriatal mosaic: multiple levels of compartmental organization. *Trends Neurosci* 15, 133–139.

Gingrich, J.A., and Caron, M.G. (1993). Recent advances in the molecular biology of dopamine receptors. *Annu Rev Neurosci* 16, 299–321.

Giros, B., Sokoloff, P., Martres, M.P., Riou, J.F., Emorine, L.J., and Schwartz, J.C. (1989). Alternative splicing directs the expression of two D_2 dopamine receptor isoforms. *Nature* 342, 923–926.

Giros, B., Martres, M.P., Pilon, C., Sokoloff, P., and Schwartz, J.C. (1991). Shorter variants of the D_3 dopamine receptor produced through various patterns of alternative splicing. *Biochem Biophys Res Commun* 176, 1584–1592.

Giros, B., Jaber, M., Jones, S.R., Wightman, R.M., and Caron, M.G. (1996). Hyperlocomotion and indifference to cocaine and amphetamine in mice lacking the dopamine transporter. *Nature* 379, 606–612.

Grandy, D.K., Marchionni, M.A., Makam, H., Stofko, R.E., Alfano, M., Frothingham, L., Fischer, J.B., Burke-Howie, K.J., Bunzow, J.R., Server, A.C., and Civelli, O. (1989). Cloning of the cDNA and gene for a human D_2 dopamine receptor. *Proc Natl Acad Sci USA* 86, 9762–9766.

Grandy, D.K., Zhang, Y.A., Bouvier, C., Zhou, Q.Y., Johnson, R.A., Allen, L., Buck, K., Bunzow, J.R., Salon, J., and Civelli, O. (1991). Multiple human D_5 dopamine receptor genes: a functional receptor and two pseudogenes. *Proc Natl Acad Sci USA* 88, 9175–9179.

Graybiel, A.M. (1990). Neurotransmitters and neuromodulators in the basal ganglia. *Trends Neurosci* 13, 244–254.

Guiramand, J., Montmayeur, J.-P., Ceraline, J., Bhatia, M., and Borrelli, E. (1995). Alternative splicing of the dopamine D_2 receptor directs specificity of coupling to G-proteins. *J Biol Chem* 270, 7354–7358.

Hersch, S.M., Ciliax, B.J., Gutekunst, C.A., Rees, H.D., Heilman, C.J., Yung, K.K., Bolam, J.P., Ince, E., Yi, H., and Levey, A.I. (1995). Electron microscopic analysis of D_1 and D_2 dopamine receptor proteins in the dorsal striatum and their synaptic relationships with motor cortico-striatal afferents. *J Neurosci* 15, 5222–5237.

Hornykiewicz, O. (1966). Dopamine and brain function. *Pharmacol Rev* 18, 925–964.

Jackson, D.J., and Westlind-Daniesson, A. (1994). Dopamine receptors: molecular biology, biochemistry and behavioural aspects. *Pharmacol Ther* 64, 291–369.

Jarvis, M.F., and Williams, M. (1989). Direct autoradiographic localization of adenosine A_2 receptors in the rat brain using the A_2-selective agonist, [^{3}H]CGS 21680. *Eur J Pharmacol* 168, 243–246.

Kurokawa, M., Kirk, I.P., Kirkpatrick, K.A., Kase, H., and Richardson, P.J. (1994). Inhibition by KF17837 of adenosine A_{2A} receptor-mediated modulation of striatal GABA and ACh release. *Br J Pharmacol* 113, 43–48.

Laprade, N., and Soghomonian, J.J. (1995). Differential regulation of mRNA levels encoding for the two isoforms of glutamate decarboxylase (GAD65 and GAD67) by dopamine receptors in the rat striatum. *Brain Res Mol Brain Res* 34, 65–74.

Ledent, C., Vaugeois, J.M., Schiffmann, S.N., Pedrazzini, T., El Yacoubi, M., Vanderhaeghen, J.J., Costentin, J., Heath, J.K., Vassart, G., and Parmentier, M. (1997). Aggressiveness, hypoalgesia and high blood pressure in mice lacking the adenosine A_{2A} receptor. *Nature* 388, 674–678.

Levesque, D., Diaz, J., Pilon, C., Martres, M.P., Giros, B., Souil, E., Schott, D., Morgat, J.L., Schwartz, J.C., and Sokoloff, P. (1992). Identification, characterization, and localization of the dopamine D_3 receptor in rat brain using 7-[^{3}H] hydroxy-N,N-di-n-propyl-2-aminotetralin. *Proc Natl Acad Sci USA* 89, 8155–8159.

Malmberg, A., Jackson, D.M., Eriksson, A., and Mohell, N. (1993). Unique binding characteristics of antipsychotic agents interacting with human dopamine D_{2A}, D_{2B}, and D_3 receptors. *Mol pharmacol* 43, 749–754.

Mayfield, R.D., Larson, G., Orona, R.A., and Zahnisser, N.R. (1996). Opposing action of adenosine A_{2A} and dopamine D_2 receptor activation of GABA release in the basal ganglia: evidence for an A_{2A}/D_2 receptor interaction in globus pallidus. *Synapse* 22, 132–138.

Meador-Woodruff, J.H., Mansour, A., Healy, D.J., Kuehn, R., Zhou, Q.Y., Bunzow, J.R., Akil, H., Civelli, O., and Watson, S.J., Jr. (1991). Comparison of the distributions of D_1 and D_2 dopamine receptor mRNAs in rat brain. *Neuropsychopharmacol* 5, 231–242.

Monsma, F.J., Mahan, L.C., McVittie, L.D., Gerfen, C.R., and Sibley, D.R. (1990). Molecular cloning and expression of a D_1 dopamine receptor linked to adenylate cyclase activation. *Proc Natl Acad Sci USA* 87, 6723–6727.

Montmayeur, J.-P., Bausero, P., Amlaiky, N., Maroteaux, L., Hen, R., and Borrelli E. (1991). Differential expression of the mouse D_2 dopamine receptor isoforms. *FEBS Lett* 278, 239–243.

Montmayeur, J.-P., and Borrelli, E. (1991). Transcription mediated by a cAMP-responsive promoter element is reduced upon activation of dopamine D_2 receptors. *Proc Natl Acad Sci USA* 88, 3135–3139.

Montmayeur, J.-P., Guiramand, J., and Borrelli, E. (1993). Preferential coupling between dopamine D_2 receptors and G-proteins. *Mol Endocrinol* 7, 161–170.

Morelli, M., Pinna, A., Wardas, J., and Di Chiara, G. (1995). Adenosine A_2 receptors stimulate c-fos expression in striatal neurons of 6-hydroxydopamine-lesioned rats. *Neurosci* 67, 49–55.

Mori, A., Shindou, T., Ichimura, M., Nonaka, H., and Kase, H. (1996). The role of adenosine A_{2A} receptors in regulating GABAergic synaptic transmission in striatal medium spiny neurons. *J Neurosci* 16, 605–611.

Ogren, S.O., and Fuxe, K. (1988). D_1 and D_2 receptor antagonist induce catalepsy via different efferent striatal pathways. *Neurosci Lett* 85, 333–338.

O'Malley, K.L., Harmon, S., Tang, L., and Todd, R.D. (1992). The rat dopamine D_4 receptor: sequence, gene structure, and demonstration of expression in the cardiovascular system. *New Biol* 4, 137–146.

Parkinson, F.E., and Fredholm, B.B. (1990). Autoradiographic evidence for G-protein coupled A_2-receptors in rat neostriatum using [^{3}H]-CGS 21680 as a ligand. *Naunyn-Schmiedeberg's Arch Pharmacol* 342, 85–89.

Picetti, R., Saiardi, A., Abdel Samad, T., Bozzi, Y. Baik, J.H., and Borrelli, E. (1997). Dopamine D_2 receptors in signal transduction and behavior. *Crit Rev Neurobiol* 11, 121–142.

Richardson, P.J., Kase, H., and Jenner, P. (1997). Adenosine A_{2A} receptor antagonists as new agents for the treatment of Parkinson's disease. *Trends Pharmacol Sci* 18, 338–344.

Rivkees, S.A., Price, S.L., and Zhou, F.C. (1995). Immunohistochemical detection of A_1 adenosine receptors in rat brain with emphasis on localization in the hippocampal formation, cerebral cortex, cerebellum, and basal ganglia. *Brain Res* 677, 193–203.

Rubinstein, M., Phillips, T.J., Bunzow, J.R., Falzone, T.L., Dziewczapolski, G., Zhang, G., Fang, Y., Larson, J.L., McDougall, J.A., Chester, J.A., Saez, C., Pugsley, T.A., Gershanik, O., Low, M.J., and Grandy, D.K. (1997). Mice lacking dopamine D_4 receptors are supersensitive to ethanol, cocaine, and methamphetamine. *Cell* 90, 991–1001.

Saiardi, A., Bozzi, Y., Baik, J.-H., and Borrelli, E. (1997). Antiproliferative role of dopamine: loss of D_2 receptors causes hormonal dysfunction and pituitary hyperplasia. *Neuron* 19, 115–126.

Schinelli, S., Paolillo, M., and Corona, G.L. (1994). Opposing actions of D_1- and D_2-dopamine receptors on arachidonic acid release and cyclic AMP production in striatal neurons. *J. Neurochem* 62, 944–949.

Schmauss, C., Haroutunian, V., Davis, K.L., and Davidson, M. (1993). Selective loss of dopamine D_3-type receptor mRNA expression in parietal and motor cortices of patients with chronic schizophrenia. *Proc Natl Acad Sci USA* 90, 8942–8946.

Seeman, P., and Niznik, H.B. (1990). Dopamine receptors and transporters in Parkinson's disease and schizophrenia. *FASEB J* 4, 2737–2744.

Seeman, P., Guan, H.-C., and Van Tol, H.H. (1993). Dopamine D_4 receptors elevated in schizophrenia. *Nature* 365, 441–445.

Selbie, L. A., Hayes, G., and Shine, J. (1989). The major dopamine D_2 receptor: molecular analysis of the human D_{2A} subtype. *DNA* 8, 683–689.

Sokoloff, P., Giros, B., Martres, M.P., Bouthenet, M.L., and Schwartz, J.C. (1990). Molecular cloning and characterization of a novel dopamine receptor (D_3) as a target for neuroleptics. *Nature* 347, 146–151.

Starke, K., Gothert, M., and Kilbinger, H. (1989). Modulation of neurotransmitter release by presynaptic autoreceptors. *Physiol Rev* 69, 864–989.

Stehle, J.H., Rivkees, S.A., Lee, J.J., Weaver, D.R., Deeds, J.D., and Reppert, S.M. (1992). Molecular cloning and expression of the cDNA for a novel A_2-adenosine receptor subtype. *Mol Endocrinol* 6, 384–393.

Sunahara, R.K., Niznik, H.B., Weiner, D.M., Stormann, T.M., Brann, M.R., Kennedy, J.L., Gelernter, J.E., Rozmahel, R., Yang, Y., Israel, Y., Seeman, P., and O'Dowd, B.F (1990). Human D_1 receptor encoded by an intronless gene on chromosome 5. *Nature* 347, 80–83.

Sunahara, R.K., Guan, H.C., O'Dowd, B.F., Seeman, P., Laurier, L.G., Ng, G., George, S.R., Torchia, J., Van Tol, H.H., and Niznik, H. (1991). Cloning of the gene for a human dopamine D_5 receptor with higher affinity for dopamine than D_1. *Nature* 350, 614–619.

Undie, A.S., Weinstock, J., Sarau, H.M., and Friedman, E. (1994). Evidence for a distinct D_1-like dopamine receptor that couples to activation of phosphoinositide metabolism in brain. *J Neurochem* 62, 2045–2048.

Vallar, L., and Meldolesi, J. (1989). Mechanisms of signal transduction at the dopamine D_2 receptor. *Trends Pharmacol Sci* 10, 74–77.

Van Tol, H.H., Bunzow, J.R., Guan, H.-C., Sunahara, R.K., Seeman, P., Niznik, H.B., and Civelli, O. (1991). Cloning of the gene for a human dopamine D_4 receptor with high affinity for the antipsychotic clozapine. *Nature* 350, 610–614.

Van Tol, H.H., Wu, CM., Guan, H.-C., Ohara, K., Bunzow, J.R., Civelli, O., Kennedy, J., Seeman, P., Niznik, H.B., and Jovanovic, V. (1992). Multiple dopamine D_4 variants in the human population. *Nature* 358, 149–152.

Xu, M., Hu, X.T., Cooper, D.C., Moratalla, R., Graybiel, A.M., White, F.J., and Tonegawa, S. (1994). Elimination of cocaine-induced hyperactivity and dopamine-mediated neurophysiological effects in dopamine D_1 receptor mutant mice. *Cell* 79, 945–955.

Xu, M., Moratalla, R., Gold, L.H., Hiroi, N., Koob, G.F., Graybiel, A.M., and Tonegawa, S. (1994). Dopamine D_1 receptor mutant mice are deficient in striatal expression of dynorphin and in dopamine-mediated behavioral responses. *Cell* 79, 729–742.

Xu, M., Koeltzow, T.E., Santiago, G.T., Moratalla, R., Cooper, D.C., Hu, X.T., White, N.M., Graybiel, A.M., White, F.J., and Tonegawa, S. (1997). Dopamine D_3 receptor mutant mice exhibit increased behavioral sensitivity to concurrent stimulation of D_1 and D_2 receptors. *Neuron* 19, 837–848.

Yang, S.N., Dasgupta, S., Lledo, P.M., Vincent, J.D., and Fuxe, K. (1995). Reduction of dopamine D_2 receptor transduction by activation of adenosine A_{2A} receptors in stably A_{2A}/D_2 (long-form) receptor co-transfected mouse fibroblast cell lines: studies on intracellular calcium levels. *Neurosci* 68, 729–736.

Yung, K.K., Bolam, J.P., Smith, A.D., Hersch, S.M., Ciliax, B.J., and Levey, A.I. (1995). Immunocytochemical localization of D_1 and D_2 dopamine receptors in the basal ganglia of the rat: light and electron microscopy. *Neurosci* 65, 709–730.

Zhou, Q.-Y., Grandy, D.K., Thambi, L., Kushner, J.A., Van Tol, H.H., Cone, R., Pribnow, D., Salon, J., Bunzow, J.R., and Civelli, O. (1990). Cloning and expression of human and rat D_1 dopamine receptors. *Nature* **347**, 76–80.

Zhou, Q.-Y., and Palmiter, R.D. (1995). Dopamine-deficient mice are severely hypoactive, adipsic, and aphagic. *Cell* **83**, 1197–1209.

CHAPTER 10

Effects of Adenosine Receptors

Experimental Models of Cognition and Motor Behavior

SHIZUO SHIOZAKI, SHUNJI ICHIKAWA, JOJI NAKAMURA, AND YOSHIHISA KUWANA

Pharmaceutical Research Institute, Kyowa Hakko Kogyo Co., Ltd., Nagaizumi-cho, Sunto-gun, Shizuoka, Japan

I. INTRODUCTION

Adenosine and adenosine analogues are remarkably active at the cellular level in altering neuronal activity, and subsequently in affecting centrally mediated behaviors. Adenosine can modulate the efficacy of synaptic transmission and affect the firing of neurons in many different brain regions. Adenosine in the central nervous system (CNS) contributes to motor function, sleep, anticonvulsant, anxiety, analgesia, and psychomotor activity. Moreover, adenosine and its analogues are reported to prevent the development of long-term potentiation in the hippocampal CA1 region of the rat. Pharmacological effects of adenosine are mediated by specific receptors initially classified into A_1 and A_2 receptors on the basis of their respective affinity for the nucleoside, and on pharmacological and biochemical criteria (e.g., inhibition $[A_1]$ or stimulation $[A_2]$ of adenylate cyclase activity) (Van Calker *et al.*, 1979). In addition, molecular cloning has led to the identification of three classes of adenosine receptors named A_1 A_2, and A_3 with A_2 receptors being further subdivided into high-affinity A_{2A} and low-affinity A_{2B} receptors (Fredholm *et al.*, 1994). The roles of A_1R and $A_{2A}R$ in the CNS have been studied extensively, whereas little is known about the effect of modulation of A_3R, mainly due to the lack of selective ligands.

In the first section of this chapter, we review the relationship of A_1R to cognitive function; in the second, the relationship of the $A_{2A}R$ to sleep and motor function is examined.

II. THE ROLE OF ADENOSINE A_1 RECEPTOR IN THE CNS IN COGNITION

A. DISTRIBUTION OF ADENOSINE A_1 RECEPTOR IN CNS

The pattern of distribution of A_1R appears to be conserved across a variety of species in specific regions of the brain (Lee and Reddington, 1986). Northern blot analysis of a variety of rat brain tissues revealed two species of mRNA (3.1 kb, 5.6 kb) for A_1R, probably produced by alternative splicing (Mahan *et al.*, 1991). The highest expression was observed in the cortex, cerebellum, and hippocampus. In particular, the hippocampus is enriched in A_1R, which are densely concentrated in the CA1 and CA3 subfields as well as in the dentate gyrus. The olfactory bulb, mesencephalon, and striatum also exhibit moderate levels of A_1R mRNAs, whereas no expression is apparent in the pituitary. *In situ* hybridization studies confirmed the tissue distribution of mRNA expression in Northern blotting. In most cases, autoradiographic labeling was restricted to neuronal but not glial nuclei. These regional distribution data are consistent with previous receptor binding studies using adenosine A_1R selective ligands, such as 8-cyclopentyl-1,3-dipropylxanthine (DPCPX).

B. COGNITION

A_1R may play a significant role in the process of cognition because it is abundantly expressed both in the hippocampus and in the cerebral cortex. Although cognitive performance is usually difficult to measure in animals and humans, there is increasing evidence that there may be some relationship between A_1R and learning or memory. However, the effect of acute administration of selective A_1R agonists and antagonists on cognition have been inconsistent. For example, although the A_1R agonists N^6-cyclopentyladenosine (CPA) and (R)-N^6-(2-phenylisopropyl)adenosine (R-PIA) impair retention in passive avoidance tasks, R-PIA has no effect on the working memory of rats. Similarly, although the selective A_1R antagonist DPCPX has no effect on responses in passive avoidance tests, another selective A_1R antagonist KFM19 (Schingnitz et al., 1991) produces an increase in memory acquisition in the Y-maze, and another A_1R antagonist MDL102503 (Dudley et al., 1994) is also reported to reverse scopolamine-induced memory deficit in rats subjected to water-maze tests (Jacobson et al., 1996).

We developed the novel selective A_1R antagonist KF15372, which efficiently crosses the blood–brain barrier making it possible to elucidate the function of the A_1R in the brain. The effects of KF15372 on amnestic syndromes in rats were investigated using passive avoidance tasks in rats treated with A_1R agonist or the acetylcholine (ACh) receptor antagonist scopolamine to cause a shortening of latency. KF15372 improved impairment of memory induced by the A_1R agonist R-PIA (1.25 mg/kg, ip) and the ACh antagonist scopolamine (1 mg/kg, ip) in the dose range of 0.31–5 mg/kg, po, and 1.25–5 mg/kg, po, respectively (Suzuki et al., 1993).

KF15372 was also effective in the amnestic models induced by basal forebrain (BF) lesions. In passive avoidance tests, the latencies in the BF-lesioned rats were significantly shorter than those in the sham-operated rats (Fig. 1).

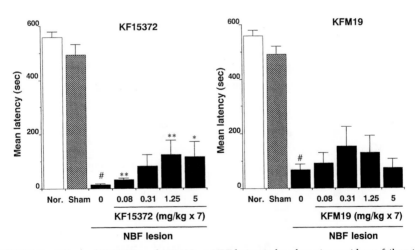

FIGURE 1   Effects of KF15372 and KFM19 on NBF lesion-induced passive avoidance failure in rats. Each drugs was repeatedly administered per os 60 min prior to the acquisition trial for 7 days. Each column and vertical bars represent the mean ± SEM ($n = 15–18$). #$p < 0.001$, Significant difference from the Sham operation group; *$p < 0.05$, **$p < 0.01$, Significant difference from the NBF lesion group (Mann–Whitney U-test).

After 7 days of repeated administration of KF15372 (0.08–5 mg/kg/day, po), the latency was significantly increased suggesting that passive avoidance response was improved (see Fig. 1). If memory could be defined as the retention of information, this information needs to be acquired, stored, and recalled when necessary. Because in this experiment, the agent was repeatedly administered before the training session, the improvement of memory is probably derived from the change in acquisition and/or store steps. The efficacy of KF15372 seems to be more potent than KFM19 as the latter was not effective at doses between 0.08 and 5 mg/kg/day in the same protocol. Moreover, KF15372 also improved the acquisition of active avoidance tasks in the basal forebrain-lesioned model (Fig. 2).

We subsequently studied the effects of KF15372 on electroencephalogram activity to elucidate the mechanism of action on cognitive improvement. Measuring rabbit cortical and hippocampal spontaneous electroencephalogram activity, KF15372 (1.25 or 5 mg/kg, po) significantly increased the appear-

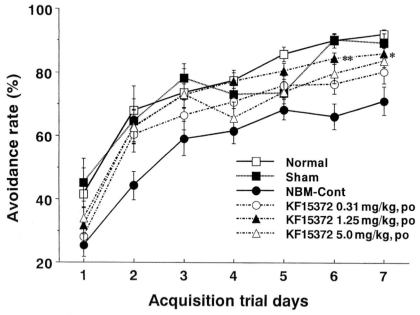

FIGURE 2   Effect of KF15372 on NBF lesion-induced acquisition failure on the conditioned avoidance response in rats. KF15372 (0.31–5 mg/kg × 7 days) was orally administered 60 min prior to the acquisition trial on each day. Acquisition trial was performed 30 trials on each day ($n = 9$–21). *$p < 0.05$, **$p < 0.01$, Significant difference vs NBF lesion group (Scheffe-type test).

ance rate of theta waves in hippocampus and alpha and beta waves in cerebral cortex (Fig. 3). This indicates that the A_1R antagonist produced an arousal effect in both cortex and hippocampus. The effect of the A_1R antagonist also suggests that activation of brain A_1R might induce drowsiness. Indeed, ip

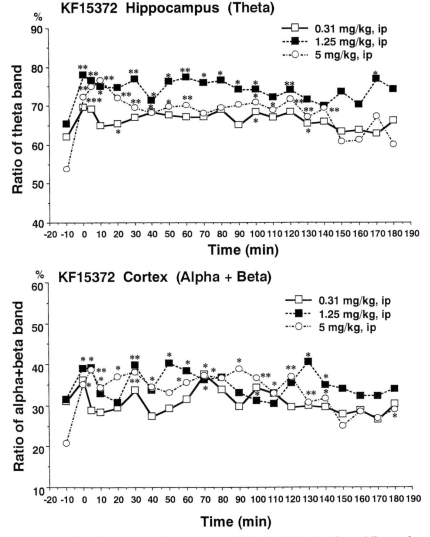

FIGURE 3   Effect of KF15372 on the spontaneous EEGs in rabbits. Significant difference from pretreatment value: *$p < 0.05$, **$p < 0.01$ (Paired t-test), $n = 5$.

injection of A_1R agonist *R*-PIA (1.25 mg/kg) decreased the ratio of theta band
in rat hippocampus, indicating desynchronization of spontaneous electroencephalogram activity. However, coadministration of KF15372 (1.25 or 5
mg/kg, po) reversed the effect of *R*-PIA (Fig. 4). Using internal capsule-le-
sioned rats, the ratio of alpha and beta waves in the total power decreased in
rats treated with KF15372. KF15372 (1.25–5 mg/kg, po) significantly increased the ratio of beta waves in cerebral cortex and produced an arousal effect not only in normal but also in impaired brain. The effect continued until
150 minutes after treatment with KF15372 (Fig. 5).

   The cholinergic system is known to be involved in learning and memory
processes. We therefore investigated adenosine control of ACh release via A_1R
as a basis of the electroencephalogram activity changes induced in the hippocampus and cerebral cortex when KF15372 is administered (Kurokawa *et
al.*, 1996a). Oral administration of KF15372 at doses comparable to those that
induced both electroencephalogram activity change and amelioration of amnesia in animal models significantly increased the extracellular levels of ACh
in rat cerebral cortex. This suggests that the extracellular level of ACh is under tonic inhibitory control of endogenous adenosine via the A_1R. Furthermore, these results indicate that A_1R antagonists may be beneficial in treating
cholinergic deficiency disorders (e.g., Alzheimer's disease).

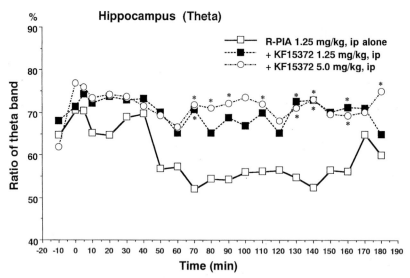

FIGURE 4   Effect of KF15372 on the *R*-PIA induced desychronization of EEGs. KF15372
was injected ip with *R*-PIA. Significant difference from *R*-PIA alone group: $^*p < 0.05$ (Steel
test), $n = 5$.

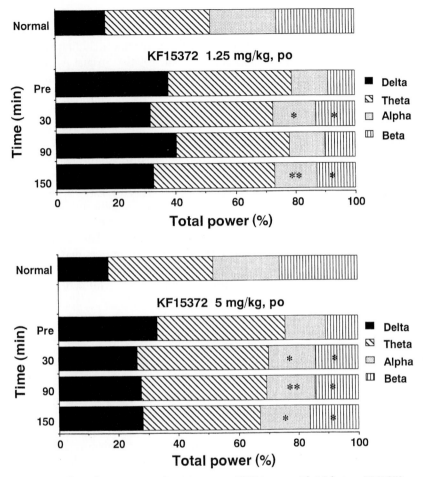

FIGURE 5 Effect of KF15372 on the spontaneous EEG in rats with IC lesion. KF15372 was administered 24 hr after internal capsule lesion. Significant difference from pretreatment value: $*p < 0.05$, $**0.01$ (Paired t-test), $n = 4-6$.

III. ROLE OF ADENOSINE A_{2A} RECEPTOR IN CNS

A. DISTRIBUTION OF A_{2A} RECEPTOR IN CNS

In contrast to the A_1R, which is widely distributed in the brain, the $A_{2A}R$ is highly localized in basal ganglia. Within basal ganglia, $A_{2A}Rs$ have been concentrated in regions that encompass the striatum, globus pallidus, nucleus accumbens, and olfactory tubercle (Schiffmann *et al.*, 1990; Schiffmann and Vanderhaeghen, 1993). Using receptor binding and *in situ* hybridization, $A_{2A}R$ protein and mRNA have been identified in many species including mice, rat, dog, monkey, and human (Nonaka *et al.*, 1994a, 1994b). Striatal A_{2A} receptor mRNA occurs exclusively in populations of GABAergic medium spiny neurons (MSN) that coexpress enkephalin and the D_2 dopamine receptor and project to the globus pallidus (Kawaguchi *et al.*, 1995). Neurochemical and electrophysiological experiments show that these A_{2A} receptors are expressed on both cell soma and presynaptic sites in the striatum. Electrophysiological experiments suggest presynaptic $A_{2A}Rs$ in striatum exist on the colateral axon terminals of MSNs to form a feedback circuit (Mori *et al.*, 1996; see Chapter 6). The mRNA encoding the A_{2A} receptor is present on at least 25 % of striatal cholinergic interneurons, although at a significantly lower level than on the MSNs (Richardson *et al.*, 1997; see Chapter 8). $A_{2A}Rs$ exist on presynaptic sites on both of these neuronal types and regulate the release of GABA and ACh in the striatum; thus, these neurotransmitters may modulate the activity of striatal efferent neurons (Kirk and Richardson, 1994; Kurokawa *et al.*, 1994, 1996b). Therefore, $A_{2A}R$ exerts a controlling influence on local and output neuronal pathways in the striatum.

B. BEHAVIORAL PHENOTYPE IN A_{2A} RECEPTOR KO MICE

The role of the $A_{2A}R$ was also investigated by disrupting the gene in mice (Ledent *et al.*, 1997). Routine histology on brain (especially striatum) and other organs did not detect any abnormalities or loss of neurons.

In $A_{2A}R$ KO mice, a decrease in both preproenkephalin and preprotachykinin transcripts was detected by *in situ* hybridization. The change of preproenkephalin gene expression was predictable because striatal preproenkephalin mRNA levels were reduced by blockade of $A_{2A}R$ with the selective antagonist, KF17837 (Richardson *et al.*, 1997). However, the direction of the change in preprotachkynin gene expression was the opposite of that expected. The authors suggested this might be due to adaptive cortical changes that could involve a reduction in the activity of glutamatergic corticostriatal projections (see Chapter 8).

As adenosine modulates motor function through the $A_{2A}R$ in basal ganglia, the KO mice were subjected to behavioral tests to investigate exploratory behavior, anxiety, and aggression. However, the results were difficult to interpret because in an open field test locomotor activity was decreased in the KO mice as opposed to the increase in locomotion seen with $A_{2A}R$ antagonists in wild-type mice.

A$_{2A}$R KO mice also appeared to be more anxious and aggressive than wild-type mice. Increased aggressiveness was confirmed in the resident–intruder test.

In conclusion, the effects of preventing A$_{2A}$R expression show several discrepancies from the consequences of blockade of A$_{2A}$R by selective antagonists, which may be due to the compensatory mechanisms brought into play during the development of the A$_{2A}$R KO mice.

C. Sleep

The A$_{2A}$R is also present in the olfactory tubercle and nucleus accumbens in the rostral basal forebrain, which is reported to be involved in the regulation of sleep. Satoh et al. (1996) reported that infusion of the A$_{2A}$R agonist CGS 21680 into the subarachnoid space just below the ventral surface region of rostral basal forebrain increased slow-wave sleep and paradoxical sleep in a dose-dependent manner. These effects of CGS 21680 were significantly suppressed by the pretreatment of A$_{2A}$R antagonist KF17837, suggesting the involvement of the A$_{2A}$R.

Prostaglandin D$_2$ (PGD$_2$) is a postulated endogenous sleep-promoting substance that increases slow-wave sleep in rats when applied into ventral surface of the rostral basal forebrain. Interestingly, this effect of PGD$_2$ was also inhibited by the pretreatment of KF17837, indicating that downstream signal transmission through the A$_{2A}$R is involved in sleep promotion by PGD$_2$. Whether PGD$_2$ enhances the synthesis of adenosine or modulates the activity of the A$_{2A}$R remains to be addressed. Thus, the A$_{2A}$R subtype appears to play a crucial role in the sleep-promoting mechanism triggered by PGD$_2$.

D. Adenosine A$_{2A}$ Receptor and Motor Function

1. Effects of A$_{2A}$R Antagonists on Drug-Induced Catalepsy

The first studies to suggest the A$_2$ receptor involvement in catalepsy were reported by Ferré et al. (1991). These studies showed that intracerebroventricular injection of the A$_{2A}$R agonist CGS 21680 produced a cataleptic response in rats that was antagonized by the methylxanthine derivative theophylline. However, because theophylline is a nonselective adenosine receptor antagonist, the contribution of A$_{2A}$R to the cataleptic response remained unknown. Subsequently, using the orally active A$_{2A}$R selective antagonist KF17837, it was possible to elucidate how the blockade of A$_{2A}$R affects catalepsy (Kanda et al., 1994; Shimada et al., 1992; Shiozaki et al., 1996). Icv injection of the A$_{2A}$R agonist CGS 21680 (10 μg) produced sedation, locomotor depression, and a severe cataleptic response. Oral administration of KF17837 reversed CGS 21680-induced catalepsy in a dose-dependent manner with an ED50 of 7.16 mg/kg, po. These results indicate that $A_{2A}R$ in brain modulates motor function in a negative manner and that orally administered KF17837 reverses the motor deficits via $A_{2A}R$ in brain. Moreover, KF17837 dose-dependently reversed haloperidol-induced catalepsy with a significant reduction being observed at doses from 0.625 mg/kg, po, and an ED50 of 2.73 mg/kg, po. To determine whether KF17837 manifests a synergistic anticataleptic effect with L-3,4-dihydroxyphenylalanine (L-DOPA) (which also reverses catalepsy) in haloperidol-treated mice, a subthreshold dose of L-DOPA (25 mg/kg, po) was combined with a subthreshold dose of KF17837 (0.156 mg/kg). The combination produced a reversal of catalepsy that was not seen with either compound alone. Reserpine pretreatment also induces catalepsy, sedation, and ptosis in mice. KF17837 dose-dependently reversed the catalepsy at doses greater than 2.5 mg/kg, po, with an ED50 of 3.53 mg/kg, po, although no effect on ptosis was evident. The more efficacious $A_{2A}R$ antagonist KW-6002, whose bioavailability is one order higher than KF17837 after oral administration (Shimada *et al.*, 1997), was also shown to reverse CGS 21680-, haloperidol-, and reserpine-induced catalepsy with ED50 value of 0.05, 0.03, and 0.26 mg/kg, po, respectively (Shiozaki *et al.*, in press).

2. Effects of Adenosine A_{2A} Receptor Ligands on Rotation of 6-OHDA-Lesioned Rats

Following destruction of the dopaminergic neurons in the substantia nigra by administration of 6-hydroxydopamine (6-OHDA), systemic administration of the dopamine agonist apomorphine causes vigorous turning behavior toward the contralateral side. This is believed to be due to preferential action on supersensitive postsynaptic dopamine receptors on the denervated side. Methylxanthine derivatives have been reported to potentiate the rotational response caused by apomorphine in rats with unilateral lesion of dopaminergic neurons in substantia nigra and this potentiation is considered to be due to blockade of A_2R (Fuxe and Ungerstedt, 1974).

This was confirmed by Brown *et al.* (1991) and by the use of $A_{2A}R$-selective agonist CGS 21680 (Koga *et al.*, 1996; Vellucci *et al.*, 1993). The ipsilateral intrastriatal administration of CGS 21680 produced a dose-related decrease in apomorphine-induced rotation in 6-OHDA-lesioned rat. This effect could be reversed by $A_{2A}R$ antagonist CP66713. In another experiment, CGS 21680 also reduced the contralateral turning induced by L-DOPA, the D_1 receptor agonist SKF38393, and the D_2 agonist LY171555 (Morelli *et al.*, 1994). Contrary to the effects seen with adenosine agonists, blockade of the $A_{2A}R$ but not the A_1R potentiates turning behavior; these results are in line with the concept that $A_{2A}R$ negatively modulates motor responses induced by dopamine agonists. It should be noted that $A_{2A}R$ antagonists such as CP66713, KF17837, and SCH58261 have no significant effects on rotation when used alone in 6-OHDA-lesioned rats.

3. Effects of A_{2A} Receptor Antagonists on Motor Function of MPTP-treated Animals

MPTP causes degeneration of the dopaminergic nigrostriatal pathway in humans, nonhuman primates, and specific mouse strains (Burns *et al.*, 1983; Heikkila *et al.*, 1984a, 1984b). In primates, MPTP-induced parkinsonism mimics the basic symptoms of idiopathic Parkinson's disease in humans (Burns *et al.*, 1983).

C57BL/6 mice is one of the strains most sensitive to the effects of MPTP. There are several reports showing that C57BL/6 mice exhibit severe dopaminergic neuron degeneration and hypoactivity following MPTP treatment (Heikkila *et al.*, 1984a, 1984b; Sundstrom *et al.*, 1990, 1994). This hypoactivity was dose-dependently reversed by L-DOPA with a therapeutic effect between 20–40 mg/kg, ip (Fredriksson *et al.*, 1990). Heikkila and colleagues (1984a, 1984b) found that repeated high doses of MPTP produced a greater than 80% depletion of striatal dopamine content with evidence for nigral cell loss. To investigate the effects of A_{2A} anatagonists in this model, a dose regimen of 30 mg/kg, ip, × 5 days was chosen as one that significantly reduces striatal dopamine levels for at least 10 days (Heikilla *et al.*, 1984a, 1984b). In our hands, this treatment regime caused severe hypoactivity 1 hour after the last injection (less than 10% of normal control activity). Mice were then subjected to behavioral testing for 30 minutes, beginning 1 hour after the last MPTP injection. L-DOPA (+ benserazide) reversed the hypolocomotion at 300 mg/kg, po (to 30% of normal control elevels), in agreement with previous findings (Fredriksson *et al.*, 1990). KF17837 also reversed the hypolocomotion caused by MPTP with a minimum effective dose of 10 mg/kg (Fig. 6).

$A_{2A}R$ antagonists such as KF17837 and KW-6002 were also shown to improve motor disability of MPTP-treated monkeys (Kanda *et al.*, 1998). Importantly, no evidence of dyskinesia was seen with the $A_{2A}R$ antagonists. A detailed description of these results can be found in Chapter 11.

4. Discussion

The ability of $A_{2A}R$ antagonists to reverse the motor deficits seen with drug-induced catalepsy and hypolocomotion caused by MPTP treatment is of

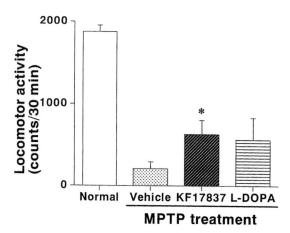

FIGURE 6 Effect of KF17837 on locomotor activity in mice pretreated with MPTP. MPTP was pretreated at the dose of 30 mg/kg/day, ip, for 5 consecutive days. KF17837 (10 mg/kg, po) or L-DOPA (300 mg/kg, po) was orally administered 30 min after the last treatment of MPTP. Data are presented total counts taken over a 30-min priod after the administration of KF17837 or L-DOPA (mean SEM, $n = 8$/group). $*p < 0.05$: Significant difference from MPTP-treated control group (Steel test).

considerable interest. In the striatum, $A_{2A}Rs$ are selectively and abundantly located on γ-aminobutyric acid (GABA)/enkephalin-containing neurons and to a lesser amount on cholinergic neurons.

$A_{2A}R$ antagonists are considered to act mainly through enhancing the release of GABA and reducing that of ACh in the striatum (Mori *et al.*, 1996; Kurokawa *et al.*, 1996b). Futhermore, A_{2A} receptor agonists are reported to reduce the binding affinity of dopamine D_2 receptors and oppose the actions of D_1 and D_2 receptors on gene expression and second messenger systems (Fenu *et al.*, 1997; Ferré *et al.*, 1997; Pinna *et al.*, 1996). Thus, inhibition of the $A_{2A}R$ would be of particular benefit in situation in which dopamine concentrations become limiting, as in Parkinson's disease.

The concept of using adenosine-related compounds in Parkinson's disease is suggested by a limited number of reports. An open trial of the nonselective adenosine receptor antagonist theophylline produced some improvement in patients with Parkinson's disease (Mally and Stone, 1994). However, theophylline is not only a nonselective adenosine receptor antagonist, but also has affinity for phosphodiesterase and guanosine receptors. Therefore, it remains to be determined through which site it produced an antiparkinsonian effect. This study has shown selective $A_{2A}R$ antagonists exhibit antiparkinsonian activity in experimental models. If these results are also applicable to humans, $A_{2A}R$ antagonists may become a novel therapeutic approach to Parkinson's disease.

IV. CONCLUSION

Adenosine is indeed a fascinating molecule whose role in physiology is varied and profound. It is conceivable from the results of preclinical studies with animal models that A_1R antagonist may be beneficial for the treatment of amnesia like Alzheimer's disease and $A_{2A}R$ antagonist for movement disorders, such as Parkinson's disease.

V. METHODS

Basal forebrain (BF) lesion-induced amnesia. The rats were anesthetized with sodium pentobarbital (40 mg/kg, ip) and fixed on a stereotaxic apparatus (Takahashi Shouten, Japan). A stainless steel injection needle (diameter 0.25 mm) was connected via a polyethylene tube to a 10 μl microsyringe mounted on a microinjector (Narishige, Japan, IM-1). A needle was inserted into the BF. The coordinates were 1.2 mm posterior to bregma and 2.7 mm lateral in the atlas of the rat brain (Paxinos and Watson, 1986). Bilateral BF lesions were produced by injection of kainic acid (0.2 μg/1 μl in saline) for 3 minutes. In the sham-operated group, the injection needle was inserted 5.5 mm from the skull. Animals were allowed to recover from the damage of neurosurgery at least 10 days and then the experiments were carried out. KF15372 or KFM-19 were administered for 7 consecutive days. The acquisition trial was carried out on the sixth day and the retention test was done on the seventh day, 1 hour after the drug administration. The apparatus and procedures for passive avoidance were the same as R-PIA-induced amnesia (Suzuki *et al.*, 1993).

A. SPONTANEOUS ELECTROENCEPHALOGRAM

The rabbits were anesthetized by sodium pentobarbital (45 mg/kg, ip) and fixed on a stereotaxic apparatus (Narishige, Japan, SN-1). Electrodes were inserted into amygdala (A:2.5, L:6.0, H:-5.0), dorsal hippocampus (P:4.0, L:4.0, H:6.0), posterior hypothalamus (P:2.0, L:1.5, H:-3.0), and mesensephalic reticular formation (P:8.0, L:2.5, H:-3.0). Electrodes were fixed on the skull by dental cement. Similarly, bipolar stainless steel electrodes were inserted into frontal, parietal, and occipital cortex, according to the atlas of the rabbit brain (Sawyer *et al.*, 1954). The animals were allowed to recover from operation damage at least 10 days, and experiments were performed after confirming that electroencephalograms (EEGs) were clearly recorded. Experiments were carried out in unanesthetized condition. Each animal was placed in a plastic cage in a soundproof room. The EEGs were recorded via electroencephalograph (EEG-5109, NIHON KOHDEN) and analyzed by a data analyzer (ATAK-450, NIHON KOHDEN). EEG power spectral analysis was performed on each epoch (2.5 sec) by means of a Fast Fourier Transformation (FFT), and the mean values for 30 seconds were displayed at every 30-second interval for 180 minutes. Moreover, the power average analysis was performed at $1-32$ Hz for a 5-minute period selected from pre- and postinjection recordings. The ratios of the beta wave ($12.4-32$ Hz) in the neocortex and of the theta wave ($3.6-7.6$ Hz) in the hippocampus were calculated as the total power of each brain region was 100%. These ratios were used as parameters of the arousal level of the animal.

B. INTERNAL CAPSULE LESION

Under sodium pentobarbital anesthesia (40 mg/kg, ip) the rats were fixed on a stereotaxic apparatus and internal capsule (IC) (P:2.0, L:3.2, H:6.5) was lesioned by a lesion generator (RFG,-4A, Radionics) at 65°C for 90 seconds, according to the atlas of the rat brain (Paxinos and Watson, 1986). Stainless steel bipolar electrodes were implanted into the cortex and the hippocampus (P:4.3, L:2.5, H:2.5) for recording of electroencephalogram activity. The electrodes were fixed to the skull by dental cement. Two days after the operation, the effects of KF15372 were investigated. The EEGs were recorded via electroencephalograph (EEG-5109, NIHON KOHDEN) and analyzed by a data analyzer (ATAK-450, NIHON KOHDEN). The power average analysis was performed at $1.6-29.6$ Hz for a 5-minute period selected from pre- and postinjection recordings. The ratios of the delta ($1.6-3.6$ Hz), theta ($3.6-7.6$ Hz), alpha 1 ($7.6-9.6$ Hz), alpha 2 ($9.6-12.4$ Hz), beta 1 ($12.4-19.6$ Hz), and beta 2 ($19.6-29.6$ Hz) waves were calculated, as the total power was 100% and each ratio compared with the preinjection value.

C. LOCOMOTOR ACTIVITY

Locomotor activity was assessed in the plastic cage with a single silent electronic counter (Automex-II; Columbus Instruments, Columbus, Ohio, USA). Automex-II works on the principle of capacitive proximity sensor. One electrode is located underneath the plastic top plate of Automex-II, whereas the second electrode constitutes the metal lid of the animal cage. Animals moving between these two electrodes change capacitance and produce pulses that are sent to the electronic counter with display on the front panel. The effect of KF17837 on MPTP-induced hypolocomotion was assessed as follows. MPTP was injected once per day with 30 mg/kg, ip, for 5 consecutive days. The effect of KF17837 on MPTP-induced hypolocomotion was measured 30 minutes after the final administration of MPTP (30 mg/kg, ip). Each mouse was administered with KF17837 and 30 minutes later placed one by one in Automex cage to measure the locomotor counts for 30 minutes.

D. DATA ANALYSIS AND STATISTICS

The effect of KF17837 on the drug-induced catalepsy was analyzed using the Kruskal–Wallis test followed by the Steel-test. The effect of KF17837 on the locomotor activity of MPTP-treated mice was analyzed by Steel-test for comparison with the control group. The difference between the MPTP-treated group and the nontreated group was analyzed by the Student's t-test or the Wilcoxon's rank sum test.

ACKNOWLEDGMENTS

The authors are grateful to Ms. T. Ohta and C. Inamura for their excellent technical assistance. They also thank Dr. Richardson for critical reading of this manuscript.

REFERENCES

Brown, S.J., Gill, R., Evenden, J.L., Iversen, S.D., and Richardson, P.J. (1991). Striatal A_2 receptor regulates apomorphine-induced turning in rats with unilateral dopamine denervation. *Psychopharmacol* 103, 78–82.

Burns, R.A., Chieuh, C.C., Markey, S.P., Ebert, M.H., Jacobowitz, D.M., and Kopin, I.J. (1983). A primate model of parkinsonism: selective destruction of dopaminergic neurons in the pars compacta of the substantia nigra by N-methyl-4-phenyl-1,2,3,6-tetrahydropyridine. *Proc Natl Acad Sci USA* 80, 4546–4550.

Dudley, M., Hitchcock, J., Sorensen, J., Chaney, S., Zwolshen, J., Leutz, N., Borcherding, D., and Peet, N. (1994). Adenosine A_1 receptor antagonists as cognition enhancers. *Drug Dev Res* 31, 266.

Fenu, S., Pinna, A., Ongini, E., and Morelli, M. (1997). Adenosine A_{2A} receptor antagonism potentiates L-DOPA-induced turning behavior and c-fos expression in 6-hydroxydopamine-lesioned rats. *Eur J Pharmacol* 321, 143–147.

Ferré S., Rubio, A., and Fuxe, K. (1991). Stimulation of adenosine A_2 receptors induces catalepsy. *Neurosci Lett* 130, 162–164.

Ferré, S., Fredholm, B.B., Morelli, M., Popoli, P., and Fuxe, K. (1997). Adenosine-dopamine receptor–receptor interactions as an integrative mechanism in the basal ganglia. *Trends Neurosci* 20(10), 482–487.

Fredholm, B.B., Abbracchio, M.P., Burnstock, G., Daly, J.W., Harden, T.K., Jacobson, K.A., Leff, P., and Williams, M. (1994). Nomenclature and classification of purinoceptors. *Pharmacological Rev* 64, 143–156.

Fredriksson, A., Plaznik, A., Sundstorm, E., Jonsson, G., and Archer, T. (1990). MPTP-induced hypoactivity in mice: reversal by L-DOPA. *Pharmacol Taxicol* 67, 295–301.

Fuxe, K., and Ungerstedt, U. (1974). Action of caffeine on supersensitive dopamine receptors: considerable enhancement of receptor response to treatment with DOPA and dopamine agonists. *Med Biol* 52, 48–54.

Heikkila, R., Cabbat, L., Manzino, L., and Duvoisin, R.C. (1984a). Effects of 1-methyl-4-phenyl-1,2,5,6-tetrahydropyridine on neostriatal dopamine in mice. *Neuropharmacol* 23, 711–713.

Heikkila, R.E., Manzino, L., Cabbat, F.S., and Duvoisin, R.C. (1984b). Protection against the dopaminergic neurotoxicity of 1-methyl-4-phenyl-1,2,5,6-tetrahydropyridine by monoamine oxidase inhibitors. *Nature* 311, 467–469.

Jacobson, K.A., von Lubitz D.K., Heikkila. J.E., Daly J.W., and Fredholm, B.B. (1996). Adenosine receptor ligands: differences with acute versus chronic treatment. *Trends Pharm Sci* 17, 108–113.

Kanda, T., Shiozaki, S., Shimada, J., Suzuki, F., and Nakamura, J. (1994). KF17837: a novel selective adenosine A_{2A} receptor antagonist with anticataleptic activity. *Eur. J Pharmacol* 256, 264–268.

Kanda, T., Jackson, M.J., Smith, L.A., Pearce, R.K.B., Nakamura, J., Kase, H., Kuwana, Y., and Jenner, P. (1998). Adenosine A_{2A} antagonist: a novel antiparkinsonian agent that does not provoke dyskinesia in parkinsonian monkeys. *Ann Neurol* 43, 507–513.

Kawaguchi, Y., Wilson, C.J., Augood, S.J., and Emson, P.C. (1995). *Trends Neurosci* 18, 527–535.

Kirk, I.P., and Richardson, P.J. (1994). Adenosine A_{2A} receptor mediated modulation of striatal [^{3}H]-GABA and [^{3}H]-ACh release. *J Neurochem* 62, 960–966.

Koga, K., Kurokawa, M., Kanda, T., Shiozaki, S., Ochi, M., Nakamura, J., and Kuwana, Y. (1996). Blockade of adenosine A_{2A} receptors potentiates dopamine agonist-induced rotation in rats with unilateral 6-hydroxydopamine lesions of nigrostriatal pathway. *Jpn J Pharmacol* 71, 95.

Kurokawa, M., Kirk, I.P., Kirkpatrick, K.A., Kase, H., and Richardson, P.J. (1994). Inhibition by KF17837 of adenosine A_{2A} receptor-mediated modulation of striatal GABA and ACh release. *Br J Pharmacol* 113, 43–48.

Kurokawa, M., Shiozaki, S., Nonaka, H., Kase, H., Nakamura, J., and Kuwana, Y. (1996a). *In vivo* regulation of acetylcholine release via adenosine A_1 receptor in rat cerebral cortex. *Neurosci Lett* 209, 181–184.

Kurokawa, M., Koga, K., Kase, H., Nakamura, J., and Kuwana, Y. (1996b). Adenosine A_{2A} receptor-mediated modulation of striatal acetylcholine release *in vivo*. *J Neurochem* 66, 1882–1888.

Kuwana, Y., Shiozaki, S., Kanda, T., Kurokawa, M., Koga, K., Ochi, M., Ikeda, K., Kase, H., Jackson, M.J., Smith, L.A., Pearce, R.K.B., and Jenner, P. (in press). Antiparkinsonian activity of adenosine A_{2A} antagonists in experimental models. *Adv Neurol*

Ledent C., Vaugeois JM., Schiffmann S.N., Pedrazzini T., Yacoubi M.E.I., Vanderhaeghen J.J., Constentin, J., Heath J.K., Vassart G., and Parmentier, M. (1997). Aggressiveness, hypoalgesia and high blood pressure in mice lacking the adenosine A_{2A} receptor. *Nature* 388, 674–678.

Lee, K.S., and Reddington, M. (1986). Autoradiographic evidence for multiple CNS binding sites for adenosine derivatives. *Neurosci* 19, 535–549.

Mahan, L.C., Mcvittie, L.D., Smyk-Randall, E.L., Nakata, H., Monsma, F.J., Gerfen, C.R., and Sibley, D.R. (1991). Cloning and expression of an A_1 adenosine receptor gene from rat brain. *Mol Pharmacol* 40, 1–7.

Mally, J., and Stone, T.W. (1994). The effect of theophylline on parkinsonian symptoms. *J Pharm Pharmacol* 46, 515–517.

Morelli, M., Fenu, S., Pinna, A., and Di Chiara, G. (1994). Adenosine A_2 receptors interact negatively with dopamine D_1 and D_2 receptors in unilaterally 6-hydroxydopamine-lesioned rats. *Eur J Pharmacol* 251, 21–25.

Mori, A., Shindou, T., Ichimura, M., Nonaka, H., and Kase, H. (1996). The role of adenosine A_{2A} receptors in regulating GABAergic synaptic transmission in striatal medium spiny neurons. *J Neurosci* **16**, 605–611.

Nonaka, H., Ichimura, M., Takeda, M., Nonaka, Y., Shimada, J., Suzuki, F., Yamaguchi, K., and Kase, H. (1994a). KF17837((E)-8-(3,4-dimethoxystyryl)-1,3-dipropyl-7-methylxanthine), a potent and selective adenosine A_2 receptor antagonist. *Eur J Pharmacol* **267**, 335–341.

Nonaka, H., Mori, A., Ichimura, M., Shindou, T., Yanagawa, K., Shimada, J., and Kase, H. (1994b). Binding of [^{3}H]KF17837S, a selective adenosine A_2 receptor antagonist, to rat brain membranes. *Mol Pharmacol* **46**, 817–822.

Paxinos, G., and Watson, C. (1986). *The Rat Bain in Stereotaxic Coordinates*. San Diego: Academic Press.

Pinna, A., Dichiara, G., Wardas, J., and Morelli, M. (1996). Blockade of A_{2A} adenosine receptors positively modulates turning behavior and c-fos expresson induced by D_1 agonists in dopamine-denervated rats. *Eur J Neurosci* **8** (6), 1176–1181.

Richardson, P.J., Kase, H., and Jenner, P.G. (1997). Adenosine A_{2A} receptor antagonists as new agents for the treatment of Parkinson's disease. *Trends Pharmacol Sci* **18**, 338–344.

Satoh, S., Matsumura, H., Suzuki, F., and Hayaishi, O. (1996). Promotion of sleep mediated by the A_{2A}-adenosine receptor and possible involvement of this receptor in the sleep induced by prostaglandin D_2 in rats. *Proc Natl Acad Sci USA* **93**, 5980–5984.

Sawyer, C.H., Everett, J.W., and Green, J.D. (1954). The rabbit diencephalon in stereotaxic coordinates. *J Comp Neurol* **101**, 801–824.

Schiffmann, S.N., Libert, F., Vassart, G., Dumont, J.E., and Vanderhaeghen, J.-J. (1990). A cloned G protein-coupled protein with a distribution restricted to striatal medium-sized neurons. Possible relationship with D_1 dopamine receptor. *Brain Res* **519**, 333–337.

Schiffmann, S.N., and Vanderhaeghen, J.-J. (1993). Adenosine A_2 receptors regulate the gene expression of striatopallidal and striatonigral neurons. *J Neurosci* **13**, 1080–1087.

Schingnitz, G., Kufner-Muhl, U., Ensinger, H., Lehr, E., and Kuhn, F.J. (1991). Selective A_1-antagonists for treatment of cognitive deficits. *Nucleoides Nucleotides* **10**, 1067–1076.

Shimada, J., Suzuki, F., Nonaka, H., Ishii, A., and Ichikawa, S. (1992). (E)-1,3-dialkyl-7-methyl-8-(3,4,5-trimethoxy-styryl) xanthines: potent and selective adenosine A_2 antagonists. *J Med Chem* **35**, 2342–2345.

Shimada, J., Koike, N., Nonaka, H., Shiozaki, S., Yanagawa, K., Kanda, T., Kobayashi, H., Ichimura, M., Nakamura, J., Kase, H., and Suzuki, F. (1997). Adenosine A_{2A} antagonists with potent anti-cataleptic activity. *Bioorg Med Chem Lett* **18**, 2349–2352.

Shiozaki, S., Ichikawa, S., Nakamura, J., Kitamura, S., Yamada, K. and Kuwana, Y. (1999). Actions of adenosine A_{2A} receptor antagonist KW-6002 on drug-induced catalepsy and hypokinesia caused by reserpine or MPTP. *Psychopharmacology*, in press.

Shiozaki, S., Nakamura, J., and Kuwana, Y. (1996). Effects of KF17837, a selective adenosine A_{2A} receptor antagonist, on drug-induced catalepsy in rodents. *Jpn J Pharmacol* **71**, 95.

Sundstrom, E., Fredriksson, A., and Archer, T. (1990). Chronic neurochemical and behavioral changes in MPTP-lesioned C57B4/6 mice: a model for Parkinson's disease. *Brain Res* **528**, 181–188.

Sundstrom, E., Henriksson, B.G., Mohammed, A.H., and Souverbie, F. (1994). MPTP-treated mice: a useful model for Parkinson's disease? In "Toxin-Induced Models of Neurological Disorders" (Woodruff, M.L., and Nonneman, A.J., eds), pp. 121–137. New York: Plenum Press.

Suzuki, F., Shimada, J., Shiozaki, S. Ichikawa, S., Ishii, A., Nakamura, J., Nonaka, H., Kobayashi, H., and Fuse, E. (1993). Adenosine A_1-antagonists. 3. Structure–activity relationships on amelioration against scopolamine- or N6-((R)-phenylisopropyl) adenosine-induced cognitive disturbance. *J Med Chem* **36**, 2508–2518.

Van Calker, D., Meuller, M., and Hamprecht, B. (1979). Adonosine regulates via two different types of receptors, accumulation of cyclic AMP in cultured brain cells. *J Neurochem* **33**, 999–1005.

Vellucci, S.V., Sirinathsinghji, D.J.S., and Richardson, P.J. (1993). Adenosine A_{2A} receptor regulation of apomorphine-induced turning in rats with unilateral striatal dapamine denervation. *Psychopharmacol* **111**, 383–388.

CHAPTER 11

Actions of Adenosine Antagonists in Primate Model of Parkinson's Disease

Tomoyuki Kanda

Department of Neurology, Pharmaceutical Research Institute, Kyowa Hakko Kogyo Co., Ltd., Sunto-Gun, Shizuoka, Japan

Peter Jenner

Neurodegenerative Diseases Research Centre, Division of Pharmacology & Therapeutics, Guy's King's & St Thomas' School of Biomedical Sciences, King's College, London, UK

I. INTRODUCTION

Adenosine regulates a variety of physiological processes in the mammalian central nervous system (CNS) [1]. Adenosine receptors are classified as A_1, A_2, and A_3. Adenosine A_2 receptors are further subdivided into two subclasses, namely A_{2A} and A_{2B} [2]. Adenosine A_{2A} receptors are highly localized in the caudate-putamen, nucleus accumbens, and olfactory tubercle. Within the caudate-putamen, the adenosine A_{2A} receptors are selectively localized on the γ-aminobutyric acid (GABA)- and enkephalin-containing medium spiny neurons, which form the indirect output pathway from the striatum to globus pallidus and bear dopamine D_2 receptors on their surface [3]. It has been suggested that the onset of parkinsonian disability and the genesis of L-3,4-dihydroxyphenylaline (L-Dopa)-provoked dyskinesia is due to alterations in the function of the indirect pathway. Thus modulation of A_{2A} receptors may undoubtedly have a profound influence on motor function, and there is considerable evidence to support such a role. For example, xanthine-derived nonspecific adenosine antagonists, such as caffeine and theophyline, modify motor activity. Caffeine produces increased locomotor activity in rodents, and this effect is blocked by dopamine receptor antagonists [4]. Similarly, turning behavior induced by the administration of selective dopamine D_1 or D_2 receptor agonists, such as quinpirole or SKF 38393, in unilateral nigrostriatal-lesioned rats is potentiated by methylxanthines [5]. Intrastriatal injection of caffeine also induces rotation, both in normal and in unilateral nigro-striatal-lesioned rats. These effects of methylxanthines are believed to be mediated at least in part by blockade of adenosine A_2 receptors, based on the behavioral effects produced by specific adenosine A_1 or A_2 agonists and the distribution of these receptors in the basal ganglia. Indeed the intracerebral injection of the adenosine A_{2A} receptor selective agonist, CGS 21680, produces catalepsy, which is a classic example of dopaminergic dysfunction, in mice and rats [6,7]. These results suggest that adenosine A_{2A} receptor stimulation exerts an inhibitory effect on motor function in rodents.

There are few commonly available ligands that show selectivity for the adenosine A_{2A} receptor. Until more recently, no selective adenosine A_{2A} receptor antagonists had been evaluated for its effects on motor function in relation to Parkinson's disease. However, modification of the xanthine nucleus led to the development of antagonists with adenosine A_{2A} receptor selectivity, such as KF17837 and KW-6002 (see Chapter 2) [8–10]. We reported that the selective adenosine A_{2A} receptor antagonist, KF17837, reduced the cataleptic response in mice induced by either the dopamine antagonist, haloperidol, or by the dopamine depletor, reserpine [7]. These initial results suggested that selective adenosine A_{2A} receptor antagonists can reverse striatal dopaminergic dysfunction [11]. However, the effects of selective adenosine A_{2A} receptor antagonists on motor function in other models of Parkinson's disease remained unknown. In this chapter, we discuss the effects of adenosine A_{2A} antagonist on motor function in MPTP-treated primates.

II. ACTION OF MPTP ON MOTOR BEHAVIOR IN COMMON MARMOSETS

In the early 1980s, the dopaminergic neurotoxin, 1-methyl-4-phenyl-1,2,3,6-tetrahydropyridine (MPTP) was shown to produce parkinsonism in young drug addicts [12]. Although MPTP treatment did not produce lesions of the substantia nigra in rodents [13–15], it caused dopaminergic cell death with the onset of parkinsonism in primates, including common marmosets (*Callithrix jaccus*) [16,17] (Fig. 1). Common marmosets exhibiting parkinsonian symptoms following MPTP treatment appear to be excellent pharmacological models of Parkinson's disease because their response to antiparkinsonian agents mimics that of human patients with similar side effects, such as vomiting, stereotyped behavior, and L-Dopa-induced dyskinesias [18,19].

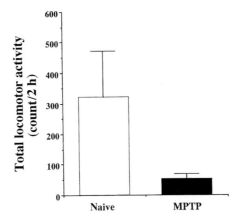

FIGURE 1   Basal locomotor activity of naive and MPTP-treated common marmosets. Total locomotor activity of MPTP-treated marmosets and normal marmosets. Each column represents the mean locomotor count/2 hour ($\pm$ SEM, $n = 4$.). $*p < 0.05$ compared with naive animal.

All studies involving primates were carried out in accordance with the U.K. legal requirements under U.K. Home Office license PPL70/3563. Common marmosets (*Callithri Jacchus*) of either sex, weighing 285–420 g and ages 2–7 years at the beginning of the study, were used. The animals were housed either in pairs or alone under standard conditions at a temperature of 24–26 and 50–60% relative humidity, using a 12 h light–dark cycle. Diet consisted of standard food pellets (Mazuri primate diet), fresh fruit, and Mazuri marmoset jelly. The animals were treated with MPTP (in sterile 0.9% physiological saline) in doses of 2 mg/kg, sc, daily for 5 days. Following MPTP treatment, the animals were allowed to recover from the acute effects over a period of 6–8 weeks. During MPTP treatment and throughout the following weeks, the animals were hand-fed with Mazuri marmoset jelly and fresh fruit puree until they were able to maintain themselves. Prior to behavioral testing, from 6–8 weeks to 8 months after exposure to MPTP, all animals showed a marked reduction of basal locomotor activity (Fig. 1), slower and less coordinated movements, abnormal postures of some parts of the body, and reduced checking movements and eye blinks. Locomotor activity was measured simultaneously in four aluminum cages (50 $\times$ 60 $\times$ 70 cm) with stainless steel grid doors (50 $\times$ 70 cm) identical to the animals' home cages but equipped with eight horizontally orientated sets of infrared photocells. The number of light beam interruptions due to the animals' movements were recorded using an IBM-compatible computer (Olivetti M290S and DEC Venturis 410). The animals were allowed to acclimatize to the test environment

TABLE I   Criteria and Indices of Motor Disability in MPTP-Treated Common Marmosets

Alertness	Normal 0, reduced 1, sleepy 2
Checking movements	Present 0, reduced 1, absent 2
Reaction to stimuli	Normal 0, reduced 1, slow 2, absent 3
Attention and eye movements	Normal 0, abnormal 1
Posture	Normal 0, abnormal trunk +1, limbs +1, tail +1, grossly abnormal 4
Balance/coordination	Normal 0, impaired 1, unstable 2, spontaneous falls 3
Vocalization	Normal 0, reduced 1, absent 2

for 30 to 60 minutes prior to drug administration. The animals were continuously monitored by trained observers. The animals were observed through a one-way mirror. During MPTP treatment and pharmacological experiments, the motor disability of the animals was scored using the rating scale in Table I [20].

III. EFFECTS OF ADENOSINE RECEPTOR LIGANDS ON MOTOR DYSFUNCTION IN MPTP-TREATED COMMON MARMOSETS

A. ADENOSINE A_1 RECEPTOR ANTAGONIST DPCPX

Oral administration of the selective adenosine A_1 receptor antagonist, 1,3-dipropyl-8-cyclopentylxanthine (DPCPX; 10 mg/kg), produced no significant effect on motor behavior in MPTP-treated marmosets, as assessed by locomotor activity and motor disability scores (Fig. 2). No abnormal oral movements, stereotyped movements of the limbs or the whole body, or other behavioral changes were observed. Furthermore, nausea and vomiting were not observed following DPCPX treatment. Thus, adenosine A_1 receptor antagonism does not appear to alter parkinsonian motor systems, even when doses of DPCPX sufficient to alter nervous system function in various species are used [21].

B. ADENOSINE A_{2A} RECEPTOR ANTAGONIST KW-6002

Oral administration of the adenosine A_{2A} receptor antagonist, KW-6002 (0.5–100 mg/kg), caused a long-lasting (up to 10 h) dose-dependent increase of locomotor activity in otherwise drug naive MPTP-treated marmosets

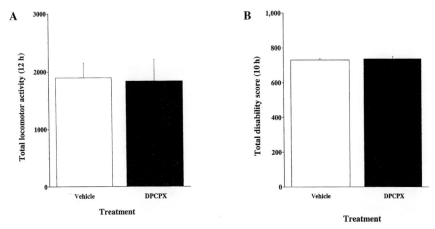

FIGURE 2   Effects of the A_1 receptor antagonist DPCPX on locomotor activity and motor disability in MPTP-treated common marmosets. (A) The effect of DPCPX (10 mg/kg, po, in 0.3% Tween 80, 10% sucrose solution) on total locomotor activity. Each column represents the mean locomotor count/12 hour $\pm$ SEM, $n = 4$). (B) The effects of DPCPX (10 mg/kg, po) on total motor disability. Each column represents the mean disability score/10 hour ($\pm$ SEM, $n = 4$). The animals were continuously monitored by trained observers. The animals were observed through a one-way mirror. During MPTP treatment and pharmacological experiments, the motor disability of the animals was scored using the rating scale shown in Table I [20].

(Fig. 3). KW-6002 (10 mg/kg, po) produced an approximate doubling of total locomotor activity over that produced by vehicle treatment. No further increase in locomotor activity was observed at higher doses of KW-6002. The effect of KW-6002 on locomotor activity was not continuous but occurred intermittently. Thus at some individual time points locomotor activity was significantly increased, whereas at other times it was not. The effects of the adenosine A_{2A} receptor antagonist on motor function differed significantly from those previously reported for L-Dopa or dopamine D_2 agonist drugs in a number of respects. For example, the adenosine A_{2A} receptor antagonist only doubled basal levels of locomotor activity and did not cause the hyperactivity that occurs following dopaminergic stimulation. In addition, locomotion was discontinuous and similar to that seen in normal animals in terms of the behavior patterns. However, L-Dopa and dopamine D_2 agonists produce a profound hyperactivity that greatly exceeds the activity of normal monkeys [22]. It is probable that the hyperactivity caused by dopaminergic agents is not indicative of therapeutic efficacy but rather a representation of drug side effects.

KW-6002 (0.5–100 mg/kg) caused a long-lasting (up to 10–11 h) and dose-dependent reduction in motor disability (Fig. 4). This was mainly due to increased checking movements and improved posture, reaction to stimuli, and alertness. No abnormal oral movements, stereotyped movements of the limbs or the whole body, or other behavioral changes were observed. In

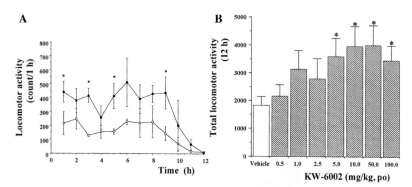

FIGURE 3   Effect of the A_{2A} receptor antagonist KW-6002 on locomotor activity in MPTP-treated common marmosets. (A) Time course of the effect of KW-6002 (10.0 mg/kg, po, 0.3% Tween 80, 10% sucrose solution) on locomotor activity. Each point represents the mean locomotor count/1 hour $\pm$ SEM, $n = 4$. Open circles show the vehicle treatment group. Closed circles show the KW-6002 treatment group. (B) Dose–response of the effects of KW-6002 (0.5–100 mg/kg, po) on locomotor activity. Each column represents the mean locomotor count/12 hour ($\pm$ SEM, $n = 4$). *$p < 0.05$ compared with control (vehicle treatment group).

addition, nausea and vomiting were not observed. Thus the pharmacological response to adenosine A_{2A} antagonists suggests that, in contrast to A_1 receptor antagonists, the A_{2A} receptor may be an important means of modifying motor behavior in Parkinson's disease.

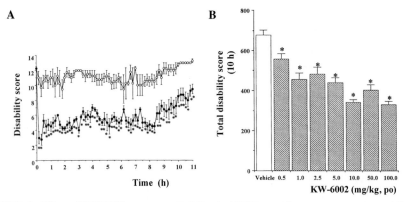

FIGURE 4   Effect of KW-6002 on motor disability in MPTP-treated common marmosets. (A) Time course of the effect of KW-6002 (10.0 mg/kg, po) on motor disability. Each point represents the mean disability score/10 minutes ($\pm$ SEM, $n = 4$). Open circles show the vehicle treatment group. Closed circles show the KW-6002 treatment group. (B) Dose–response of the effects of KW-6002 (0.5–100 mg/kg, po) on motor disability. Each column represents the mean disability score/10 hour ($\pm$ SEM, $n = 4$). *$p < 0.05$ compared with control (vehicle treatment group).

C. ADENOSINE A$_{2A}$ RECEPTOR AGONIST APEC

In rodents, intracerebroventricular injection of the adenosine A$_{2A}$ agonist, CGS 21680, reduced locomotor activity [23]. A similar depression of locomotor activity occurred in mice following systemic administration of 2-[(2-amino-ethylamino)-carbonylethylphenylethylamino]-5'N-ethylcarboxamido adenosine (APEC), which efficiently penetrates into brain and thus is convenient to use in primate studies where intracerebroventricular injection is not feasible. In MPTP-treated common marmosets, administration of APEC (2.5 mg/kg, ip) produced a significant decrease of locomotor activity, accompanied by salivation, prostration, reduced alertness, and muscle relaxation. At a low dose of APEC (0.625 mg/kg, ip), no significant effect on locomotor activity or other actions was observed (Fig. 5).

The administration of a low dose of the selective high-affinity adenosine A$_{2A}$ receptor agonist APEC; 0.625 mg/kg, ip [24] completely blocked the increase

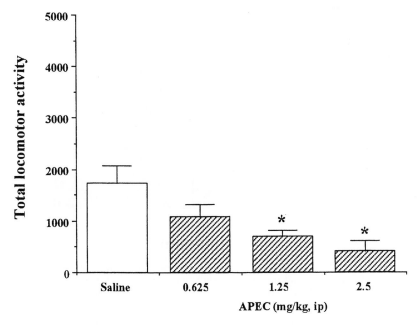

FIGURE 5 Effect of the A$_{2A}$ receptor agonist APEC on locomotor activity in MPTP-treated common marmosets. Dose–response of the effects of APEC on locomotor activity. Each column represents the mean locomotor count/12 hour ($\pm$ SEM, $n = 4$). *$p < 0.05$ compared with control (saline treatment group).

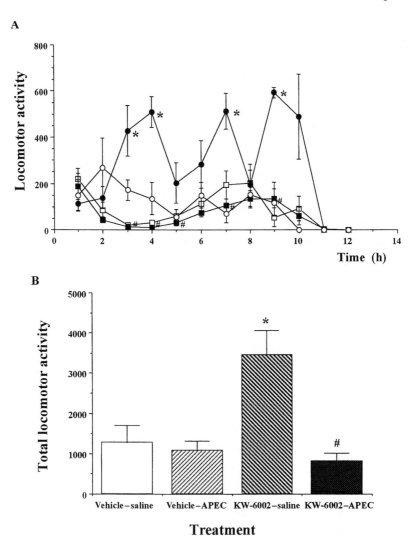

FIGURE 6 The effects of APEC and KW-6002 on locomotor activity in MPTP-treated common marmosets. (**A**) Time course of the effects of APEC and KW-6002 on locomotor activity. Each value represents mean (± SEM) of four animals. Each symbol represents as follows: circles, vehicle- and saline-treated group; square, vehicle and APEC (0.625 mg/kg, ip)-treated group; solid circles, KW-6002 (10 mg/kg, po) and saline-treated group; solid square, KW-6002 (10 mg/kg, po)- and APEC (0.625 mg/kg, ip)-treated group, respectively. (**B**) Effects of APEC and KW-6002 on total locomotor activity. Each value represents mean locomotor activity counts/12 hours (± SEM) of four animals. *$p < 0.05$ compared with the value of vehicle- and saline-treated group. #$p < 0.05$ compared with the value of KW-6002- and saline-treated group.

in locomotor activity caused by KW-6002 (Fig. 6). In contrast, administration of the adenosine A_1 receptor antagonist, DPCPX, did not affect either locomotor activity or motor disability in MPTP-treated common marmosets. Thus these findings strongly suggest that the effects of KW-6002 on locomotor activity in MPTP-treated common marmosets can be attributed to the blockade of adenosine A_{2A} receptor [25].

IV. EFFECT OF ADENOSINE A_{2A} RECEPTOR ANTAGONIST KW-6002 ON L-DOPA-INDUCED DYSKINESIAS

Administration of L-Dopa (10 mg/kg, po, twice daily) plus benserazide (2.5 mg/kg, po, twice daily) for 21 days induces limb and trunk dyskinesias in MPTP-treated marmosets [19]. After 6–10 days of L-Dopa treatment,

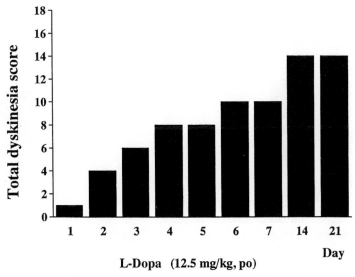

L-Dopa (12.5 mg/kg, po)

FIGURE 7   Induction of L-Dopa-induced dyskinesia on MPTP-treated common marmosets. L-Dopa (12.5 mg/kg po) treated twice daily. Carbidopa (12.5 mg/kg, po) treated 30 minutes before L-Dopa treatment. Each column represents the total dyskinesia score for four animals. Animals were observed for the presence or absence of stereotypy, the degree of motor stimulation or inhibition, the incidence of head twitches, wet dog shakes or grooming, oral movements, or other motor disturbance. The presence of dyskinesias was scored employing a semiquantitative rating system in Table II [s20]. Abnormal movements were described according to classically defined criteria: chorea—rapid random flicking movements, athetosis—sinuous writhing limb movements, dystonia—abnormal sustained posturing, and stereotypy–repetitive purposeless or semi-purposive movement.

dyskinetic movements appeared in all animals, initially with chorea, choreoathetosis, and stereotypies in the upper extremities. After 2–3 weeks of L-Dopa treatment, the dyskinesias became more severe and generalized with chorea, dystonia, and distal flicking and waving movements. After 3 weeks of L-Dopa treatment, all animals showed marked dyskinesia that could be consistently evoked by L-Dopa treatment (Fig. 7).

Oral administration of the A_{2A} receptor antagonist KW-6002 (10 mg/kg/day) for 21 days induced little or no dyskinesias in these L-Dopa-primed MPTP-treated marmosets (Fig. 8). Some mild athetosis and stereotyped reaching movements were observed in both the antagonist- and the vehicle-treated animals.

These results show that administration of an adenosine A_{2A} receptor antagonist fails to induce dyskinesia in animals previously exposed to L-Dopa. Even the repeated administration of an effective dose of KW-6002 for 21 days did not induce abnormal movement in otherwise drug naive MPTP-treated common marmosets. Dyskinesia is a common complication of the chronic treatment of Parkinson's disease with L-Dopa, but the mechanisms

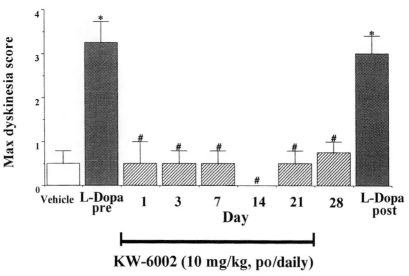

FIGURE 8   Effect of KW-6002 administered daily for 21 days on dyskinesia in MPTP-treated common marmosets primed with L-Dopa to exhibit dyskinesia. The animals previously received 21 days chronic L-Dopa (10 mg/kg, po, in 10% sucrose twice daily) plus benserazide (2.5 mg/kg, po, twice daily) for induction of dyskinesia. Each column represents the mean maximum dyskinesia score for four animals. *$p < 0.05$ compared with control (vehicle treatment group). #$p < 0.05$ compared with L-Dopa-treated group.

responsible for its induction have not been fully elucidated. Current concepts suggest that dyskinesia results from an imbalance between the indirect striopallidal output pathway and the direct striopallidal/nigral pathway. In particular, the indirect pathway has been implicated as becoming dysfunctional, indirectly causing alterations in pallidothalamic output [26–30]. Adenosine A_{2A} receptor antagonists may be able to modify the balance between the direct and indirect output pathways from striatum, producing antiparkinsonian activity without provoking dyskinesias (see Chapter 5).

V. EFFECT OF CHRONIC ADMINISTRATION OF ADENOSINE A_{2A} RECEPTOR ANTAGONIST KW-6002

Acute oral administration of KW-6002 (10 mg/kg) caused a two-fold increase of locomotor activity and a corresponding reduction in motor disability score in MPTP-treated marmosets. Repeated administration of KW-6002 (10 mg/kg, po) for up to 21 days did not diminish the antiparkinsonian activity of KW-6002 on locomotor activity or motor disability in MPTP-treated marmosets (Fig. 9; Table II). Acute administration of KW-6002 (10 mg/kg, po) 1 week following the end of a chronic dosage regime again produced an identical

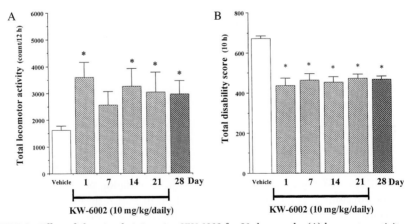

FIGURE 9 Effect of chronic administration KW-6002 for 21 days on the (A) locomotor activity and (B) motor disability of MPTP-treated common marmosets. KW-6002 (10 mg/kg, po) was administered once per day. In Figure 5A, each column represents the mean locomotor count/12 hour (± SEM, $n = 4$), and in Figure 5B the mean disability score/10 hour (± SEM, $n = 4$). *$p < 0.05$ compared with control (vehicle treatment group).

TABLE II   Dyskinesia Rating Scale

Score	Symptoms
0, Absent	No dyskinetic posture or movements
1, Mild	Fleeting and rare dyskinetic postures and movements
2, Moderate	More prominent abnormal movements, not interfering significantly with normal behavior
3, Marked	Frequent and at times continuous dyskinesias intruding upon normal activity
4, Severe	Virtually continuous dyskinetic activity, disabling to animal and replacing normal movement

increase in locomotor activity and a decrease in disability score to that observed initially (see Fig. 9). Again, no dyskinesias were observed. The antiparkinsonian activity of KW-6002 was maintained both during and after 21 days of chronic treatment. In contrast, the repeated administration of dopamine agonist drugs can induce tolerance to the reversal of motor deficits in MPTP-lesioned primates [28]. The fact that KW-6002 is an antagonist and does not stimulate receptors may be the reason it does not cause downregulation and the onset of tolerance.

VI. COMPARISON OF THE ANTIPARKINSONIAN ACTIVITY OF L-DOPA AND A_{2A} ANTAGONIST KW-6002

A comparison of the effects of KW-6002 or L-Dopa on locomotor activity in MPTP-treated common marmosets with the basal locomotor activity in normal common marmosets showed different effects of the drug treatments (Fig. 10). Locomotor activity of MPTP-treated marmosets was increased to the level observed in normal animals by the administration of KW-6002. In contrast, administration of L-Dopa (10 mg/kg, po) plus benserazide (2.5 mg/kg, po) induced locomotor hyperactivity in these animals. Administration of L-Dopa (10 mg/kg, po) plus benserazide (2.5 mg/kg, po) similarly reduced motor disability. The extent of the reduction in motor disability produced by L-Dopa was not different from that produced by KW-6002 (Table III).Thus the effects of the adenosine A_{2A} receptor antagonist on motor function differ significantly from those previously reported for L-Dopa or dopamine D_2 agonist drugs in a number of respects.

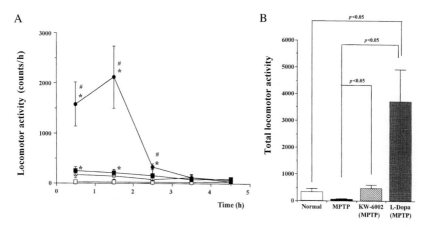

FIGURE 10 Effect of KW-6002 or L-Dopa on locomotor activity in MPTP-treated common marmosets and the basal locomotor activity of naive and MPTP-treated common marmosets. (**A**) Time course of the effect of KW-6002 (10.0 mg/kg, po) or L-Dopa (10 mg/kg, po plus benser-azide 2.5 mg/kg, po) on locomotor activity in MPTP-treated common marmosets and the loco-motor activity of vehicle-treated normal common marmosets. Each point represents the mean lo-comotor count/1 hour ($\pm$ SEM, $n = 4$). Open circles show the vehicle-treated normal marmosets. Open squares show the vehicle-treated MPTP-lesioned marmosets. Closed circles show the L-Dopa treatment group. Closed squares show the KW-6002 treatment group. (**B**) Total locomotor activity of MPTP-treated marmosets administered with vehicle, KW-6002, or L-Dopa, and normal marmosets administered with vehicle. Each column represents the mean locomotor count/2 hour ($\pm$ SEM, $n = 4$). *$p < 0.05$ compared with naive animal (vehicle treatment group). #$p < 0.05$ compared with MPTP-treated control group (MPTP-treated marmoset administered with vehicle).

Table III   Maximum Reduction of Motor Disability Score by KW-6002 or L-Dopa

Animal	Treatment	Disability score ($\pm$ SEM)	N
Normal	Vehicle	2.00 ± 1.35^{a}	4
MPTP-treated	Vehicle	11.75 ± 0.41	4
MPTP-treated	KW-6002	4.00 ± 0.49^{a}	4
MPTP-treated	L-Dopa	4.25 ± 0.75^{a}	4

The maximum reduction of motor disability score represents average of minimum score recorded for each animal during an observation period at each preparations. $^{a}p < 0.05$ compare with MPTP-treated animals value. There are no significant differences among vehicle-treated normal group, L-Dopa-treated, MPTP-treated group, and KW-6002-treated, MPTP-treated group.

VII. CONCLUSION

MPTP-treated primates represent the most effective animal model of Parkinson's disease because the motor changes and the responses to drug treatments closely resemble those observed with Parkinson's disease. In addition, the effects of antiparkinsonian drugs are closely related to those observed in clinical use. The effects of a selective adenosine A_{2A} receptor agonist and antagonist, and an adenosine A_1 receptor antagonist, on motor symptoms in MPTP-treated common marmosets show that the adenosine A_{2A} receptor, but not the adenosine A_1 receptor, is involved in the improvement of motor symptoms. The mechanism by which adenosine A_{2A} receptor antagonists produce antiparkinsonian activity is of interest, and the selective expression of adenosine A_{2A} receptors reported on striatal GABA/enkephalin-containing neurons and cholinergic interneurons provides a major clue. Adenosine A_{2A} receptor mRNA is coexpressed with that of dopamine D_2 receptors in GABA/enkephalin-containing neurons of the indirect pathway. Previously, the actions of adenosine in striatum were explained by a direct interaction of D_2 and A_2 receptors in 6-OHDA-lesioned rats [31]. However, many studies conducted both *in vivo* and *in vitro* have demonstrated adenosine A_{2A} receptor-mediated control of the release of GABA and acetylcholine (ACh) by [32,33; see Chapter 7]. Specifically, adenosine A_{2A} receptors regulate the GABAergic inhibitory synaptic transmission in striatal medium-size spiny neurons. This suggests that adenosine A_{2A} receptor antagonists exert an inhibitory effect on the GABAergic output pathway. Thus adenosine A_{2A} receptor antagonists may exert a direct action on medium spiny neurons of the striatum to produce antiparkinsonian effects [34].

Interestingly, it has been shown that degeneration of dopaminergic neurons in the substantia nigra did not affect adenosine A_{2A} receptor binding in the striatum, and the number of adenosine A_{2A} receptors in parkinsonian patients are not different from those in "normal" individuals [35]. The concept of using adenosine compounds in Parkinson's disease has been suggested by some previous reports. An open trial of the nonselective adenosine receptor antagonist theophylline produced some improvement in patients with Parkinson's disease [36]. However, theophylline is not only a nonselective adenosine receptor antagonist, but it also inhibits phosphodiestsrases and/or guanosine receptors. The failure of KW-6002 to induce dyskinesias is of considerable interest. Dyskinesia is a common and serious complication of chronic treatment with L-Dopa. The mechanism responsible has not been fully elucidated, although there are several hypotheses. L-Dopa-induced dyskinesia was initially considered to be related to D_1 receptor stimulation, but the D_2 receptor agonists (+)-4-propyl-9-hydroxy-naphthoxazine (PHNO) and quinpirole were also found to cause dyskinesia in MPTP-lesioned primates

[26]. Consequently, dyskinesias are now often attributed to an imbalance between D_1 and D_2 receptor-mediated control of the direct and indirect output pathways [29].

Adenosine A_{2A} receptors modulate the release of GABA in the striatum, which possibly regulates the activity of medium spiny neurons constituting the indirect and direct pathways [37]. Thus, adenosine A_{2A} receptor antagonists might maintain the balance between the pathways, producing antiparkinsonian activity without provoking dyskinesias.

ACKNOWLEDGMENTS

This study was supported by a grant from Kyowa Hakko Kogyo Co. Ltd. P. Jenner thanks the Parkinson's Disease Society, the National Parkinson Foundation, Miami, and the Medical Research Council for their support. The authors are thankful for consistent support from collaborators in the Pharmacology Group, Biomedical Sciences Division, King's College London, and collaborators in the Pharmaceutical Research Institute of Kyowa Hakko Kogyo Co., Ltd. The authors thank Drs. J. Shimada and F. Suzuki for providing KW-6002 and Ms. T. Tashiro for excellent technical assistance.

REFERENCES

1. Dunwiddie, T.V. (1985). The Physiological role of adenosine in the central nervous system. *Int Rev Neurobiol* 27, 63–139.
2. Fredholm, B.B., Abbracchio, M.P., Burnstock, G., Daly, J.W., Harden, T.K., Jacobson, K.A., Leff, P., and Williams, M. (1994). Nomenclature and classification of purinoceptor. *Pharmacol Rev* 46, 143–156.
3. Schiffmann, S.N., Jacobs, O., and Vanderhaeghen, J.-J. (1991). Striatal restricted adenosine A_2 receptor (RDC8) is expressed by enkephalin but not by substance P neurons: an *in situ* hybridization histochemistry study. *J Neurochem* 57, 1062–1067.
4. Josselyn, S.A., and Beninger, R.J. (1991). Behavioral effects of intrastriatal caffeine mediated by adenosinergic modulation of dopamine. *Pharmacol Biochem Behav* 39, 97–103.
5. Fuxe, K., and Ungerstedt, U. (1974). Action of caffeine and theophyllamine on supersensitive dopamine receptors: considerable enhancement of receptor response to treatment with DOPA and dopamine receptor agonists. *Med Biol* 52, 48–54.
6. Ferre, S., Rubio, A., and Fuxe, K. (1991). Stimulation of adenosine A_2 receptors induces catalepsy. *Neurosci Lett* 130, 162–164.
7. Kanda, T., Shiozaki, S., Schimada, J., Suzuki, F., and Nakamura, J. (1994). KF17837: a novel selective adenosine A_{2A} receptor antagonist with anticataleptic activity. *Eur J Pharmacol* 256, 263–268.
8. Shimada, J., Suzuki, F., Nonaka, H., Ishii, A., and Ichikawa, S. (1992). (E)-1,3-dialkyl-7-methyl-8-(3,4,5-trimethoxystyryl) xanthines: potent and selective adenosine A_2 antagonists. *J Med Chem* 35, 2342–2345.
9. Nonaka, H., Ichimura, M., Takeda, M., Nonaka, Y., Shimada, J., Suzuki, F., Yamaguchi, K., and Kase, H. (1994). KF17837(E)-8-(3,4-dimethoxystyryl) 1,3-dipropyl-7-methylxanthine), a potent and selective adenosine A_2 receptor antagonist. *Eur J Pharmacol* 267, 335–341.

10. Shimada, J., Koike, N., Nonaka, H., Shiozaki, S., Yanagawa, K., Kanada, T., Kobayashi, H., Ichimura, M., Nakamura, J., Kase, H., and Suzuki, F. (1997). (E)-1,3-diethyl-8-(3,4-dimethoxystyryl)-7-methlxanthine: a potent adenosine A_2 antagonist with anti-cataleptic activity. *Bioorg Med Chem Lett* 7, 2349–2352.

11. Richardson, P.J., Kase, H., and Jenner, P.G. (1997). Adenosine A_{2A} receptor antagonists as new agents for the treatment of Parkinson's disease. *Trends Pharmacol Sci* 18, 338–344.

12. Langston, J.W., Ballaerd, P., Tetrud, J.W., and Irwin, I. (1983). Chronic parkinsonism in human due to a product of meperidine analog synthesis. *Science* 219, 979–980.

13. Heikkila, R.E., Cabbat, F.S., Manzino, L., and Duvoisin, R.C. (1984). Effects of 1-methyl-4-phenyl-1,2,3,6-tetrahydropyridine on neostriatal dopamine in mice. *Neuropharmacol* 3, 711–713.

14. Johannessen, J.N., Chiueh, C.C., Herkenham, M.A., and Markey, S.P. (1986). Relationship of the *in vivo* metabolism of MPTP to toxicity. In MPTP: Aneurotoxin Producing a Parkinsonian Syndrome (Markey, S.P., Castagnili, N., Jr., Trevor, A.J., and Kopin, I.J., eds.), pp. 173–189. London: Academic Press.

15. May, T., Pawlik, M., and Rommelspacher, H. (1991). [^{3}H] Harman binding experiments. II: regional and subcellular distribution of specific [^{3}H] harman binding and monoamine oxidase subtypes A and B activity in marmoset and rat. *J Neurochem* 56, 500–508.

16. Burns, R.S., Chiueh, C.C., Markey, S.P., Ebert, M.H., Jacobowitz, D.M., and Kopin, I.J. (1983). A primate model of parkinsonism: selective destruction of dopaminergic 1,2,3,6-tetrahydropyridine. *Proc Natl Acad Sci USA* 80, 4546–4550.

17. Jenner, P., Rupniak, N.M.J., Rose, S., Kelly, E., Kilpatrick, G., Less, A., and Marsden, C.D. (1984). 1-Methyl-4-phenyl-1,2,3,6-tetrahydropyridine-induced parkinsonism in the common marmoset. *Neurosci Lett* 50, 85–90.

18. Loschmann, P.A., Smith, L.A., Lange, K.W., Jenner, P., and Marsden, C.D. (1992). Motor activity following the administration of selective D-1 and D-2 dopaminergic drugs to MPTP treated common marmosets. *Psychopharmacol* 109, 49–56.

19. Pearce, R.K.B., Jackson, M.J., Smith, L.A., Jenner, P., and Marsden, C.D. (1995). Chronic L-DOPA administration induces dyskinesia in the MPTP-treated common marmoset (*Callithrix jacchus*). *Movement Disord* 10, 731–740.

20. Kanda, T., Jackson, M.J., Smith, L.A., Pearce, R.K.B., Nakamura, J., Kase, H., Kuwana, Y., and Jenner, P. (1998). Adenosine A_{2A} antagonist: a novel antiparkinsonian agent that does not provoke dyskinesia in parkinsonian monkey. *Ann Neurol* 43, 507–513.

21. Griebel, G., Saffroy-Spittler, M., Misslin, R., Remmy, D., and Vogel, E. (1991). Comparison of the behavioural effects of an adenosine A_1/A_2-receptor antagonist, CGS15943A, and an A_1-selective antagonist, DPCPX. *Psychopharmacol* 103, 541–544.

22. Akai, T., Yamaguchi, M., Mizuta, E., and Kuno, S. (1993). Effects of terguride, a partial D_2 agonist, on MPTP-lesioned parkinsonian cynomolgus monkeys. *Ann neurol* 33, 507–511.

23. Nikodijevic, O., Daly, J.W., and Jacobson, K.A. (1990). Characterization of the locomotor depression preoduced by an A-2-selective adenosine agonist. *FEBS Lett* 261, 67–70.

24. Nikodijevic, O., Sarges, R., Daly, J.W., and Jacobson, K.A. (1991). Behavioral effects of A_1-and A_2-selective adenosine agonists and antagonists: evidence for synergism and antagonism. *J Pharmacol Exp Ther* 259, 286–294.

25. Kanda, T., Tashiro, T., Kuwana, Y., and Jenner, P. (1998). Modulation of motor function by adenosine A_{2A} receptors in parkinsonian common marmosets. *Neuroreport* 9, 2857–2860.

26. Mouradian, M.M., Heuser, I.J.E., Baronti, F., Fabbrini, G., Juncos, J.L., and Chase, T.N. (1989). Pathogenesis of dyskinesias in Parkinson's disease. *Ann Neurol* 25, 523–526.

27. Blanchet, P., Bedard, P.J., Britton, D.R., and Kebabian, J.W. (1993). Differential effect of selective D-1 and D-2 dopamine receptor agonists on levodopa-induced dyskinesia in 1-methyl-4-phenyl-1,2,3,6-tetrahydropyridine-exposed monkeys. *J Pharm Exp Ther* 267, 275–279.

28. Blanchet, P.J., Grondin, R., and Bedard, P.J. (1996). Dyskinesia and wearing-off following dopamine D_1 agonist treatment in drug-naive 1-methyl-4-phenyul-1,2,3,6-tetrahydropyridine-lesioned primates. *Movement Disord* **11**, 91–94.

29. Balanchet, P.J., Gomez-Mancilla, B., Di Paolo, T., and Bedard, P.J. (1995). Is striatal dopaminergic receptor imbalance responsible for levodopa-induced dyskinesia? *Fundam Clin Pharm* **9**, 434–442.

30. Calon, F., Goulet, M., Blanchet, P.J., Martel, J.C., Piercey, M.F., Bedard, P.J., and Di Paolo, T. (1995). Levodopa or D_2 agonist induced dyskinesia in MPTP monkeys: correlation with changes in dopamine and $GABA_A$ receptors in the striatopallidal complex. *Brain Res* **680**, 43–52.

31. Ferré, S., Herrera-Marschitz, M., Grabowska-Anden, M., Ungerstedt, U., Cacas, M., and Anden, N.-E. (1991). Postsynaptic dopamine/adenosine interaction: I. Adenosine analogues inhibit dopamine D2-mediated behaviour in short-term reserpinized mice. *Eur J Pharmacol* **192**, 25–30.

32. Kurokawa, M., Kirk, I.P., Kirkpatrick, K.A., Kase, H., and Richardson, P.J. (1994). Inhibition by KF17837 of adenosine A_{2A} receptor-mediated modulation of striatal GABA and ACh release. *Br J Pharmacol* **113**, 43–48.

33. Kurokawa, M., Koga, K., Kase, H., Nakamura, J., and Kuwana, Y. (1996). Adenosine A_{2A} receptor-mediated modulation of striatal actylcholine release *in vivo*. *J Neurochem* **66**, 1882–1888.

34. Mori, A., Shindou, T., Ichimura, M., Nonaka, H., and Kase, H. (1996). The role of adenosine A_{2A} receptors in regulating GABAergic synaptic transmission in striatal medium spiny neurons. *J Neurosci* **16**, 605–611.

35. Martines-Mir, M.I., Probst, A., and Palacios, J.M (1991). Adenosine A_2 receptors: selective localization in the human basal ganglia and alterations with disease. *Neurosci* **42**, 697–706.

36. Maliy, J., and Stone, T.W. (1994). The effect of theophylline on parkinsonian symptoms. *J Pharm Pharmacol* **46**, 515–517.

37. Kawaguchi, Y., Wilson, C.J., Augood, S.J., and Emson, P.C (1995). Striatal interneurons: chemical, physiological and morphological characterization. *Trends Neurosci* **18**, 527–535.

CHAPTER 12

Selective Adenosine A_{2A} Receptor Antagonism as an Alternative Therapy for Parkinson's Disease
A Study in Nonhuman Primates

A. Hadj Tahar, R. Grondin, L. Grégoire, and P.J. Bédard
Neuroscience Research Unit, Laval University Research Center, Ste-Foy, Quebec, Canada

A. Mori and H. Kase
Pharmaceutical Research and Development Center, Kyowa Hakko Kogyo Co., Ltd., Tokyo, Japan

I. INTRODUCTION

Parkinson's disease (PD), a neurodegenerative disease of the central nervous system (CNS) characterized by bradykinesia, rigidity, tremor, and loss of postural reflexes, still presents therapeutic challenges. Long-term treatment with L-3,4-dihydroxyphenylalanine (L-Dopa), the cornerstone of PD therapy, is often associated with motor complications over time (Marsden, 1994). Indeed some adverse effects such as L-Dopa-induced dyskinesias offset the therapeutic benefit that can be achieved. Hence, there is a pressing need to find alternative methods to treat PD. In the search for rational, improved, or alternative therapies, one possibility that has become apparent is to modify the activity of adenosine within the brain.

The nucleoside adenosine is a widely distributed biological compound released from most tissues, including neurons and glia, as a result of metabolic activity, and it mediates a variety of physiological responses in mammalian systems (Fredholm, 1995; Linden, 1994; Stone *et al.*, 1990). In the brain, adenosine acts as neuromodulator and the normal extracellular levels of adenosine are in the low micromolar range, although this concentration can rise several hundred-fold as a result of repeated stimulation or limitations of oxygen supply, as during hypoxia or ischemia. However, adenosine can also be released from neurons under nonhypoxic conditions and independently of the transporters. Neuronal activity leads to release of adenosine triphosphate (ATP) into the extracellular space, which can be degraded to adenosine. The low basal level of extracellular adenosine can influence the activity of those central neurons bearing abundant adenosine A_1 and A_{2A} receptors.

Adenosine exerts its effects by acting on specific membrane-bound receptors belonging to the G-protein coupled receptor superfamily, which has been classified into at least four subtypes, of which the most is understood of the A_1 and A_2 subtypes (Fredholm, 1995; Williams, 1995). By acting on the A_1 receptor, which is negatively coupled to adenylyl cyclase, adenosine exerts a potent depressant effect on neurons by reducing transmitter release from presynaptic nerve terminals and increasing potassium conductance in the postsynaptic cell (Corradetti *et al.*, 1984; Stone and Bartrup, 1991). Excitatory actions of adenosine, mediated by the activation of the A_{2A} receptor subtype, which is positively coupled to the adenylyl cyclase, have also been shown in the CNS. Using selective agonists and antagonists for adenosine A_{2A} receptors, their role in the modulation of several neurotransmitters (acetylcholine [ACH], dopamine, glutamate, γ-aminobutyric acid [GABA]) has been extensively studied in the striatum, cortex, and hippocampus (see Daval *et al.*, 1996; Latini *et al.*, 1996).

The distribution of adenosine receptor subtypes in the mammalian brain has been extensively studied (Goodman and Snyder, 1982; Jarvis, 1988). Contrasting with A_1 sites, which are widely distributed throughout the brain, the distribution of A_{2A} receptors is highly localized in the striatum, nucleus accumbens, and olfactory tubercle, as demonstrated by the binding assay of the A_{2A} selective agonist, CGS 21680 (Hutchison *et al.*, 1989), and by analysis of the A_2 receptor mRNA localization with *in situ* hybridization histochemistry (Schiffmann *et al.*, 1990, 1991a, 1991b; see Chapter 2). However, adenosine A_{2A} receptors, albeit at lower levels, are also localized in other brain regions, such as the cortex and the hippocampus (Dixon *et al.*, 1996; Svenningsson *et al.*, 1997a). The selective distribution of A_{2A} receptor in regions known to be a critical component of subcortical circuits involved in the processing of motor activity, such as the striatum, suggests a possible implication in the control of motor activity. In fact, in the striatum, the A_{2A} receptor is coexpressed in the same medium spiny neurons as those bearing DA D_2 receptors (Fink *et al.*, 1992; Pollack *et al.*, 1993), containing enkephalin (Augood and Emson, 1994; Schiffmann *et al.*, 1991a) and projecting to the external segment of the pallidum (GPe) (indirect pathway).

Moreover, A_{2A} receptor density is significantly decreased in basal ganglia of Huntington's chorea patients but unaltered in PD. Such findings confirm the receptor localization on neurons that have their cell bodies in the striatum and are selectively destroyed in Huntington's disease (Martinez-Mir *et al.*, 1991). Similarly, dopamine denervation also had no effect on A_{2A} binding sites as observed in the striatum of 6-hydroxydopamine (6-OHDA) rats (Morelli *et al.*, 1994). These data suggest an implication of adenosine A_{2A} receptors in basal ganglia functions and offer an anatomical basis for dopamine (D_2 receptor) and adenosine (A_{2A} receptor) interactions in the brain as seen at behavioral, neuronal function, and cellular levels (see Ferré *et al.*, 1997).

In behavioral studies, nonselective adenosine receptor antagonists such as caffeine and theophylline induce motor activation, and this is counteracted by dopamine depletion or dopamine D_1 or D_2 receptor blockade (see Ferré *et al.*, 1992, 1997). Moreover, adenosine receptor agonists inhibit and adenosine receptor antagonists potentiate the motor activation effect of dopamine agonists (Ferré *et al.*, 1992, 1997). Using selective adenosine receptor antagonists, it has been shown that although selective A_1 receptor antagonists potentiate only D_1 agonist-induced motor activation, selective A_{2A} receptor antagonists potentiate both D_1 and D_2 stimulation of motor behavior (Fenu *et al.*, 1997; Pinna *et al.*, 1996; Popoli *et al.*, 1996). Moreover, the xanthine selective A_{2A} receptor antagonist, KF17837, reverses catalepsy induced by CGS 21680, haloperidol, and reserpine in mice (Kanda *et al.*, 1994). Significantly, a synergistic effect between L-Dopa and KF17837 was observed under both dopamine depletion and D_2 receptor blockade (Kanda *et al.*, 1994). KF17837 also antagonizes hypomobility induced by MPTP in mice and reverses the effects of CGS 21680 in 6-OHDA-lesioned rats (Ongini and Fredholm, 1996). Using positron emission tomography (PET), it was found that the xanthine KF17837 labeled with [^{11}C] passes into the brain, albeit sluggishly (Stone-Elander *et al.*, 1997). Similar to caffeine and CGS 15943, the nonxanthine selective A_{2A} receptor antagonist, SCH58261 stimulates motor behavior and increases wakefulness duration (for review see Ongini and Fredholm, 1996).

Hence, there is good reason to believe that blockade of the adenosine A_{2A} receptor could help restore the balance of striatal function and could be of value in the treatment of PD. The aim of this study was to evaluate, in MPTP exposed monkeys having a stable parkinsonian syndrome and exibiting dyskinesias to levodopa, both the antiparkinsonian and dyskinetic effects upon challenge with the selective adenosine A_{2A} receptor antagonist: [(E)-8-[2-(3,4-dimethoxyphenyl)ethenyl]-1,3-diethyl-3,7-dihydro-7-methyl-1h-puri-ne-2,6-dionel (KW-6002). KW-6002 is a newly developed adenosine receptor antagonist showing high affinity for the rat striatal A_{2A} receptor with a K_i

value of 2.2 nM and about 68-fold selectivity for the A_{2A} receptor over the A_1 receptor (Nonaka *et al.*, 1997).

II. MATERIALS AND METHODS

A. ANIMALS

Six female cynomolgus monkeys (*Macaca fascicularis*) weighing 3–4 kg were used in this study in accordance with the standards of the Canadian Council on Animal Care. The animals were housed separately in individual observation cages in a temperature-controlled room and exposed to a 12-hour light–dark cycle. They were fed with certified primate chow with fruit supplements, and water was provided *ad libitum*.

B. DRUG TREATMENTS

All animals were initially treated with the neurotoxin MPTP dissolved in sterile water and injected subcutaneously at an initial dose of 0.6 mg/kg. Injections were repeated weekly until a clear and stable parkinsonian syndrome developed (i.e., same score of 5 or more on the disability scale over a month). At that stage, all animals were treated once daily with oral administration of one capsule containing both L-Dopa (50 mg) and benserazide (12.5 mg) (Hoffmann-La Roche, Mississauga, Ontario) until dyskinesia had developed, which was thereafter reproducible by subsequent challenge of L-Dopa/benserazide or dopamine receptor agonists.

KW-6002 (Kyowa Hakko Kogyo Co., Ltd., Tokyo) was then administered, alone or in combination with oral L-Dopa/benserazide (50/12.5), using two different preparations of KW-6002. The first preparation of KW-6002 was suspended in 30 mL of a sucrose (10%)/Tween 80 solution and administered orally at 10 and 30 mg/kg using an esophageal tube coupled to a syringe. The second formulation (10 mg pure substance/210 mg excipients) of KW-6002 was given orally at 10 mg/kg in 2–3 gelatin capsules. Doses of KW-6002 administered alone and in combination with L-Dopa/benserazide were separated by a drug-free period of 24 hours (washout). On control days, each animal was administered with vehicle (30 ML sucrose (10%)/Tween 80 solution or empty capsule). L-Dopa/benserazide (50/12.5) was also administered orally as a single capsule together with vehicle. On study days, the animals were observed in their home cage through a one-way screen and scored every 30 minutes for up to 6 hours without being disturbed.

C. MOTOR ASSESSMENT

1. Disability Scale

The parkinsonian syndrome following MPTP exposure and the relief of parkinsonism following KW-6002 and/or L-Dopa administration were rated according to a disability scale for MPTP-treated monkeys used previously in our laboratory (Grondin *et al.*, 1997). The rating scale assessed posture, mobility, climbing, gait, grooming, vocalization, social interaction, and tremor. The maximal disability representing a score of 10. In addition, stereotypies, hyperactivity, somnolence, and vomiting were each evaluated qualitatively.

2. Dyskinesia Scale

The severity of dyskinesia was also rated for the face, neck, trunk, arms, and legs on a scale of None = 0 to Severe (continuous) = 3. The dyskinetic score obtained was the sum of the scores for all body segments for a maximal score of 21 points.

3. Locomotion

The gross locomotor activity was monitored continuously throughout the experiment using photocell activity counters fixed on each home cage. A light beam was interrupted by the movements of the animal, and these signals were accumulated by a computer that provided a mobility count every 15 minutes.

D. STATISTICAL ANALYSIS

The improvement in disability and the dyskinetic scores recorded individually at peak effect, after a given drug administration, were averaged for all six animals. They were then compared using the nonparametric Friedman's test. The total mobility counts recorded individually during a 6-hour period following a given treatment were also averaged for all six monkeys and compared using an analysis of variance (ANOVA) followed by a Fisher's probability of least significant difference (PLSD) test.

III. RESULTS

A. LOCOMOTION

L-Dopa/benserazide (50/12.5 mg) administered alone produced a stimulatory effect on locomotion as indicated by the mean mobility counts, which were significantly increased compared with the mean vehicle control values (Fig. 1A and 1B, black bars). At the dosage used, the effect on locomotor

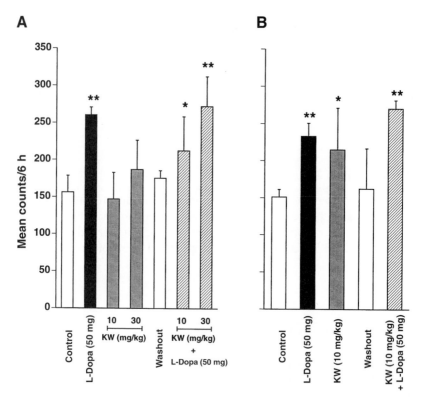

FIGURE 1   Locomotion counts after acute administration of KW-6002 (**A**) in suspension and (**B**) in gelatin capsules. The total mobility counts recorded individually during a 6-hour period following each treatment were averaged for all six animals. The values were compared using ANOVA followed by a Fisher's PLSD test. Due to technical difficulties, four of the six animals were considered for statistical analysis. Counts $\pm$ SEM ($*p < 0.05$ and $**p < 0.01$ vs control).

activity occurred 45 minutes after the oral administration of L-Dopa/benserazide and lasted 90 minutes average.

When given alone in suspension, KW-6002 produced no (at 10 mg/kg) or little (at 30 mg/kg) improvement in the motor behavior on average (Fig. 1A, gray bars). Indeed we observed in one monkey a very short locomotor response for approximately 15 minutes, which occurred 90 minutes after the administration of the lower dose of KW-6002 tested. At 30 mg/kg, this response occurred 60 minutes after the administration of KW-6002 and lasted 45 minutes in this animal. In contrast, when given alone in gelatin capsules at 10 mg/kg, KW-6002 produced a clear locomotor response in all animals that reached statistical significance (Fig. 1B, gray bars). The response occurred 60 minutes after the administration of KW-6002 and lasted approximately 75 minutes on average.

Doses of KW-6002 administered alone and in combination with L-Dopa/benserazide were separated by a drug-free period of 24 hours. On such washout days, the locomotor activity was back to control levels (Fig. 1A and 1B, open bars) as well as the parkinsonian symptoms. KW-6002 coadministered with L-Dopa/benserazide was found to slightly increase (+10%) the effect of L-Dopa/benserazide on motor activity at 10 mg/kg (Fig. 1B, hatched bars). No clear potentiation was observed relative to the duration of action of L-Dopa/benserazide.

B. Improvement in Disability and Dyskinesias

The monkeys had a stable parkinsonian score of 5.3 ± 0.1 on average on the disability scale. L-Dopa/benserazide alone significantly improved the parkinsonian symptoms by more than 2 points on average on the disability scale (Fig. 2A and 2B, top). However, this was linked to moderate to severe dyskinesias, either choreic or dystonic in nature (Fig. 2A and 2B, bottom).

When given in suspension at 10 and 30 mg/kg, KW-6002 slightly improved the parkinsonian symptoms (less than 2 points on the scale) (Fig. 2A, top). At these dosages, no dyskinesias were seen except in one animal where mild dyskinesias were observed compared with severe dyskinesias under L-Dopa/benserazide therapy (Fig. 2A, bottom). However, when administered in capsules at 10 mg/kg, KW-6002 significantly improved the parkinsonian symptoms on the disability scale, respectively (Fig. 2B, top). Interestingly, virtually little or no dyskinesias were observed contrary to L-Dopa/benserazide given alone (Fig. 2A, bottom).

Coadministration of KW-6002 with L-Dopa/benserazide produced a small increase (not significant) in L-Dopa improvement of motor disability without excacerbation of L-Dopa-induced dyskinesias (Fig. 2A and 2B). KW-6002 was

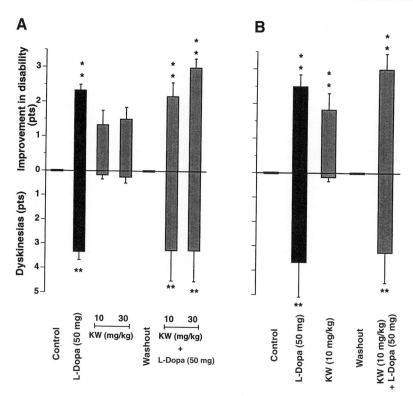

FIGURE 2   Antiparkinsonian (top) and dyskinetic (bottom) response after acute administration of KW-6002 (**A**) in suspension and (**B**) in gelatin capsules. The improvement in disability (top) and the dyskinetic scores (bottom) recorded individually at peak effect for each treatment were averaged for all six animals. The values were compared using the nonparametric Friedman's test. Improvement in disability $\pm$ SEM (**$p < 0.01$ vs control). Dyskinetic scores $\pm$ SEM (**$p < 0.01$ vs control).

well tolerated by all animals because it did not induce abnormal behaviors (stereotypies, hyperactivity) or other clinically observable adverse effects (somnolence, vomiting) at any of the doses tested.

IV. DISCUSSION

Our data show that selective adenosine receptor antagonism, by KW-6002 administered alone, increases locomotion and improves parkinsonian symptoms in a significant manner in MPTP-treated monkeys (Figs. 1B and 2B).

Furthermore, when coadministered with L-Dopa, KW-6002 tended to increase L-Dopa response (Fig. 1A and 1B). These results fit well with other behavioral studies on 6-OHDA-lesioned rats (Ferré *et al.*, 1992, 1997; Fuxe and Ungerstedt, 1974; Garrett and Holtzman, 1995; Herrara-Marschitz *et al.*, 1988; Ungerstedt *et al.*, 1981) and MPTP-treated monkeys (Kanda *et al.*, 1998). Indeed it has been shown in these studies that adenosine antagonists induce turning behavior in 6-OHDA-lesioned rats and have an antiparkinsonian action in primates. Significantly, a similar synergism is observed between L-Dopa and A_{2A} antagonist under conditions of both dopamine depletion by reserpine and dopamine receptor blockade by haloperidol. In fact, the xanthine KF17837 potentiates the anticataleptic effects of L-Dopa in both models (Kanda *et al.*, 1994). Similarly, KF17837 was shown to antagonize hypomobility induced by MPTP in mice (Ongini and Fredholm, 1996) and to improve the motor disability in MPTP-treated marmosets with no evidence of dyskinesias (Kanda *et al.*, 1998). In addition, a synergistic interaction has been observed between A_{2A} receptor antagonists and dopamine D_1 and D_2 receptor agonists in 6-OHDA-lesioned rats (Fenu *et al.*, 1997; Jiang *et al.*, 1993; Pinna *et al.*, 1996). Finally, in humans, the nonselective adenosine receptor antagonist, theophylline, causes an improvement in both subjective and objective parkinsonian scores (Mally and Stone, 1994).

The mechanism(s) of action of KW-6002 is probably related to adenosine A_{2A} receptor antagonism. Indeed Svenningsson and colleagues (1997b) provided evidence that the stimulatory effects of caffeine are due to inhibition of the tonic stimulatory actions of endogenous adenosine at A_{2A} receptors on striatopallidal GABAergic neurons. In support of this model, it has been shown that caffeine no longer increases spontaneous locomotor activity in A_{2A} receptor knockout mice (Ledent *et al.*, 1997). Furthermore, the GABA-enkephalin-containing striato-GPe neurons of the indirect pathway are excited by cortical inputs and inhibited by recurrent collaterals (via $GABA_A$ receptors). In Parkinson's disease, the feedback inhibition of the indirect pathway by the recurrent collaterals may be insufficient to control the overactivity of these neurons. It is postulated that A_{2A} receptor stimulation decreases GABA release (Kurokawa *et al.*, 1994; see Chapter 6) and that consequently a A_{2A} receptor antagonist, by relieving this antagonism, would enhance recurrent GABA inhibition, thereby reducing the activity of the GABA-containing striatopallidal neurons. In addition, these effects would be expected to occur when the striato-GPe neurons are firing, having relatively little effect the neurons are inactive. In fact, it has been reported by Mori and colleagues (1994), in an electrophysiological study, that presynaptic A_{2A} receptors localized in collateral axons of striatal GABAergic neurons exert an inhibitory modulation of GABA release in the striatum (see Chapter 4). Moreover, A_{2A} antagonists of the same family as KW-6002, increase GABA release in the striatum, suggesting that such modulation may be involved in the control of movement.

Hence, since inhibition of GABA release onto striatopallidal neurons is likely to increase their activity, antagonists of adenosine A_{2A} receptors should mimic the behavioral effect of a D_2 agonist (Richardson *et al.*, 1997).

It should be noted here that there is evidence that A_{2A} receptor activation enhanced GABA release in both striatum and globus pallidus (Mayfield *et al.*, 1993; Mayfield *et al.*, 1996). However, A_{2A} receptor agonists inhibit GABA release from nerve terminals derived from both of these areas (Kirk and Richardson, 1994; Kurokawa *et al.*, 1994; see Chapter 5).

The coexpression of adenosine A_{2A} and DA D_2 receptors on the same neurons could also account for an interaction at the second messenger level because A_{2A} receptor activation stimulates adenylate cyclase whereas DA D_2 receptor activation inhibits it (Ongini and Fredholm, 1996). Indeed the A_{2A}/D_2 receptors interact at the level of neuron function, and it has been shown, using *in vivo* microdialysis studies, that the striatal infusion of the selective A_{2A} agonist, CGS 21680, counteracts the decrease of GABA release, in the globus pallidus, induced by D_2 receptor stimulation (Ferré *et al.*, 1993). In contrast, the infusion of theophylline, a nonselective adenosine antagonist, in the striatum potentiate the D_2-mediated inhibition of pallidal GABA release (Ferré *et al.*, 1993). In agreement with these results, the haloperidol-induced increase in striatal c-fos expression can be partially counteracted by the administration of A_{2A} receptor antagonists (Boegman and Vincent, 1996). Similarly, the increase in c-fos expression induced by CGS 21680 in the dopamine-denervated striatum is conteracted by a selective D_2 receptor agonist (Morelli *et al.*, 1995). Moreover, following acute reserpine pretreatment, A_{2A} receptor antagonism potentiates a D_2 agonist-mediated increase in c-fos expression in the striatopallidal neurons (Pollack and Fink, 1995).

Interestingly, the administration of low dose of caffeine induces a decrease in the striatal expression of some IEGs that have a high basal expression; an effect that could be mimicked by the D_2 agonist quinpirole (Svenningsson *et al.*, 1995). The effect of caffeine is only observed in the striatopallidal neurons and is not blocked by the administration of raclopride, a D_2 antagonist (Svenningsson *et al.*, 1995). This suggests that striatal A_{2A} receptors are tonically activated by endogenous adenosine and that A_{2A} receptor antagonism could induce some functional effects independent of D_2 receptor transduction mechanisms (Ferré *et al.*, 1997).

Furthermore, antagonistic intramembrane $A_{2A}-D_2$ interactions were suggested as important mechanisms of action responsible for the motor effects of adenosine receptor agonists and antagonists (Ferré *et al.*, 1992, 1997; Ferré *et al.*, 1994a). In fact, both receptors are expressed on striatal GABA/enkephalin-containing output neurons providing an anatomical basis for functional interaction between adenosine and dopamine (Fink *et al.*, 1992; Pollack *et al.*, 1993). It has been shown, using the rat striatal membranes or a mouse fibroblast cell line stably cotransfected with A_{2A} and D_2 receptors, that stimulation of A_{2A} receptors decreases the affinity of the D_2 receptor for agonists but does not change the affinity for antagonists (Ferré et al., 1991). Such interaction was enhanced by dopamine denervation or chronic dopamine D_2 receptor blockade (Ferré and Fuxe, 1992; Ferré et al., 1994b). In fact, after striatal dopamine denervation or chronic treatment with haloperidol, an upregulation of both A_{2A} and D_2 receptors has been found in the rat striatum (Abbracchio et al., 1987; Parsons et al., 1995). Moreover, in the A_{2A}/D_2 cotransfected cells, stimulation of A_{2A} receptors specifically counteracted a D_2 receptor-mediated Ca^{2+} influx from the extracellular medium (Yang et al., 1995). However, intramembrane A_{2A}–D_2 interactions would be expected to occur mainly in intact systems where nigrostriatal projection is preserved. When dopamine was depleted, which is the case in Parkinson's disease patients or in MPTP-exposed monkeys, the antiparkinsonian actions of adenosine antagonists seems to be mediated directly by adenosine antagonism rather than by an antagonist interaction with endogenous dopamine.

There are still controversies about the importance of the expression of A_{2A} receptor in the striatal cholinergic interneurons (Dixon et al., 1996; Fink et al., 1992; Schiffmann et al., 1991a; Svenningsson et al., 1997a). Kirkpatrick and Richardson (1994), by evaluating the effect of the more selective agonist CGS 21680 and antagonists CP66713 and CGS 15943A on the veratridine-evoked release of $[^3H]$-acetylcholine from rat striatal synaptosomes, have confirmed the existence of A_{2A} receptors on striatal cholinergic nerve terminals and their stimulatory action on acetylcholine release. In fact, stimulation of A_{2A} receptors most probably localized in the striatal cholinergic interneurons has been reported to induce acetylcholine (ACh) release in the striatal synaptosomal preparations (Brown et al., 1990; Kirk and Richardson, 1994; Kurokawa et al., 1994) and a similar effect was also observed in vivo (Kurokawa et al., 1996). Such findings were not seen in striatal slices (Jin et al., 1993); however, in the latter preparation the D_2 receptor-mediated inhibition of ACh release was completely reversed by CGS 21680 (Jin et al., 1993). Moreover, blockade of muscarinic ACh receptors has been shown to partially counteract the increase in c-fos expression observed in the dopamine-denervated striatum (Morelli et al., 1995) and the inhibition of a dopamine-mediated behavior induced by CGS 21680 (Vellucci et al., 1993). Consequently, ACh neurotransmission could mediate some effects of A_{2A} receptor stimulation and A_{2A} receptor antagonists could assist in the therapy of Parkinson's disease by reducing the influence of ACh (Ferré et al., 1997; Richardson et al., 1997).

The results also showed that selective blockade of adenosine A_{2A} receptors is less likely to reproduce dyskinesias than L-Dopa at doses that produce comparable antiparkinsonian benefit. The reasons for this advantage are not entirely clear. Piccini and colleagues (1997) found an increase in neuropeptide transmission in basal ganglia of dyskinetic parkinsonian patients compared with those without dyskinesias. Interestingly, after the loss of dopamine or levodopa therapy, the increase in preproenkephalin mRNA requires both A_{2A} and muscarinic ACh receptor activation (for review see Richardson *et al.*, 1997, Pollack and Wooten, 1992). Prevention of this increase in preproenkephalin expression by A_{2A} receptor blockade is consistent with a reduction in the activity of the striato-GPe neurons that are overactive in experimental models of Parkinson's disease (Henry and Brotchie, 1996). However, in spite of the fact that chronic treatment by caffeine reverses the alterations of enkephalin gene expression i striatopallidal neurons of 6-OHDA-lesioned rats (Schiffmann and Vanderhaeghen, 1993), It is not certain that acute treatment by adenosine A_{2A} antagonists can do the same. Chronic study with KW-6002 is still needed to evaluate such findings.

An other explanation is the possibility that adenosine A_{2A} receptors may positively modulate the activity of striatal output neurons bearing DA D_1 receptors (Le Moine *et al.*, 1997; Pinna *et al.*, 1996) and that this could account for the antidyskinetic effects of KW-6002. In fact, we have reported that selective DA D_1 receptor agonists displayed a better profile of clear antiparkinsonian activity with very little dyskinesia in MPTP-treated parkinsonian monkeys (Blanchet *et al.*, 1993; Grondin *et al.*, 1997). Alternatively, increases in GABA-mediated collateral inhibition in the striatum by A_{2A} receptor antagonism could focus the activity of striatal neurons and sharpen the intrastriatal message, resulting in a precise motor command not plagued by dyskinesia.

V. CONCLUSION

Our results clearly show that selective adenosine A_{2A} receptor blockade is capable of restoring the balance of striatal function and improving parkinsonian symptoms in a primate model of PD. Hence, selective A_{2A} receptor antagonists might be a potential future nondopaminergic approach to treat Parkinsonian patients, either alone or as adjuncts to levodopa or dopamine agonist therapy. Understanding the exact mode of action of KW-6002 could help to elucidate the mechanism(s) underlying abnormal involuntary movements such as levodopa-induced dyskinesias.

REFERENCES

Abbracchio, M.P., Colombo, F., Di Luca, M., Zaratin, P., and Cattabeni, F. (1987). Adenosine modulates the dopaminergic function in the nigro-striatal system by interacting with striatal dopamine dependent adenylate cyclase. *Pharmacol Res Commun* 19(4), 275–286.

Augood, S.J., and Emson, P.C. (1994). Adenosine A_{2A} receptor mRNA is expressed by enkephalin cells but not by somatostatin cells in rat striatum: a co-expression study. *Mol Brain Res* 22, 204–210.

Blanchet, P., Bédard, P.J., Britton, D.R., and Kebabian, J.W. (1993). Differential effect of selective D-1 and D-2 dopamine receptor agonists on levodopa-induced dyskinesia in 1-methyl-4-phenyl-1,2,3,6-tetrahydropyridine-exposed monkeys. *J Pharmacol Exp Ther* 267(1), 272–279.

Boegman, R.J., and Vincent, S.R. (1996). Involvement of adenosine and glutamate receptors in the induction of c-fos in the striatum by haloperidol. *Synapse* 22, 70–77.

Brown, S.J., James, S., Reddington, M., and Richardson, P.J. (1990). Both A_1 and A_{2A} purine receptors regulate striatal acetylcholine release. *J Neurochem* 55, 31–38.

Corradetti, R., Lo Conte, G., Moroni, F., Passani, M.B., and Pepeu, G. (1984). Adenosine decreases aspartate and glutamate release from rat hippocampal slices. *Eur J Pharmacol* 104, 19–26.

Daval, J.L., Nicolas, F., and Doriat, J.F. (1996). Adenosine physiology and pharmacology: how about A_2 receptors? *Pharmacol Ther* 71, 325–335.

Dixon, A.K., Gubitz, A.K., Sirinathsinghji, D.J., Richardson, P.J., and Freeman, T.C. (1996). Tissue distribution of adenosine receptor mRNAs in the rat. *Br J Pharmacol* 118(6), 1461–1468.

Fenu, S., Pinna, A., Ongini, E., and Morelli, M. (1997). Adenosine A_{2A} receptor antagonism potentiates L-DOPA-induced turning behavior and c-*fos* expression in 6-hydroxydopamine-lesioned rats. *Eur J Pharmacol* 321, 143–147.

Ferré, S., and Fuxe, K. (1992). Dopamine denervation leads to an increase in the intramembrane interaction between adenosine A_2 and dopamine D_2 receptors in the neostriatum. *Brain Res* 594, 124–130.

Ferré, S., Fredholm, B.B., Morelli, M., Popoli, P., and Fuxe, K. (1997). Adenosine-dopamine receptor–receptor interactions as integrative mechanism in the basal ganglia. *Trends Neurosci* 20, 482–492.

Ferré, S., Fuxe, K., von Euler, G., Johanson, B., and Fredholm, B.B (1992). Adenosine-depamine interactions in the brain. *Neurosci* 51, 501–512.

Ferré, S., O'Connor, W.T., Fuxe, K., and Ungerstedt, U. (1993). The striopallidal neuron: a main locus for adenosine–dopamine interactions in the brain. *J Neurosci* 13(12), 5402–5406.

Ferré, S., Popoli, P., Gimenez-Llort, L., Finnman, U.B., Martinez, E., Scotti de Carolis, A., and Fuxe, K. (1994a). Postsynaptic antagonistic interaction between adenosine A_1 and dopamine D_1 receptors. *Neuroreport* 6, 73–76.

Ferré, S., Schwarcz, R., Li, X.M., Snaprud, P., Ogren, S.O., and Fuxe, K. (1994b). Chronic haloperidol treatment leads to an increase in the intramembrane interaction between adenosine A_2 and dopamine D_2 receptors in the neostriatum. *Psychopharmacol (Berl)* 116(3), 279–284.

Ferré S., von Euler, G., Johanson, B., Fredholm, B.B., and Fuxe, K. (1991). Stimulation of high-affinity adenosine A_2 receptors decreases the affinity of dopamine D_2 recceptors in rat striatal membranes *Proc Natl Acad Sci* USA 88, 7237–77241.

Fink, J.S., Weaver, D.R., Rivkees, S.A., Peterfreund, R.A., Pollack, A.E., Adler, E.M., and Reppert, S.M. (1992). Molecular cloning of the rat A_2 adenosine receptor: selective co-expression with D_2 dopamine receptors in rat striatum. *Mol Brain Res* 14, 186–195.

Fredholm, B.B. (1995). Adenosine receptors in the central nervous system. *News Physiol Sci* 10, 122–1228.

Fuxe, K., and Ungerstedt, U. (1974). Action of caffeine and theophylline on supersensitive dopamine receptors: considerable enhancement of receptor response to treatment with dopa and dopamine receptor agonists. *Med Biol* 52, 48–54.

Garrett, B.E., and Holtzman, S.G. (1995). Does adenosine receptor blockade mediate caffeine-induced rotational behavior? *J Pharmacol Exp Ther* 274, 207–214.

Goodman, R.R., and Snyder, S.H. (1982). Autoradiographic localisation of adenosine receptors in rat brain using [^{3}H]cyclohexyladenosine. *J Neurosci* 2, 1230–1241.

Grondin, R., Bédard, P.J., Briton, D.R., and Shiosaki, K. (1997). Potential therapeutic use of selective dopamine D_1 receptor agonist, A-86929: an acute study in parkinsonian levodopa-primed monkeys. *Neurology* 49, 421–426.

Henry, B., and Brotchie, J.M. (1996). Potential of opioid antagonists in the treatment of levodopa-induced dyskinesias in Parkinson's disease. *Drugs Ageing* 9(3), 149–158.

Herrara-Marschitz, M., Casas, M., and Ungerstedt, U. (1988). Caffeine produces controlateral turning in rats with unilateral dopamine denervation: comparison with apomorphine induced responses. *Psychopharmacol* 94, 38–45.

Hutchison, A.J., Webb, R.L., Oei H.H., Ghai, G.R., Zimmerman, M.B., and Williams, M., (1989). CGS 21680C, an A_2 selective adenosine receptor agonist with preferential hypotensive activity. *J Pharmacol Exp Ther* 251(1), 47–55.

Jarvis, M.F. (1988). Autoradiographic localization and characterization of brain adenosine receptor subtypes. In "Receptor Localization: Ligand Autoradiography", (Leslie, F., and Alter, C.A. eds.), pp. 95–113. New York: Alan R. Liss.

Jiang, H., Jackson-Lewis, V., Muthane, U., Dollison, A., and Ferreira, M. (1993). Adenosine receptor antagonists potentiate dopamine receptor agonist-induced rotational behavior in 6-hydroxydopamine-lesioned rats. *Brain Res* 613, 347–351.

Jin, S., Johansson, B., and Fredholm, B.B. (1993). Effects of adenosine A_1 and A_2 receptor activation on electrically evoked dopamine and acetylcholine release from rat striatal slices. *J Pharmacol Exp Ther* 267(2), 801–808.

Kanda, T., Shiozaki, S., Shimada, J., Suzuki, F., and Nakamura, J., (1994). KF17837: a novel selective adenosine A_{2A} receptor antagonist with anticataleptic activity. *Eur J Pharmacol* 256(3), 263–268.

Kanda, T., Jackson, M.J., Smith, L.A., Pearce, R.K., Nakamura, J., Kase, H., Kuwana, Y., and Jenner, P. (1998). Adenosine A_{2A} antagonist: a novel antiparkinsonian agent that does not provoke dyskinesia in parkinsonian monkeys. *Ann Neurol* 43, 507–513.

Kirk, I.P., and Richardson, P.J. (1994). Adenosine A_{2A} receptor-mediated modulation of striatal [^{3}H]GABA and [^{3}H]acetylcholine release. *J Neurochem* 62(3), 960–966.

Kurokawa, M., Kirk, I.P., Kirkpatrick, K.A., Kase, H., and Richardson, P.J. (1994). Inhibition by KF17837 of adenosine A_{2A} receptor-mediated modulation of striatal GABA and ACh release. *Br J Parmacol* 113, 43–48.

Kurokawa, M., Koga, K., Kase, H., Nakamura, J., and Kuwana, Y. (1996). Adenosine A_{2A} receptor-mediated modulation of striatal acetylcholine release *in vivo*. *J Neurochem* 66, 1882–1888.

Latini, S., Pazzagli, M., Pepeu, G., and Pedata, F. (1996). A_2 adenosine receptors: their presence and neuromodulatory role in the central nervous system. *Gen Pharmacol* 27, 925–933.

Le Moine, C., Svenningsson, P., Fredholm, B.B., and Bloch, B. (1997). Dopamine-adenosine interactions in the striatum and the globus pallidus: inhibition of striatopallidal neurons through either D_2 or A_{2A} receptors enhances D_1 receptor-mediated effects on c-fos expression. *Neurosci* 17(20), 8038–8048.

Ledent, C., Vaugeois, J.M., Schiffmann, S.N., Pedrazzini, T., El Yacoubi, M., Vanderhaeghen, J.J., Costentin, J., Heath, J.K., Vassart, G., and Parmentier, M. (1997). Aggressiveness, Hypoalgesia and high blood pressure in mice lacking the adenosine A_{2A} receptor. *Nature* 388, 674–678.

Linden, J. (1994). Purinergic systems. In "Basic Neurochemistry" (Siegel, G.J., *et al*, eds. 5th ed.), pp. 401–416. New York: Raven Press.

Mally, J., and Stone, T.W. (1994). The effect of theophylline on parkinsonian symptoms. *J Pharm Pharmacol* 46(6), 515–517.

Marsden, C.D. (1994). Problems with long-term levodopa therapy for Parkinson's disease. *Clin Neuropharmacol* 17(suppl. 2), S32–S44.

Martinez-Mir, M.I., Probst, A., and Palacios, J.M. (1991). Adenosine A_2 receptors: selective localization in the human basal ganglia and alterations with disease. *Neurosci* 42, 697–706.

Mayfield, R.D., Larson, G., Orona, R.A., and Zahniser, N.R. (1996). Opposing actions of adenosine A_{2A} and dopamine D_2 receptor activation on GABA release in the basal ganglia: evidence for an A_{2A}/D_2 receptor interactions in globus pallidus. *Synapse* 22, 132–138.

Mayfield, R.D., Suzuki, F., and Zahniser, N.R. (1993). Adenosine A_{2A} receptor modulation of electrically evoked endogenous GABA release from slices of rat globus pallidus. *J Neurochem* 60(6), 2334–2337.

Morelli, M., Fenu, S., Pinna, A., and Di Chiara, G. (1994). Adenosine A_2 receptors interact negatively with dopamine D_1 and D_2 receptors in unilaterally 6-hydroxydopamine-lesioned rats. *Eur J Pharmacol* 251, 21–25.

Morelli, M., Pinna, A., Wardas, J., and Di chiara, G. (1995). Adenosine A_2 receptors stimulate c-fos expression in striatale neurons of 6-hydroxydopamine-lesioned rats. *Neurosci* 67, 49–55.

Mori, A., Shindou, T., Ichimura, M., Nonaka, H., and Kase, H. (1996). The role of adenosine A_{2A} receptors in the regulating GABAergic synaptic transmission in striatal medium spiny neurons. *J Neurosci* 16, 605–611.

Nonaka, H., Saki, M., Ichimura, M., Kase, H. (1997). Novel potent adenosine A_{2A} receptor antagonists. *Move Disord* 12(Suppl. 1), 120.

Ongini, E., and Fredholm, B.B. (1996). Pharmacology of adenosine A_{2A} receptors. *Trends Pharmacol Sci* 17, 364–372.

Parsons, B., Togasaki, D.M., Kassir, S., and Przedborski, S. (1995). Neuroleptics up-regulate adenosine A_{2A} receptors in rat striatum: Implications for the mechanism and treatment of tardive dyskinesia. *J Neuro Chem* 65, 2057–2064.

Piccini, P., Weeks, R.A., and Brooks, D.J. (1997). Alterations in opioid receptor binding in Parkinson's disease patients with levodopa-induced dyskinesias. *Ann Neurol* 42, 720–726.

Pinna, A., Di Chiara, G., Wardas, J., and Morelli, M. (1996). Blockade of A_{2A} adenosine receptors positively modulates turning behaviour and c-fos expression induced by D_1 agonists in dopamine-denervated rats. *Eur J Neurosci* 8, 1176–1181.

Pollack, A.E., and Fink, J.S. (1995). Adenosine antagonists potentiate D_2 dopamine-dependent activation of fos in the striatopallidal pathway. *Neurosci* 68(3), 721–728.

Pollack, A.E., Harrison, M.B., Wooten, F.G., and Fink, S.J. (1993). Differential localization of A_{2A} adenosine receptor mRNA with D_1 and D_2 dopamine receptor mRNA in striatal output pathways following a selective lesion of striatonigral neurons. *Brain Res* 631, 161–166.

Pollack, A.E., and Wooten, G.F. (1992). D_2 dopaminergic regulation of striatal preproenkephalin mRNA levels is mediated at least in part through cholinergic interneurons. *Brain Res Mol Brain Res* 13(1–2), 35–41.

Popoli, P., Gimenez-Llort, L., Pezzola, A., Reggio, R., Martinez, E., Fuxe, K., and Ferré, S. (1996). Adenosine A_1 receptor blockade selectively potentiates the motor effects induced by dopamine D_1 receptor stimulation in rodents. *Neurosci Lett* 218(3), 209–213.

Richardson, P.J., Kase, H., and Jenner, P.G. (1997). Adenosine receptor antagonists as new agents for the treatment of Parkinson's disease. *Trends Pharmacol Sci* 18(9), 338–344.

Schiffmann S.N., Libert, F., Vassart, G., Dumont, J.E., and Vanderhaegen, J.-J. (1990). A cloned G protein-coupled protein with a distribution restricted to striatal medium-sized neurons. Possible relationship with D_1 dopamine receptor. *Brain Res* 519, 333–337.

Schiffmann, S.N., Libert, F., Vassart, G., and Vanderhaegen, J.-J. (1991a). Distribution of adenosine A_2 receptor mRNA in the human brain. *Neurosci Lett* 130, 177–181.

Schiffmann, S.N., Jacobs, O., and Vanderhaeghen, J.-J. (1991b). Striatal restricted adenosine receptors (RDC8) is expressed by enkephalin by substance P neurons: an *in situ* hybridization histochemistry study *J Neurochem* 57, 1062–1067.

Stone, T.W., and Bartrup, J.T. (1991). Electropharmacology of adenosine. In "Adenosine in the Nervous System" (Stone, T., ed.), pp. 197–216. London; Academic Press.

Stone, T.W., Newby, A.C., and Lloyd, H.G.E. (1990). Adenosine release. In "Adenosine and Adenosine Receptors" (Williams, M., ed.), pp. 173–224. New York: Humana Press.

Stone-Elander, S., Thorell, J.O., Eriksson, L., Fredholm, B.B., and Ingvar, M. (1997). *In vivo* biodistribution of [N-11C-methyl]KF 17837 using 3-D-PET: evaluation as a ligand for the study of adenosine A_{2A} receptors. *Nucl Med Biol* 24, 187–191.

Svenningsson, P., Hall, H., Sedvall, G., and Fredholm, B.B. (1997a). Distribution of adenosine receptors in the post mortem human brain: an extended autoradiographic study. *Synapuase* 27(4), 322–335.

Svenningsson, P., Nomikos, G.G., and Fredholm, B. (1995). Biphasic changes in locomotor behavior and in expression of mRNA for NGFI-A and NGFI-B in rat striatum following acute caffeine administration. *J Neurosci* 15(11), 7612–7624.

Svenningsson, P., Nomikos, G.G., Ongini, E., and Fredholm, B.B. (1997b). Antagonism of adenosine A_{2A} receptors underlies the behavioural activating effect of caffeine and is associated with reduced expression of messenger RNA for NGFI-A and NGFI-B in caudate-putamen and nucleus accumbens. *Neurosci* 79(3), 753–764.

Ungerstedt, U., Herrara-Marschitz, M., and Casas, M. (1981). Are apomorphine, bromocriptine, and the methylxanthine agonists at the same dopamine receptors? In "Apomorphine and Other Dopaminomimetics: Basic Pharmacology" (Gessa, G.L., and Corsini, G.U., eds.), Vol. 1, pp. 85–93. New York: Raven Press.

Vellucci, S.V., Sirinathsinghji, D.J., and Richardson, P.J. (1993). Adenosine A_2 receptor regulation of apomorphine-induced turning in rats with unilateral striatal dopamine denervation. *Psychopharmacol (Berl)* 111(3), 383–388.

Williams, M. (1995). Purinoceptors in central nervous system function: targets for therapeutic intervention. In. "Psychopharmacology: The Fourth Generation of Progress" (Bloom, F.E., and Kupfer, D.J., Eds.), pp. 643– 655. New York; Raven Press.

Yang, S.N., Dasgupta, S., Lledo, P.M., Vincent, J.D., and Fuxe K. (1995). Reduction of dopamine D_2 receptor transduction by activation of adenosine A_{2A} receptors in stably A_{2A}/D_2 (long-form) receptor co-transfected mouse fibroblast cell lines: studies on intracellular calcium levels. *Neurosci* 68, 729–736.

CHAPTER 13

Neurobiology of Adenosine Receptors

Adenosine and Its Metabolites in Movement Disorders

MASAHIRO NOMOTO

Department of Pharmacology and Clinical Pharmacology,
Kagoshima University School of Medicine, Kagoshima, Japan

I. INTRODUCTION

Adenosine acts as a neurotransmitter or neuromodulator in peripheral tissues, especially in the cardiovascular and respiratory systems. Adenosine also occurs in the central nervous system (CNS) and is involved in neurotransmitter release (1). Methylxanthines such as caffeine modify locomotor activity induced by l-Dopa or amphetamine in 6-OHDA-lesioned rats (2–6). Because methylxanthines are adenosine receptor antagonists (7), these findings suggest that adenosine may modify motor function in the CNS. Adenosine receptors are classified into four subtypes (A_1, A_{2A}, A_{2B}, and A_3), based on the agonist actions of adenosine. A_1 and A_2 receptors are antagonized by xanthines, whereas A_3 receptors are not. A_1 receptors are associated with the inhibition of adenylate cyclase, whereas A_2 receptors stimulate cyclic-AMP (cAMP) formation. Adenosine A_2 receptors are subdivided into two subtypes, A_{2A} and A_{2B}. A_{2A} receptors are localized to the striatum, nucleus accumbens, and the olfactory tubercle (8–10). Previous studies have demonstrated that the administration of adenosine A_{2A} receptor agonists induces catalepsy and reduces locomotor activity (11,12). In contrast, adenosine receptor A_{2A}

antagonists reduce catalepsy induced by haloperidol and reverse parkinson-ism induced by 1-methyl-4-phenyl-1,2,3,6-tetrahydropyridine (MPTP) in monkeys (13,14). These reports suggest that adenosine is involved in the control of motor function in the striatum through adenosine A_{2A} receptors.

In this chapter, manipulations of the adenosine system in the treatment of movement disorders are reviewed.

A. Adenosine in the Basal Ganglia

Adenosine is found throughout the entire brain. In the striatum, the choliner-gic neuron is a main sources of adenosine (15), and A_{2A} receptors are local-ized on these and GABA neurons projecting to the external segment of the globus pallidus (GPe). Striatopallidal neurons express both adenosine A_{2A} and dopamine D_2 receptors, and these receptors act in an antagonistic manner. The stimulation of A_{2A} receptors inhibits the effects of dopamine on GABA neurons, resulting in akinesia or catalepsy (16). Striatal cholinergic neurons (17,18) are normally inhibited by nigrostriatal dopaminergic neurons. Consequently, in Parkinson's disease, the release of acetylcholine (ACh) is increased as the inhibitory input from nigrostriatal dopaminergic neurons diminishes. It is probable that the release of adenosine in the striatum increases after the degeneration of dopamine neurons in the substantia nigra. In fact, the extracellular concentration of adenosine in the striatum increases in MPTP(1-methyl-4-phenyl-1,2,3,6-tetrahydropyridine)-treated common marmosets that have lost most of the dopaminergic neurons projecting to the caudate and putamen (19,20). The increased release of adenosine in the striatum may contribute to the akinesia occurring in parkinsonism. This concept is compatible with the ability of dipyridamole, an inhibitor of adenosine transport that increases interstitial levels of adenosine, to decreased locomotor activity (21).

B. Effects of Caffeine or Other Methylxanthines on Parkinson's Disease

Caffeine is contained in tea or coffee, and it is the most commonly and widely used social drug worldwide. Caffeine and other methylxanthines inhibit the activity of phosphodiesterase, which hydrolyzes cyclic nucleotides, and this inhibition results in a higher concentration of intracellular cAMP (22). Dopamine can also induce cAMP production by activation of D_1 receptors. Attempts have been made to use methylxanthines in the treatment of Parkinson's disease, with the expectation that they would potentiate the effects of dopamine or dopamine agonists. Indeed, caffeine potentiated the action of L-Dopa or dopamine receptor agonists, such as apomorphine, piribedil, or bromocriptine in 6-OHDA-lesioned rats (2–6). In patients with Parkinson's disease, caffeine has also been reported to potentiate the effects of chlorphenoxamine, an anticholinergic agent (23). However, caffeine and other methylxanthines are also adenosine A_1 and A_2 receptor antagonists, and this may better account for the phamacological effects of methylxanthines in the doses that are administered therapeutically (22). In other studies, however, caffeine did not improve the motor activity of patients with Parkinson's disease, even at a dose of 1400 mg per day (24,25). Indeed these high doses of caffeine often caused insomnia, restlessness, anxiety, or palpitations (22), and these effects may exacerbate parkinsonism symptoms. In fact, caffeine produces detrimental effects on performance skill in some individuals (26). Caffeine has also been used for patients with neuroleptic-induced parkinsonism but again with no effect (27). However, more specific inhibitors of adenosine receptors may produce greater benefit in the manipulation of the nigostriatal dopaminergic system and the striatal outflow pathways in patients with Parkinson's disease.

Activation of the adenosine A_{2A} receptor causes a decrease in locomotor activity, whereas antagonists cause motor activation (28). In patients with Parkinson's disease, theophyllamine (theophylline-ethylenediamine) an adenosine A_{2A} receptor antagonist, produced significant improvements in motor disability score and a subjective improvement at a dose of 150 mg/day when combined with L-Dopa therapy. It has also been suggested that theophylline might be a useful adjunct to therapy for Parkinson's disease (29). However, when theophylline was administered to eight patients with idiopathic Parkinson's disease in combination with L-Dopa, it was without effect (30) even though high concentrations were found in blood.

In experimental studies, theophylline and caffeine produced a marked potentiation of dopaminergic function, but in patients with Parkinson's disease, some studies have only shown useful effects of theophylline, not caffeine. This may be because theophylline produces more potent effects on the CNS than caffeine (22). Caffeine and theophylline have effects on motor function and cause the previously listed side effects, which are unpleasant for patients with Parkinson's disease and reported as common adverse reactions. Such side effects may also exacerbate the symptoms of Parkinson's disease. Because caffeine and theophylline do not distinguish between adenosine receptors (31), they may not be the most appropriate agents for determining the potential of adenosine receptor antagonism in the treatment of Parkinson's disease. The adenosine A_{2A} receptor is selectively localized in the striatum, the nucleus accumbens, and the tuberculum olfactorium (see Chapter 2), all of which are involved in the control of motor function

(9,10). Thus more selective agents, such as A_{2A} receptor antagonists, to modulate motor function may give more positive results in clinical trials in Parkinson's disease.

C. Effects of Caffeine or Other Methylxanthines on Essential Tremor

Caffeine has been assessed as a treatment for essential tremor; however, it is not effective, and possibly even worsens the tremor (32,33). Caffeine sometimes, but not often, induces or exacerbates tremor in "normal" people (34,35). In an epidemiological study, habitual caffeine consumption was found to cause palpitations, tremor, headache, and insomnia, and one quarter of these symptoms were attributable to caffeine (36). It has been proposed that considerable benefits may be achieved by the reduction of caffeine consumption in patients presenting with tremor, insomnia, or headache. However, caffeine does not usually exacerbate pathological tremors, such as essential or parkinsonian tremor (32). Yet pathological tremors are intensified by insomnia, excitement, or restlessness, which can be induced by caffeine. The potentiation of tremor by caffeine presumably occurs through action on the CNS.

In a double-blind study, Mally and Stone (37,38) showed that theophylline was effective in treating essential tremor at doses of 150–300 mg/day. Ongoing treatment with theophylline increased the sensitivity of GABA receptors, which may be involved in theophylline's suppression of essential tremor. Theophyllamine has also been useful in the treatment of essential tremor at a dose of 300 mg/day (39). However, the evidence remains controversial because theophylline is also reported to induce tremor (40). Methylxanthines have many effects on the central and peripheral tissues. Some effects, such as inducing anxiety, may worsen tremor; and this may contribute to the existing controversy.

D. Effects of Caffeine and Other Methylxanthines on Other Movement Disorders

Caffeine may worsen or intensify paroxysmal movement disorders, including paroxysmal dystonia choreoathetosis, familial paroxysmal choreoathetosis, or paroxysmal dystonic choreoathetosis (41,42). Dyskinesia and/or dystonia in these disorders can be induced by emotional stress or excitement. Thus the effects of caffeine on the sympathetic nervous system may intensify involuntary movements in these disorders. Familial paroxysmal choreoathetosis of the Mount and Reback type can be Provoked by alcohol and intensified by caffeine or emotional excitement. L-Dopa also provokes the choreoathetosis, and the dopamine receptor antagonist haloperidol is the most effective means of reducing the attacks. Consequently, dopaminergic function appears to modify the frequency and intensity of choreoathetosis, and caffeine may increase the intensity of the attacks by modification of dopaminergic function (43).

Xanthines cause insomnia, restlessness, and excitement, and in high doses, delirium, emesis, cardiac arrythmia, or convulsions may be induced (22). Caffeine and theophylline cause seizures in genetically epilepsy-prone rats (44). In humans theophylline may also cause seizures in toxically high concentrations (45). A more selective antagonism of adenosine receptors subtypes may eliminate the epileptogenicity of xanthines.

Adenosine is believed to have a function in the sensory system within the spinal cord (46). It is possible that adenosine is also involved in some types of restless leg syndromes with pain (47). More cases of sensory disorders need to be examined to investigate the potential involvement of adenosine in such disorders in humans.

E. LEVELS OF ADENOSINE AND OTHER NUCLEOSIDES IN NEUROLOGICAL DISORDERS

The concentration of adenosine in the cerebrospinal fluid (CSF) is approximately 63 nM, ranging from 39 to 106 nM in patients with minor neurological disorders, such as muscle contraction headache, or neuropathy (47). Patients with status epilepticus show similar CSF concentrations of adenosine ranging from 27 to 120 nM; however, concentrations of the metabolites inosine and hypoxanthine are higher in these patients (48) (Table I). The concentration of adenosine in the CSF in progressive myoclonic epilepsy is 16 nM, which is similar to that of controls (49). We studied the concentration of adenosine in CSF taken from the lateral ventricles of four patients with essential tremor. The concentration was 13.3 nM (9.3–17.4). These data suggest that concentrations of adenosine in the CSF are in the nM range.

Extracellular concentrations of inosine and hypoxanthine have been measured using microdialysis techniques in the thalamus of patients with Parkinsons's disease at the time of stereotactic surgery to relieve tremor (50). In this study, the concentrations of inosine and hypoxanthine in the perfusates were approximately 10 pmol/10 μL (1000 nM) 60 min after the start of perfusion with a physiological solution. In experimental animals, adenosine levels

TABLE I   Concentrations of Adenosine and the Metabolites in the Cerebrospinal Fluid

CSF[a]	Case and number	Adenosine (nM)	Inosine (nM)	Hypoxanthine (μM)	Authors
Lumbar	Neuropathy, headache, multiple sclerosis 11	63	410	2.36	48
Lumbar	Headache and dizziness 10	17	570	6.06	49
Lateral ventricle	Essential tremor 4	13.3	104	—	68

[a]CSF, cerebrospinal fluid.

also appear to be in the nM range in the CSF. The extracellular levels of adenosine in 3- and 22-month-old rats were 66.8 ± 0.7 and 71.6 ± 1.0 nM, respectively (51). We also studied the extracellular levels of adenosine and inosine in the striatum of MPTP-treated and normal control monkeys (19). The extracellular output of adenosine during the 2–4 h after the start of dialysis was 6.06 ± 0.93 pmol/2 h (50.5 nM) in MPTP-treated animals, and 3.81 ± 1.13 (31.8 nM) in normal control animals. The extracellular output of inosine was 31.61 ± 3.57 pmol/2 h (263.4 nM) in MPTP-treated animals, and 19.3 ± 1.64 pmol/2 h (160.8 nM) in normal control animals. Interestingly, the output of adenosine and inosine were higher in the striatum of MPTP-treated common marmosets exhibiting the motor symptoms of Parkinson's disease than in that of normal control animals (see Tables I and II).

Other investigations have implicated changes in adenosine metabolism in Parkinson's disease. For instance, serum adenosine deaminase, which

TABLE II   Extracellular Concentration of Adenosine and the Metabolites

Brain	Species and treatment	Adenosine (nM)	Inosine (nM)	Hypoxanthine (nM)	Authors
Thalamus	Human Parkinson's disease	—	1000	1000	50
Striatum	Rat 3 and 21 month old	66.8 ± 0.7 and 71.6 ± 1.0	—	—	51
Striatum	Monkey Parkinsonism and control	50.5 ± 7.8 and 31.8 ± 9.4	263.4 ± 29.8 and 160.8 ± 13.7	—	19

metabolizes adenosine to inosine, has been reported to be higher in patients with Parkinson's desease than in controls (57). The authors suspected that higher adenosine deaminase activity may be involved in the pathogenesis of Parkinson's disease through peripheral T lymphocyte activation. In addition, it has been reported that administration of S-adenosylmethionine (SAM) induces parkinsonism in rodents and that chronic L-Dopa treatment significantly increases methionine adenosyl transferase (MAT) activity, which increases the production of SAM (58). Finally, urinary cAMP is lower in patients with tremor-type Parkinson's disease than in hospitalized controls. L-Dopa treatment decreases cAMP excretion in the patient subgroup with akinesia or rigidity (59). These findings seem to indicate that urinary cAMP may reflect the locomotor activity of patients with Parkinson's disease.

F. Effects of Xanthines or L-Dopa on Other Neurological Disorders

Ephedrine and caffeine in combination are effective in treating obesity, whereas caffeine or ephedrine separately are not. This finding is analogous to the results of animal studies (60). L-Dopa has a tendency to reduce body weight in ongoing administration for the treatment of Parkinson's disease. Caffeine may have the same tendency in the control of body weight.

Caffeine reduces theta or alpha waves in electroencephalograph (EEG) and increases alertness self-ratings. The rating of tiredness is also decreased (61). Patients with Parkinson's disease have been shown to be easily tired and to be inert or inactive. The administration of caffeine may provide some benefit to patients with these kinds of symptoms.

SAM, a methyl group donor, has also been reported to be effective as a treatment for depression. SAM crosses the blood–brain barrier in humans (62–64). SAM is also one of the precursors of adenosine (21), and the injection of SAM into the brain causes tremor and hypokinesia in rats (66,67). An increase of extracellular adenosine induces hypokinesia or sedation (21). There are, however, no data to show the relationship between administered SAM and adenosine in the brain.

REFERENCES

1. Richardson, P.J., Brown, S.J., Bailyes, E.M., and Luzio, J.P. (1987). Ectoenzymes control adenosine modulation of immunoisolated cholinergic synapses. *Nature* 327:232–234.
2. Corrodi, H., Fuxe, K., and Jonsson, G. (1972). Effects of caffeine on central monoamine neurons. *J Pharm Pharmacol* 24:155–158.

3. Fuxe, K., and Ungerstedt, U. (1974). Action of caffeine and theophyllamine on supersensitive dopamine receptors: considerable enhancement of receptor response to treatment with dopa and dopamine receptor agonists. *Med Biol* 52:48–54.

4. Waldeck, B. (1972). Increased accumulation of [³H]catecholamines formed from [³H]dopa after treatment with caffeine and aminophylline. *J Pharm Pharmacol* 24:654–655.

5. Stromberg, U., and Waldeck, B. (1973). Behavioural and biochemical interaction between caffeine and l-DOPA. *J Neural Transm* 34: 61–72.

6. Klawans, H.L., Moses, H., and Beaulieu, D.M. (1974). The influence of caffeine on d-amphetamine and apomorphine-induced stereotyped behavior. *Life Sci* 14:1493–1500.

7. Rall, T.W. (1990). Drugs used in the treatment of asthma. In "Goodman & Gilman's The Pharmacological Basis of Therapeutics" 8th ed. (A.G. Gilman, T.W. Rall, A.S. Nies, and P. Taylor, eds.), pp. 618–637. Pergamon Press, New York.

8. Daly, J.W., Butts-Lamb, P., and Padgett, W. (1983). Subclasses of adenosine receptors in the central nervous system: interactions with caffeine and related methylxanthines. *Cell Mol Neurobiol* 3:69–80.

9. Jarvis, M.F., and Williams, M. (1989). Direct autoradiographic localization of adenosine A₂ receptors in the rat brain using the A₂-selective agonist, [³H]CGS 21680. *Eur J Pharmacol* 168:243–246.

10. Schiffmann, S.N., Libert, F., Vassart, G., and Vanderhaeghen, J.-J. (1991). Distribution of adenosine A₂ receptor mRNA in the human brain. *Neurosci Lett* 130:177–181.

11. Ferré, S., Rubio, A., and Fuxe, K. (1991). Stimulation of adenosine A₂ receptor induced catalepsy. *Neurosci Lett* 130:162–164.

12. Coffin, V.L., Taylor, J.A., Phillis, J.W., Altman, H.J., and Barraco, R.A. (1984). Behavioral interaction of adenosine and methylxanthines on central purinergic systems. *Neurosci Lett* 47: 91–98.

13. Kanda, T., Shiozaki, S., Shimada, J., Suzuki, F., and Nakamura, J. (1994). KF17837: a novel selective adenosine A₂ₐ receptor antagonist with anticataleptic activity. *Eur J Pharmacol* 256:263–268.

14. Kanda, T., Jackson, M.J., Smith, L.A., Pearce, R.K.B., Nakamura, J., Kase, H., Kuwana, Y., and Jenner, P. (1998). Adenosine A₂ₐ antagonist: a novel antiparkinsonian agent that does not provoke dyskinesia in parkinsonian monkeys. *Ann Neurol* 43:507–513.

15. James, S., and Richardson, P.J. (1993). Production of adenosine from extracellular ATP at the striatal cholinergic synapse. *J Neurochem* 60:219–227.

16. Richardson, P.J., Kase, H., and Jenner, P.G. (1997). Adenosine A₂ₐ receptor antagonists as new agents for the treatment of Parkinson's disease. *Trends in Pharmacological Sciences* 18: 338–344.

17. Damsma, G., Tham, C.S., Robertson, G.S., and Fibiger, H.C. (1990). Dopamine D₁ receptor stimulation increases striatal acetylcholine release in the rat. *Eur J Pharmacol* 186: 335–338.

18. Bertorelli, R., and Consolo, S. (1990). D¹ and D² dopaminergic regulation of acetylcholine release from striata of freely moving rats. *J Neurochem* 54:2145–2148.

19. Nomoto, M., Shimizu, T., Iwata, S.-I., Kaseda, S., Mitsuda, M., and Fukuda, T. (in press). The metabolism of adenosine increased in the striatum of parkinsonism in common marmosets induced by 1-methyl-4-phenyl-1,2,3,6-tetrahydropyridine. *Adv Neurol*

20. Nomoto, M., Iwata, S.-I., Kaseda, S., Fukuda, T., and Nakagawa, S. (1997). Increased dopamine turnover in the putamen after MPTP treatment in common marmosets. *Brain Res* 767:235–238.

21. Linden, J. (1994). Purinergic systems. In "Basic Neurochemistry" 5th ed. (G.L. Siegel, B.W. Agranoff, R.W. Albers, and P.B. Molinoff, eds.), pp. 401–416. Raven Press, New York.

22. Serfin, W.E. (1996). Drugs used in the treatment of asthma. In "Goodman & Gilman's The Pharmacological Basis of Therapeutics" 9th ed. (J.G. Hardman, L.E. Limbird, P.B. Molinoff, R.W. Ruddeon, and A.G. Gilman, eds.), pp. 659–682. McGraw-Hill, New York.

23. Strang, R.R. (1967). A clinical evaluation of chlorphenoxamine with caffeine in the treatment of Parkinson's disease, including a comparison with methixene. *J Clin Pharmacol* 7:214–220.
24. Shoulson, I., and Chase, T. (1975). Caffeine and the antiparkinsonian response to levodopa or piribedil. *Neurology* 25:722–724.
25. Kartzinel, R., Shoulson, I., and Calne, D.B. (1976). Studies with bromocriptine: III. Concominat administration of caffeine to patients with idiopathic parkinsonism. *Neurology* 26:741–743.
26. Jacobson, B.H., Winter Roberts, K., and Gemmell, H.A. (1991). Influence of caffeine on selected manual manipulation skills. *Percept Mot Skills* 72:1175–1181.
27. Arushanian, E.B., Stoliarov, G.V., and Tolpyshev, B.A. (1973). Effect of caffeine on drug-induced parkinsonism and the caudal reaction of arrest. *Zh Nevropatol Psikahiatr* 73:759–761.
28. Barraco, R.A., Martens, K.A., Parizon, M., and Normile, H.J. (1993). Adenosine A_{2A} receptors in the nucleus accumbens mediate locomotor depression. *Brain Res Bull* 31:397–404.
29. Mally, J., and Stone, T.W. (1994). The effect of theophylline on parkinsonian symptoms. *J Pharm Pharmacol* 46:515–517.
30. Magnussen, E., Dupont, E., and Jakobsen, P. (1977). Theophylline and the antiparkinsonian response to levodopa treatment. *Acta Neurol Scandinav* 56:29–36.
31. Daly, J.W., Padgett, W.L., and Shamim, M.T. (1986). Analogues of caffeine and theophylline: effect of structural alterations on affinity at receptors. *J Med Chem* 29:1305–1308.
32. Koller, W., Cone, S., and Herbster, G. (1987). Caffeine and tremor. *Neurology* 37:169–172.
33. Humayun, M.U., Rader, R.S., Pieramici, D.J., Awh, C.C., and de-Juan, E., Jr. (1997). Quantitative measurement of the effects of caffeine and propranolol on surgeon hand tremor. *Arch Ophthalmol* 115:371–374.
34. Mattila, M., Seppala, T., and Mattila, M.J. (1988). Anxiogenic effect of yohinbine in healthy subjects: comparison with caffeine and antagonism by clonidine and diazepam. *Int Clin Psychopharmacol* 3:215–229.
35. Wharrad, H.J., Birmingham, A.T., Macdonald, I.A., Inch, P.J., and Mead, J.L. (1985). The influence of fasting and of caffeine intake on finger tremor. *Eur J Clin Pharmacol* 29:37–43.
36. Shirlow, M.J., and Mathers, C.D. (1985). A study of caffeine consumptions, indigestion, palpitations, tremor, headache and insomnia. *Int J Epidemiol* 14:239–248.
37. Mally, J., and Stone, T.W. (1991). The effect of theophylline on essential tremor: the possible role of GABA. *Pharmacol Biochem Behav* 39:345–349.
38. Mally, J., and Stone, T.W. (1995). Efficacy of an adenosine antagonist, theophylline, in essential tremor: comparison with placebo and propranolol. *J Neurol Sci* 132:129–132.
39. Mally, J. (1989). Aminophylline and essential tremor. *Lancet* 2:278–279.
40. Reinhardt, D., Berdel, D., Heinmann, G., Kusenbach, G., von Berg, A., Johnson, E., Steinijans, V.W., and Staudinger, H. (1987). Steady state pharmacokinetics, metabolism and pharmacodynamics of theophylline in children after unequal twice-daily dosing of a new sustained-release formulation. *Chronobiol Int* 4:369–380.
41. Nakano, T., Kondo, K., Oguchi, K., Yanagisawa, N., and Nakano, T. (1983). A late onset case of paroxysmal dystonic choreoathetosis induced by caffeine and aminophylline. *Rinsho Shinkeigaku* 23:199–202.
42. Fink, J.K., Hedera, P., Mathay, J.G., and Albin, R.L. (1997). Paroxysmal dystonic choreoathetosis linked to chrmosome 2q: clinical analysis and proposed pathophysiology. *Neurology* 49:177–183.
43. Przuntek, H., and Monninger, P. (1983). Therapeutic aspects of kinesiogenic paroxysmal choreoathetosis and familial paroxysmal choreoathetosis of the Mount and Reback type. *J Neurol* 230:163–169.
44. De Sarro, A., Grasso, S., Zappala, M., Nava, F., and De Sarro, G. (1997). Convulsant effects of some xanthine derivatives in genetically epilepsy-prone rats. *Naunyn-Schmiedeberg's Arch Pharmacol* 356:48–55.

45. (1993). Theophylline. In "Martindale The Extra Pharmacopoeia" 13th ed. (J.E.F. Reynolds, ed.), p. 1319. Pharmaceutical Press, London.

46. Salter, M.W., and Henry, J.L. (1987). Evidence that adenosine mediates the depression of spinal dorsal horn neurons by peripheral vibration in the cat. *Neurosci* 22:631–650.

47. Guieu, R., Sampieri, F., Pouget, J., Guy, B., and Rochat, H. (1994). Adenosine in painful legs and moving toes syndrome. *Clin Neuropharmacol* 17:460–469.

48. Chin, J.H., Wiesner, J.B., and Fijitaki, J. (1995). Increase in adenosine metabolites in human cerebrospinal fluid after status epilepticus. *J Neurol Neurosurg Psychiatry* 58:513–514.

49. Ohisalo, J.J., Murros, K., Fredholm, B., and Hare, T.A. (1983). Concentrations of gamma-aminobutyric acid and adenosine in the CSF in progressive myoclonus epilepsy without Lafora's bodies. *Arch Neurol* 40:623–625.

50. Meyerson, B.A., Linderoth, B., Kalsson, H., and Ungerstedt, U. (1990). Microdialysis in the human brain: Extracellular measurements in the thalamus of parkinsonian patients. *Life Sci* 46:301–308.

51. Pazzaglia, M., Corsi, C., Fratti, S., Pedata, F., and Pepeu, G. (1995). Regulation of extracellular adenosine levels in the striatum of aging rats. *Brain Res* 684:103–106.

52. Covickovic-Sternic, N., Kostic, V.S., Djericic, B.M., Bumbasirevic-Beslac, L., Nikolic, M., and Mrsulja, B.B. (1987). Cyclic nucleotides in cerebrospinal fluid of drug-free Parkinson patients. *Eur Neurol* 27:24–28.

53. Volicer, L., Beal, M.F., Direnfeld, L.K., Marquis, J.K., and Albert, M.L. (1986). CSF cyclic nucleotides and somatostatin in Parkinson's disease. *Neurology* 36:89–92.

54. Rudman, D., Fleischer, A., and Kutner, M.H. (1976). Concentration of 3′, 5′ cyclic adenosine monophosphate in ventricular cerebrospinal fluid of patients with prolonged coma after head trauma or intracranial hemorrhage. *N Engl J Med* 295:635–638.

55. Vapaatalo, H., Myllyla, V., Heikkinen, E., and Hokkanen, E. (1976). Cyclic AMP in CSF of patients with neurologic disease. *N Engl J Med* 296:691–692.

56. Wolberg, G., Zimmerman, T.P., Hiemstra, K., Winston, M., and Chu, L.C. (1975). Adenosine inhibition of lymphocyte-mediated cytolysis: possible role of cyclic adenosine monophosphate. *Science* 187:957–959.

57. Chiba, S., Matsumoto, H., Saitoh, M., Kasahara, M., Matsuya, M., and Kashiwagi, M. (1995). A correlation study between serum adenosine deaminase activities and peripheral lymphocyte subsets in Parkinson's disease. *J Neurol Sci* 132:170–173.

58. Benson, R., Crowell, B., Hill, B., Doonquah, K., and Charlton, C. (1993). The effects of L-dopa on the methionine adenosyltransferase: relevance to L-dopa therapy and tolerance. *Neurochem Res* 18:325–330.

59. Markianos, M., and Hadjikonstantinou, M. (1981). Urinary homovanilic acid and c-AMP in drug-free Parkinson patients: effects of L-dopa treatment. *Eur Neurol* 20:118–124.

60. Astrup, A., Breum, L., Toubro, S., Hein, P., and Quaade, F. (1992). The effect and safety of an ephedrine/caffeine compound compared to ephedrine, caffeine and placebo in obese subjects on an energy restricted diet. A double blind trial. *Int J Obs Relat Metab Disord* 16:269–277.

61. Bruce, M., Scott, N., Lader, M., and Marks, V. (1986). The psychopharmacological and electrophisiological effects of single doses of caffeine in healthy human subjects. *Br J Clin Pharmacol* 22:81–87.

62. Smythies, J.R. (1984). The role of the one-carbon cycle in neuropsychiatric disease. *Biol Psychiatry* 19:755–758.

63. Carney, M.V.P., Martin, R., Bottiglieri, T., Reynolds, E.H., Nussenbaum, H., Toone, B.K., and Sheffield, B.F. (1983). Switch mechanism in affective illness and S-adenosyl-methionine. *Lancet* 18:820–521.

64. Bottilieri, T., Godfrey, P., Flynn, T., Carney, M.W., Toone, B.K., and Reynolds, E.H. (1990). Cerebrospinal fluid S-adenosylmethionine in depression and dementia: effects of teatment with parenteral and oral S-adenosylmethionine. *J Neurol Neurosurg Psychiatry* **53**:1096–1098.
65. Kagan, B.L., Sultzer, D.L., Rosenlicht, N., and Gerner, R.H. (1990). Oral S-adenosylmethionine in depression: a randomized, double-blind, placebo-controlled trial. *Am J Psychiatry* **147**:591–595.
66. Charlton, C.G., and Crowell, B., Jr. (1992). Parkinson's disease-like effects of S-adenosyl-L-methionine: effects of L-dopa. *Pharmacol Biochem Behav* **43**:423–432.
67. Charlton, C.G. (1997). Depletion of nigrostriatal and forebrain tyrosine hydroxylase by S-adenosylmethionine: a model that may explain the occurrence of depression in Parkinson's disease. *Life Sci* **61**:495–502.
68. Nomoto, M., Shimizu, T., Fukuda, T., Hirato, M. and Ohye, C. unpublished data.

CHAPTER 14

The Relevance of Adenosine A_{2A} Antagonists to the Treatment of Parkinson's Disease: Concluding Remarks

Peter Jenner

Neurodegenerative Diseases Research Centre, Division of Pharmacology & Therapeutics, Guy's King's & St Thomas' School of Biomedical Sciences, King's College, London, UK

INTRODUCTION

The primary pathology of Parkinson's disease is the degeneration of dopaminergic neurons in the zona compacta of the substantia nigra, leading to a marked fall in caudate-putamen dopamine content which is held responsible for the onset of motor symptoms (Hornykiewicz, 1982). For the past 35 years treatment of Parkinson's disease has been available in the form of L-DOPA replacement therapy, and more recently, in the use of dopamine agonist drugs, such as pergolide, ropinirole, and pramipexole to provide post-synaptic receptor stimulation in the striatum (see Hagan *et al.*, 1987). The introduction of dopaminergic therapy is accompanied by an acute side effect profile involving both peripheral and central dopaminergic stimulation leading to nausea, vomiting, and orthostatic hypotension. Such effects make the introduction of L-DOPA and particularly dopamine agonist drugs difficult in this patient population. Dopamine replacement therapy is highly effective in the early stages of Parkinson's disease; but with time, efficacy declines such that the duration of action of each dose of L-DOPA becomes shorter and more unpredictable (Poewe, 1993). Other long term complications of treating Parkinson's disease are also a serious issue. In particular, some elderly patients become sensitive to the ability of L-DOPA and dopamine agonists to induce psychosis, and the occurrence of prolonged psychotic episodes can prevent the continuation of drug treatment (Koller, 1994). Commonly, patients treated with L-DOPA develop involuntary abnormal movements comprising dystonic and choreic components collectively termed dyskinesia, which appear due to a combination of nigral pathology and drug treatment (Jankovic and Marsden, 1993; Nutt, 1990). The incidence of dyskinesia has declined in recent years due to the use of lower doses of L-DOPA, but still some 20–30% of patients develop involuntary movements which can be particularly severe in patients with a younger onset of disease (Schrag et al., 1998). This again leads to a situation that makes dopaminergic approaches to therapy difficult to maintain. Besides the obvious motor abnormalities that occur in Parkinson's disease, the illness is also characterized by a range of other symptoms such as bladder dysfunction, profuse sweating, drooling, and postural instability, none of which respond to current therapy (Jankovic, 1990). So, while the dopaminergic drugs available are useful in providing symptomatic treatment for the motor symptoms of Parkinson's disease, their effects are not ideal and there is considerable room for the improvement of therapy. The ideal profile for a novel approach to treating Parkinson's disease would provide symptomatic relief for all manifestations of the illness without producing acute or chronic side effects. In addition, novel therapeutic approaches would also deal with the issue of continuing disease progression, which is not addressed by dopaminergic approaches to treatment.

A consequence of the imperfections of the current treatment of Parkinson's disease is the concept of moving beyond the damaged dopaminergic system to target neuronal receptors localized on striatal output pathways. Indeed, there is a growing literature based largely on attempts at manipulation of motor function in 1-methyl-4-phenyl-1,2,3,6-tetrahydropyridine (MPTP)-treated monkeys which would suggest that such nondopaminergic approaches might provide both symptomatic relief of Parkinson's disease coupled with the avoidance or reversal of dyskinetic movements (Brotchie, 1998; Blanchet et al., 1998; Schneider, et al., 1998). However, the manipulation of A_{2A} adenosine receptors has attracted particular attention because of their highly selective localization to cholinergic interneurones in the striatum and to the indirect striopallidal GABA output pathway (Dixon et al., 1996). The positioning of the A_{2A} receptors offers an opportunity to manipulate those neuronal pathway that are currently thought to be primarily responsible for the onset of motor deficits in Parkinson's disease and subsequently for the occurrence of dyskinetic movements (Parent and Cicchetti, 1998).

STRIATAL OUTPUT PATHWAYS AND
PARKINSON'S DISEASE

The two major striatal output pathways are the indirect strio-external segment of globus pallidus (GPe) pathway and the direct strio-internal segment of globus pallidus (GPi) nigral pathway (Gerfen *et al.*, 1990, 1991). The indirect striopallidal pathway is a GABA-containing pathway which contains enkephalin and has largely D-2 receptors on its cell bodies in the striatum. The direct output pathway is also a GABA-containing pathway but it contains substance P and dynorphin and it mainly has D-1 receptors on its surface. It is an imbalance between these output pathways which is currently believed to lead to motor dysfunction in Parkinson's disease. Following destruction of the nigro-striatal pathway, in either Parkinson's disease or following MPTP treatment of primates, altered activity of the indirect striopallidal pathway develops following removal of inhibitory dopaminergic control (Wichmann and DeLong, 1996; but see Levy *et al.*, 1997; Parent and Cicchetti, 1998). In contrast, the direct striopallidal nigral pathway becomes underactive since it is normally under excitatory dopaminergic tone. It is these changes which then lead to a series of events culminating in alterations in the activity of the subthalamic nucleus and output pathways to the thalamus, and subsequently to premotor and motor cortex.

The selective localization of adenosine A_{2A} receptors to striatal cholinergic interneurones and to the cell bodies of the GABAergic striopallidal indirect output pathway provides a unique opportunity to manipulate acetylcholine and GABA release in this disorganized pathway in Parkinson's disease (see Richardson and Kurokawa, this volume). Indeed, as has been demonstrated in previous chapters, occupation of the A_{2A} receptors by the selective antagonist KW6002 alters GABAergic transmission directly, and through collateral interactions affects the activity of striatal cholinergic interneurones (Mori *et al.*, 1996; Kurokawa *et al.*, 1994). The overall effect of the action of KW6002 is to produce suppression of GABAergic inhibitory synaptic processes, which translates *in vivo* into the production of increased locomotor activity in both rodent and primate models of Parkinson's disease (see Kuwana *et al.*, this volume; Kanda *et al.*, this volume; Hadj Tahar *et al.*, this volume). In particular, KW6002 can induce increasd locomotor activity in reserpinized mice, reverse haloperidol-induced catalepsy in rodents, and initiate circling behavior in 6-hydroxydopamine lesioned rats (Kanda *et al.*, 1994; Brown *et al.*, 1991). However, it is the effects of KW6002 in the MPTP treated primate model of Parkinson's disease that is of greatest interest since this model is highly predictive of drug action in man (Kanda *et al.*, 1998; Hadj Tahar *et al.*, this volume). As reported earlier in this volume, administration of KW6002 to MPTP-treated common marmosets leads to a modest increase in locomotor activity coupled to a significant reversal of motor disability, which is not accompanied by nausea or vomiting or other obvious peripheral side effects. While these effects are not qualitatively different from those one might expect with a dopaminergic approach to Parkinson's disease, there is considerable interest in the failure of KW6002 to provoke abnormal involuntary movements in MPTP-treated common marmosets previously exposed to L-DOPA, and which exhibit dyskinesia in response to all dopaminergic drugs. In the marmoset model, KW6002 has a long duration of effect, although this is not seen in all primate species (see Hadj-Tahar *et al.*, this volume), but importantly, on repeated administration this does not result in tolerance to its antiparkinsonian effects. KW6002 also produces additive effects when administered in combination with L-DOPA or selective D-1 and D-2 agonist drugs (Kanda *et al.*, 1999). Significantly, 24 and 48h after the administration of KW6002, when it alone produces no obvious behavioral effect, there is a synergism or sensitization to the effects of an acute challenge with selective D-1 or D-2 agonists. All of these data suggest that KW6002 may be useful in the symptomatic treatment of Parkinson's disease by providing an approach which may be effective as monotherapy, and which may be useful later in the disease as adjunct therapy, by producing additional benefit to that seen with dopaminergic compounds with the avoidance of dyskinesia established by prior L-DOPA exposure.

ALTERATIONS IN STRIATAL OUTPUT PATHWAYS FOLLOWING THE OCCURRENCE OF DYSKINESIA

A key question related to the role of A_{2A} antagonists in the treatment of Parkinson's disease is the status of these receptors following nigrostriatal denervation and the onset of L-DOPA induced dyskinesia. Recently, we have undertaken a study of alterations in A_{2A} receptor mRNA in MPTP-treated common marmosets subsequently exposed to L-DOPA to produce priming for the expression of dyskinesia (unpublished data). The effect of MPTP treatment is to produce a decrease in mRNA for preprotachykinin (PPT) as an index of altered activity in the direct output pathway and to produce an increase in preproenkephalin (PPE-A) mRNA as a reflection of changes in the activity of the indirect striopallidal pathway (Jolkkonen *et al.*, 1995). Treatment with MPTP produced no alterations in the density of D-1 receptor mRNA in striatum, but despite an increase in D-2 receptor mRNA, A_{2A} receptor mRNA was unaltered in agreement with previous studies utilizing postmortem tissues from patients dying with Parkinson's disease and 6-OHDA-lesioned rats (Martinez-Mir *et al.*, 1991; Przedborski *et al.*, 1995). Following chronic treatment of MPTP lesioned marmosets with L-DOPA to induce dyskinesia, there was a reversal of the decreased PPT mRNA in striatum without a change in the elevated level of PPE-A or D-2 receptor mRNA, while A$_{2A}$ receptor mRNA again was not altered. However, in normal monkeys treated chronically with L-DOPA in very high doses (80 mg/kg po plus carbidopa), both PPE mRNA and A$_{2A}$ receptor mRNA—but not PPT mRNA—were increased, but only in those animals showing involuntary movements (unpublished data). These results support the concept that KW6002 as an A$_{2A}$ receptor antagonist may alter adenosine receptor function within the disorganized indirect output pathway, thus producing symptomatic benefit and potentially reversing those changes associated with the onset of dyskinesia.

FINAL COMMENTS

The current dopaminergic treatment of Parkinson's disease is highly effective in producing an initial reversal of the motor deficits associated with this disorder. Indeed, the availability of such treatment separates Parkinson's disease from all other neurodegenerative diseases where currently such symptomatic therapy is not available. However, treatment remains problematic particularly in terms of the long-term complications associated with chronic drug therapy in the face of continuing neuronal degeneration. A move to produce therapies that act beyond the damaged dopaminergic system would seem to provide a credible alternative approach if the targets attacked are selectively localized within the basal ganglia output systems responsible for controlling motor activity. In this respect the A$_{2A}$ antagonist approach meets many of the criteria that one would ideally want in a novel treatment for Parkinson's disease. The receptor system to be manipulated has a highly selective localization to the indirect output pathway from the striatum. The acute administration of KW 6002 leads to a mild symptomatic improvement in Parkinson's disease but coupled with an inability to provoke an established dyskinesia. KW6002 administration is not associated with the occurrence of nausea or vomiting nor obvious cardiovascular changes. It is unlikely that an approach based on A$_{2A}$ antagonists would provoke psychosis. Interestingly, in the animal experiments carried out so far there is no indication of tolerance to the actions of the drug, although such experimental situations do not reflect the ongoing progressive nature of Parkinson's disease nor the very long treatment periods used in man. It will be interesting to discover whether A$_{2A}$ antagonists benefit symptoms of Parkinson's disease which are not controlled by dopaminergic drugs. There may also be an opportunity for A$_{2A}$ antagonists to be effective against neuropsychiatric complications of Parkinson's disease by exerting antidepressant or anxiolytic activity through populations of A$_{2A}$ receptors present in the hippocampus and limbic regions of brain. Finally there is increasing evidence that A_{2A} antagonists may exert neuroprotective actions and so slow the progress of neurodegenerative diseases, such as Parkinson's disease (Monopoli *et al.,* 1998).

The future treatment of Parkinson's disease is dependent on further insight into the mechanisms responsible for the motor symptoms and the targeting of neuronal systems other than those acted on by dopaminergic drugs. Greater understanding of the mechanisms underlying dyskinesia and the role played by the striatal output pathways will also lead to the development of drugs which do not initiate dyskinesia or provoke established involuntary movements. The use of A_{2A} antagonists would seem to be a novel and fundamental step in achieving these objectives.

ACKNOWLEDGEMENTS

This study was supported by the Parkinson's Disease Society and the National Parkinson Foundation, Miami.

REFERENCES

Blanchet PJ, Konitsiotis S, and Chase TN. (1998). Amantadine reduces levodopa-induced dyskinesias in parkinsonian monkeys. *Movement Disorders* 13, 798–802.

Brotchie JM. (1998). Adjuncts to dopamine replacement: A pragmatic approach to reducing the problem of dyskinesia in Parkinson's disease. *Movement Disorders* 13, 871–876.

Brown SJ, Gill R, Evenden J, Iversen SD, and Richardson PJ. (1991). Striatal A_2 receptor regulates apomorphine induced turning in rats with unilateral dopamine denervation *Psychopharmacology* 103, 78–82.

Dixon AK, Gubitz AK, Sirinathsinghji DJS, Richardson PJ, and Freeman TC. (1996). Tissue distribution of adenosine receptor messenger-RNAs in the rat. *Br J Pharmacol* 118, 1461–1468.

Gerfen CR, Engber TM, Mahan LC, Susel Z, Chase TN, Monsma FF Jr, and Sibley DR. (1990). D-1 and D-2 dopamine-receptor regulated gene expression of striato-GPi/nigral and striatopallidal neurones. *Science* 250, 1429–1432.

Gerfen CR, McGinty JF, and Young SW III. (1991). Dopamine differentially regulates dynorphin, substance P and enkephalin expression in striatal neurones: *in situ* hybridisation histochemical analysis. *J Neurosci* 11, 1016–1031.

Hagan JJ, Middlemiss DN, Sharpe PC, and Poste GH. (1997). Parkinson's disease: prospects for improved drug therapy. *TiPS* 18, 156–157.

Hornykiewicz O. (1981). Brain neurotransmitter changes in Parkinson's disease. In: *Movement Disorders*. Eds. Marsden CD and Fahn S. Butterworth & Co., London, pp 41–58.

Jankovic J. (1990). Clinical aspects of Parkinson's disease. In: *The Assessment and Therapy of Parkinsonism*. Eds. Marsden CD and Fahn S. Parthenon Publishing Group, Carnforth, pp 53–75.

Jankovic J and Marsden CD. (1993). Therapeutic strategies in Parkinson's disease. In: *Parkinson's Disease and Movement Disorders*. Eds. Jankovic J and Tolosa E. Williams & Wilkins, Baltimore, pp 115–144.

Jolkkonen J, Jenner P, and Marsden CD. (1995). L-DOPA reverses altered gene expression of substance P but not enkephalin in the caudate-putamen of common marmosets treated with MPTP. *Mol Brain Res* 32, 297–307.

Kanda T, Shiozaki S, Schimada J, et al. (1994). A novel selective adenosine A$_{2A}$ receptor antagonist with anticataleptic activity. *Eur J Pharmacol* 256, 263–268.

Kanda T, Jackson MJ, Smith LA, Pearce RKB, Nakamura J, Kase H, Kuwana Y, and Jenner P. (1998). Adenosine A$_{2A}$ antagonist: A novel antiparkinsonian agent that does not provoke dyskinesia in parkinsonian monkeys. *Ann Neurol* 43, 507–513.

Kanda T, Jackson MJ, Smith LA, Pearce RKB, Nakamura J, Kase H, Kuwana Y, and Jenner P. (1999). Combined use of the adenosine A$_{2A}$ antagonist KW6002 with L-DOPA or with selective D-1 or D-2 dopamine agonists increases antiparkinsonian activity but not dyskinesia in MPTP treated monkeys. *Exp Neurol* (in press).

Koller WC. (1994). Adverse effects of levodopa and other symptomatic therapies: impact on quality of life of the Parkinson's disease patients. In: *Beyond the Decade of the Brain*. Ed. Stern MB. Wells Medical, Royal Tunbridge Wells, pp 31–46.

Kurokawa M, Kirk IP, Kirkpatrik A, et al. (1994). Inhibition by KF17837 of adenosine A$_{2A}$ receptor-mediated modulation of striatal GABA and ACh release. *Br J Pharmacol* 113, 43–48.

Levy R, Hazrati L-N, Herrero M-T, Vila M, Hassani OK, Mouroux M, Ruberg M, Aseni H, Agid Y, Feger J, Obeso JA, Parent A, and Hirsch EC. (1997). Re-evaluation of the functional anatomy of the basal ganglia in normal and parkinsonian states. *Neuroscience* 76, 335–343.

Martinez-Mir MI, Probst A, and Palacios JM. (1991). Adenosine A$_{2A}$ receptors: selective localisation in the human basal ganglia and alterations with disease. *Neuroscience* 42, 697–706.

Monopoli Angela, Lozza G, Forlani A, Mattavelli A, and Ongini E. (1998). Blockade of adenosine A$_{2A}$ receptors by SCG 58261 results in neuroprotective effects in cerebral ischaemia in rats. *NeuroReport* 9, 3955–3959.

Mori A, Shindou T, Ichimura M, Nonaka H, and Kasa H. (1996). The role of adenosine A$_{2A}$ receptors in regulating GABAergic synaptic transmission in striatal medium spiny neurones. *J Neurosci* 16, 605–611.

Nutt JC. (1990). Levodopa induced dyskinesia. *Neurology* 40, 340–345.

Parent A and Cicchetti F. (1998). The current model of basal ganglia organisation under scrutiny. *Movement Disorders* 13, 199–202.

Poewe W. (1993). L-DOPA in Parkinson's disease: Mechanisms of action and Pathophysiology of late failure. In: *Parkinson's Disease and Movement Disorders*. Eds. Jankovic J and Tolosa E. Williams & Wilkins, Baltimore, pp 103–113.

Przedborski S, Levivier M, Jiang H, Ferreira M, Jackson-Lewis V, Donaldson D, and Togasaki DM. (1995). Dose-dependent lesions of the dopaminergic nigrostriatal pathway by intrastriatal injection of 6-hydroxydopamine. *Neuroscience* 67, 631–647.

Schneider JS, Pope-Coleman A, Van Velson M, Menzaghi F, and Lloyd K. (1998). Effects of SIB-1508Y, a novel neuronal nicotinic acetylcholine receptor agonist, on motor behaviour in parkinsonian monkeys. *Movement Disorders* 13, 637–642.

Schrag A, Ben-Shlomo Y, Brown R, Marsden CD, and Quinn N. (1998). Young-onset Parkinson's disease revisited—Clinical features, natural history and mortality. *Movement Disorders* 13, 885–894.

Wichmann T and DeLong MR. (1996). Functional and pathophysiological models of the basal ganglia. *Curr Opin Neurobiol* 6, 751–758.

INDEX

Note: t = table and f = figure after page numbers in index.